SCREAMING
TO BE HEARD

SCREAMING TO BE HEARD

HORMONAL CONNECTIONS WOMEN SUSPECT . . . AND DOCTORS IGNORE

ELIZABETH LEE VLIET, M.D.

M. Evans and Company, Inc.
New York

M. Evans and Company, Inc.
216 East 49th Street
New York, NY 10017

Permissions

Gambrell, R. D., Jr. "Breast Disease in the post-menopausal years." *Seminar Reprod Endocrinol* 1983; 1:27. Copyright © 1983 by R. Don Gambrell, Jr., M.D. Reprinted by permission of the author.

"Figure Problems" by Allison Joseph. Reprinted from *I Am Becoming the Woman I've Wanted*, edited by Sandra Haldeman Martz, Papier-Mache Press, 1994. Copyright © 1994 by Allison Joseph. Reprinted by permission of the author.

"Of Mountains and Women" from *Spirit Walker* by Nancy Wood. Illustrations by Frank Howell. Copyright © 1993 by Nancy Wood. Used by permission of Doubleday, a division of Bantam Doubleday Dell Publishing Group, Inc.

From *Preventing Osteoporosis* by Kenneth H. Cooper. Copyright © 1989 by Kenneth H. Cooper. Used by permission of Bantam Books, a division of Bantam Doubleday Dell Publishing Group, Inc.

Cartoons and the original artwork for diagrams used in this book are by Gordon Vliet.

Library of Congress Cataloging-in-Publication Data

Vliet, Elizabeth Lee, 1946–
    Screaming to be heard : hormonal connections women suspect . . . and doctors ignore /
Elizabeth Lee Vliet. — 1st ed.
        p. cm.
    Includes bibliographical references and index.
    ISBN 0-87131-784-2 (cloth) : $24.95
    1. Women—Health and hygiene.   I. Title.
RA778.V55 1995
613′.04244—dc20

94-49419
CIP

Design by Bernard Schleifer

Typeset by Classic Type, Inc.

Manufactured in the United States of America

9 8 7 6 5 4 3 2

This book is dedicated to:

♦ The courage of my women patients—and their partners—who listened to their inner voice of knowing, and who persisted in seeking answers to their health questions in spite of traditional medical teachings contradicting women's wisdom and insights. As I have listened, you have taught me; your experiences will now benefit others who are seeking answers.

♦ My mother and her mother: women of strength and faith in the face of adversity, women of intellect and wisdom, and women who taught me to believe in my abilities and to listen well to the voice of wisdom.

♦ My husband, Gordon Vliet, who from the beginning encouraged and nurtured me in my pursuit of a medical career, even though it has meant many sacrifices for both of us.

♦ Our Creator, who has given us this incredible blessing of life, and has provided guidance and insights throughout my life.

ACKNOWLEDGMENTS

This book has been the culmination of many years of experience and input from my teachers. It would be impossible to name all of you. For the men and women friends, teachers, mentors, guides who have given of your knowledge, my heartfelt gratitude for the insights and wisdom you have shared with me.

In medicine, several of my teachers stand out as true practitioners of the art and science of being a physician: Robert Manning, M.D., Desmond Hayes, M.D., Jerome Frank, M.D., Paul Mozley, M.D., Michael Kaminsky, M.D., Phillip Slavney, M.D., James Dorsey, M.D., and Dan Kay, M.D. Sadly, in my medical career, there have not been many women mentors ahead of me, and almost no role models of women physicians during my medical school and residency days. I am rewarded by my part in changing that situation for the upcoming generation of physicians.

Friends who have urged me on in writing this book, and who have reviewed early drafts deserve special mention: Dr. Bernie Halbur, Jenifer Jones, Dr. Virginia Armstrong, Roslyn and Robert Brown, Carol Minker (your cards and cartoons kept me going!), Gillian Ford, Gloria King, Donna Gilson, Risa Waldt and my wonderful family.

To Jerry Cohen in Tucson, Jerry Petersen and George Kemble, M.D. in Ft. Worth, thanks for giving me the opportunity to develop the Women's Program in settings that broaden the impact of my vision.

I will also be forever grateful to three people who saw me through the trials and tribulations of learning to use the computer to write this book: Victoria Hahn who devoted hours of volunteer time to set up the system and figure out the new word processing, Tom Wadkins who taught me that backing up computer files is just like the preventive medicine I teach, and Virginia Davis who showed that women over sixty-five can not only learn the computer but also push the limits of Word Perfect in writing a manuscript. I could not have survived the process without your help! And speaking of help, my office staff through the years have contributed much to my efficiency with patients, and to the patients' feeling of connection with their physician—to all of you, my deepest thanks.

I thank two special spiritual teachers: Dr. Lewis Galloway and Curtis Kee-kah-bah. Your wisdom and spiritual depth have enriched my life greatly.

Contents

Speaking Out: A Woman Physician's Experience • Women's Traditional Healing Wisdom: Devalued and Ignored • Challenges and Controversies in Women's Health • Behind the Headlines: Alarming Facts You Don't Hear • Why Women Aren't Heard • Shocking Facts in Women's Health: Risks You Are Not Told • Setting the Stage for Change

What Are Hormones? • The Endocrine System: A Look at Key Hormones and What They Do • Brain–Body Hormonal Communication Pathways • The Menstrual Cycle RHYTHM of Changes • What Happens When Estrogen Declines: Hormone Changes Through the Decades • The Thyroid: The Great Imitator Often Missed in Women

The Brain: Master Conductor of Our Body's Orchestra • New Understandings of the Brain's Chemical Messengers • It's NOT All in Your Imagination! The Biology of Mood Changes • Clarification: Depression and Anxiety Symptoms versus Psychiatric Disorders • Estrogen Effects on Serotonin and Other Mood Regulators • The Brain's Alarm Center: Hormone Triggers of "Anxiety," "Racing Heart," and "Flutters" • Progesterone and the Brain • Testosterone and the Brain • Future Directions

The Use of "Doctors" in the Title

When I use the word *doctors* in the title of my book, I am *not* referring just to physicians, or medical doctors. Indeed, it is doctorate level professionals in many fields who, as teachers and researchers, have ignored the biological gender differences that are the focus of this book. In its original meaning, doctor meant "teacher" or "great teacher." Historically, the first "doctor" degree was *doctor of philosophy* (Ph.D.), not doctor of medicine (M.D.) *Philosophy* is derived from Greek words meaning "love of wisdom." Individuals who loved learning and gaining wisdom enough to continue their studies for an advanced degree were then awarded the doctor of philosophy. The new "doctors" typically then became "teachers" of others. The *doctor of medicine* degree actually came later in time than did the doctor of philosophy; and today we have a variety of doctorate level degrees in diverse fields: osteopathy (D.O.), education (Ed.D.), social work (D.S.W.), science (Sc. D.), Ministry/Theology (D. Min.), and many others.

An example came up recently illustrating ways in which doctorate level professionals in diverse fields have failed to consider the crucial biological differences in women's health. In attending the Society of Menstrual Cycle Research annual meeting at which my paper was presented on "Hormonal Relationships in Perimenopausal Mood Changes," many of the Ph.D.s, Ed.D.s, and doctorate level nurses (all of whom were women) seemed to discount the *biological* hormonal connections. One presenter in another session said: "Forget all this stuff about serotonin and estrogen; we all know that mood problems at menopause are caused by life stresses. The medical industry is just trying to medicalize everything." Think about the ramifications of this comment.

I ask you: which is more stigmatizing? To think that suddenly, when you reach menopause, you can't cope with life stress and so become depressed or anxious? To think that hormonal changes and decreases may be *adversely affecting* how you feel and your usual coping strategies? To acknowledge that brain chemistry is impacted by changing body chemistry? Why should it be difficult to acknowledge and accept the last two possible explanations?

The presenter I just described was a *woman*, speaking to an audience of women professionals. We can't blame only the men for these attitudes. My husband happened to be the only male in the audience when these comments were made discounting the potential impact of biological hormonal changes women experience. I find these *either-or* attitudes even more disheartening coming from women healthcare professionals who seem to be in denial about these important biological differences! Perhaps I am even more disappointed when *women* aren't any more sensitive to other women's needs than are the male physicians who have borne the brunt of criticism so far. Clearly, *medical doctors* are not the only ones who fail to see the integrated picture of women's health in its totality. In my view, such *either-or* attitudes are indicative of my point: *doctors* in many field ignore these crucial biological links which is the reason we are still missing so much crucial research to answer the questions I am raising in this book; questions women consumers have been raising for decades.

To the physicians reading this: keep in mind, my comments are not meant to be an indictment of medicine; they are intended to stimulate a broader view of the integration needed in women's health research, clinical care, and the teaching of our wisdom. I also hope to help all health professionals reading this book to gain ways of "seeing" women patients with new insights about important *overlooked* hormonal connections, and to listen to the wisdom our patients have been trying to teach us. We all have much we can learn and share to improve the way women's health services are conceptualized and delivered. Our patients can teach all of us a great deal, if we just stop to listen to their voices of experience.

ELIZABETH LEE VLIET, M.D.
Founder, *HER Place: The Women's Center for Health Enhancement and Renewal, Inc.*
Tucson, Arizona, and Ft. Worth, Texas

Introduction

Women are not being listened to, not just in doctors' offices, but everywhere. Women's wisdom is ignored. Women's body knowledge is dismissed as "neurotic," "hypochondriacal," "hysterical." Women suffer in silence, alone with their fears: "Am I crazy? I know something is different about my body, but the doctors keep saying there's nothing wrong."

It's not just *male* physicians who don't listen or who discount women's ideas about what may be wrong. *Women* physicians aren't necessarily more understanding because they are women. All physicians have been taught by the same flawed system of education that does not fully *hear* women's voices, does not adequately address women's body differences or value women's insights and women's experiences. Women physicians have been taught the same negative stereotypes of female patients as have male doctors. I will never forget a woman family physician I was trying to recruit to join my Women's Center medical practice some time back. She said, quite disdainfully, "I don't want to just work with *women* patients; they're so neurotic and complain all the time. I'd rather have male patients." I was shocked by her comments. There is a vast undercurrent of stigma women face when they enter the health care system as patients, and this stigma permeates all levels, from doctors to nurses to insurance claims case managers who see women as "over-utilizers of services." Actually, I think the primary reason women utilize medical services more often than men is due to their body awareness, and the fact that their questions and problems often go unresolved.

Historically, women have been socialized to be passive, to accept without question what the authority figure, in this case the physician, tells them to do. In the last thirty years, there has been a great deal of emphasis on teaching women to be more assertive.

Standing up for yourself and asking questions is not "bitchy" or aggressive; it just makes good sense when your health is at stake. We have seen in recent years that women have made a difference when they ask questions and demand appropriate attention to the gender difference in health needs. At first, just a few women's voices speak out, then more join in as realizations hit full awareness. Finally, whispers become louder, more women are talking, finding that others have similar experiences. Gail Sheehy publishes *The Silent Passage*, and now the M word is out of the closet, and women begin to share experiences. The Women's Health Initiative in clinical research is launched. Women's health is a *hot topic*, finally gaining national attention. BUT. And it is a big BUT. Trying to find help amid the confusing information and media hype becomes even more frustrating. Fears mount: "Am I getting Alzheimer's?" "Will I get breast cancer?" "What to do?" "Do I take hormones?" "What about alternatives?" "Will someone give me some answers?" Blank stares from physicians.

Silence again. The voices quiet down as women once again discover that there are no set answers to their questions and concerns and often not even much interest. "There, there, dearie, it's just menopause. Everyone goes through it. Why are you so upset? Just live with it and it will pass." Meanwhile, the sleepless nights continue, that previously abundant energy level seems to fade more quickly; the memory seems less sharp; the work demands pile up; family needs have to be met; tempers flare; the crying spells hit for no reason; joint aches and pains get worse. Then the doctor says "You can't be in menopause; you're too young. It's just stress. Take it easy. Take a vacation. Don't get so wrought up. (Men are "concerned;" women are "wrought up.") See a therapist. You just need to get a grip on things." Then another betrayal: Women leaders who have previously spoken out for women's issues trivialize menopause and accuse those women who have negative experiences of being afraid to face the reality of aging. One feminist activist was heard to describe her own menopause this way: "I think it lasted about an hour. I don't see what all the fuss is about." Menopause is *not* another "should" that a woman has to *do right* or she is somehow *less* of a woman.

Once again, women are led to doubt themselves and *their* perceptions of their reality. The voices of inner knowing scream inside a woman's head: "Wait a minute. I used to handle stress in life just fine. Why *now*, when I have everything going for me, does it seem to get me down? I don't have reasons to cry like this. I *know* there is something changing with my hormones, but I'm told there's no connection. I'm told I'm fine. What is happening? It *is* real. I *know* it. Will *someone* just listen to me?"

Is it any wonder, then, that women today feel disenfranchised, devalued, and discounted by the medical professionals and turn to alternative therapies for help? Women are angry. Women are becoming increasingly proactive in seeking *anyone* who will listen, anyone who will take into account the needs of the whole person. But are they getting women getting *all* the care they may need from these nonmedical options?

As a physician who has been listening to women's voices and experiences for many years, I have felt a deepening disquiet as I have found, over and over again, the unrecognized medical problems that are overlooked or ignored because the wisdom and knowledge of the women patients are not being heard and heeded. The scream inside my own mind was barely audible to me at first: "she's describing it so thoroughly. Why haven't her other doctors listened to what she is saying?" But the screams became louder and more insistent as the years went on, as I grew in wisdom and experience as a woman physician and was better able to trust *my own intuition* about what women were telling me. Day in and day out, women continued to tell me stories of not being listened to and the patterns repeated.

How did I branch out from internal medicine and psychiatry to begin working with the hormonal aspects of women's health that are usually addressed by gynecologists? During my residency days, and ever since, physicians would frequently refer women to me for "psychogenic" problems, anxiety, stress-related illness, or depression. I would see the person, expecting to help with those issues. But after a thorough history and evaluation, I often found myself saying to the woman and her physician, "The problems you are describing have a clear pattern related to your menstrual cycle, and I don't think you have a major depression (or whatever happened to be in question). I do not find a *psychiatric* disorder; I think you are experiencing *hormonal* changes that are affecting your moods." I thought the referring physician would be glad to have the information. The woman typically was relieved that she now had some answers that made sense *to her*. What I discovered, however, was that most commonly their physician didn't listen to me either! I struggled for many years to get other physicians to understand and accept that hormonal shifts can effect brain chemistry and trigger changes in mood, anxiety, pain, headaches…you name it.

Finally, I decided I had had enough of this battle. I *knew* the women were right, and I could relate what they told me directly to the normal physiology of a woman's body rhythms. I undertook more a systematic study of endocrinology and reproductive hormones, attended many Continuing Medical Education programs on menopause and gynecology, read journals, and whatever else I could find in these areas. Much of the scientific work I could locate came from the international menopause journals and research done in Europe, Australia, and Canada over many years, in addition to the pioneering work in this country by Dr. Robert Greenblatt and Dr. Edward Klaiber. I learned more and more about the differences in the various types of hormones and saw how well these differences fit with what women were describing to me. I was finding the pieces of the puzzle that had been overlooked and these pieces were fitting beautifully with other pieces of the puzzle discovered at Johns Hopkins, where extraordinary neuroscience research was happening during my residency. It was exciting and rewarding for me at both the personal and the professional levels. And the improvement women described as a result of fine-tuning of their hormonal balance further validated my belief that I was heading in the right direction.

Early in my career in medicine, I began speaking around the country, doing what I could to educate women and groups of physicians about these health issues. But still, women had so many questions and so many stories of not being heard or their questions not being answered in health care settings. They kept asking me, "Is there a book on this anywhere? Is there something I can read about what you are saying? It makes so much *sense*." I gave the usual references, but the bottom line was that there really wasn't a book I had seen on the market that addressed the *integration* of all these women's health issues.

I could not ignore the "screams" any longer. I *had* to write this book. *Screaming to Be Heard* is an outgrowth of many years of clinical work taking an *integrated* approach to the multiplicity of factors affecting women's health: from the biological to the spiritual. My book is the tapestry woven of women's experiences as I listened to them over my twenty years in medicine; the voices of women's wisdom as patients, family members, friends, colleagues; the voice of my own experiences through several ordeals as a patient; the voices of women who have not been heard; and the voices of our ancestors, whose writings gave us the legacy of *their* wisdom, pain, joys, struggles, and achievements in the face of adversity.

I have had my own adversities. I was a patient who was not listened to until I lost the function of my left leg, bladder, and bowel and had reached a point requiring emergency back surgery for a fully ruptured disk compressing my spinal cord. I know first-hand the pain, suffering, fear, self-doubt (*"Imustbecrazy. NO. I'mNOT!"*), the helplessness of not being listened to or believed, the frustrations of wanting to be well and not being able to make progress. I was a physician; I was the patient. And when the *patient* is female, the old stereotypes and patterns of relating take precedence over her *professional* status.

As the patient, I *knew* something crucial had happened. I had followed directions and stayed in bed for a month; yet, I wasn't getting better. In fact, my ability to stand up for more than three or four minutes was getting progressively worse. My brain felt like it was in a fog; I couldn't even think clearly enough to focus on my medical reading. I began to berate myself, lying there telling myself that I must be lazy or something; that I really *should* be using this time to catch up on my medical journals. I would start to read, and I couldn't focus on the pages. Several years later, while at Johns Hopkins, I found out that I had not been imagining this "foggy brain" feeling. It was real, and a side effect of the Valium that had been prescribed four times a day for muscle relaxation. There was something *terribly wrong* with my body, but my doctors were telling me there was *nothing wrong*. I began to think I *was* going crazy!

"*Nothing wrong?* Nothing? What do you *mean*? I collapse when I try to stand. I can't go to the bathroom. What *is* this? How could it be something in my mind? I just don't understand." I went back for a checkup. The neurologist thought I "might" have a worsening herniation of the disk and sent me to his partner, a neurosurgeon. This doctor did not re-examine me. He just patted me on the shoulder saying, "Now, you're just fine. You're just too anxious. All you have is a back strain, and it will be fine if you just get out of bed and go on about your business. It's time for you to get back to work." I felt like I had been chastised for avoiding my work responsibilities. So, having been raised in the southern tradition of responding like a dutiful little girl to an older male authority figure, (even though at the time this happened, I was an adult woman, a physician through medical school and internship), I went back to work at the hospital.

I lasted half a day before my legs collapsed once again and I couldn't stand. I was getting really frightened by this time, although I tried not to show it. "Remember, Lee, physicians don't cry. If you cry, they'll just think you're anxious and neurotic," I said to myself. My internal medicine doctor, a friend and mentor during medical school, said he thought I should be admitted to the hospital and try a week of traction to see if that would help. So I did that. As the week went on, I could barely walk well enough to go to the bathroom; once I got there, I had trouble urinating, and I became unable to have a bowel movement. Thinking I was constipated from inactivity, my physician ordered regular daily doses of Metamucil as a stool softener. But the problem wasn't constipation; it was nerve damage to the bowel from spinal cord compression. I *couldn't* have a bowel movement on my own. My abdomen was blowing up like a balloon from the Metamucil and no *movement*. It was awful. I must have looked like a snake that had swallowed a pig. But I still did what I was told, like the proverbial "good girl." I didn't know what else to do, and no one seemed to be listening. My confusion and fear were compounded by the fact that I was reminded I was the patient, not the doctor, and to follow directions. As I write this in 1994, I can see the humor in this picture; in 1979, when it happened, I was terrified.

Finally, *I* asked for a psychiatric consultation from one of my former professors. He was concerned and sympathetic but astutely said, "Lee, I'll be happy to see you professionally, but I don't really think you have a psychiatric disorder. I think you should get a second opinion *from a back surgeon*."

Two days later, Dr. Henry Wilde, from Houston, Texas, came to Williamsburg for a business meeting with my husband, who mentioned that I was in the hospital with unexplained back problems that weren't getting better. When Henry, an orthopedic surgeon who specialized in back surgery, came to my hospital room, I felt a sense of relief. I just knew he would take me seriously. He listened to my description of what had happened, did a thorough neurological examination, and said, "Lee, you don't have a muscle strain, you have a centrally herniated lumbar disk with compression of the end of the spinal cord. You have lost function in your leg, bladder, and bowel because of the nerve compression over such a long time. You need surgery, and you need it *now* in order for there to be any chance of the function coming back."

Needless to say, I felt an overwhelming sense of relief at finally having *confirmation* that something *was* wrong, what it was, and what needed to be done. I wasn't imagining what was happening, and it wasn't some unknown psychological conflict I was avoiding. This physician listened, did a thorough examination, and gave me a diagnosis that explained all that I had been experiencing. I certainly wasn't at all eager to go through major surgery, but I felt a tremendous weight lifted from my shoulders because I now knew what was wrong and what had to be done. I could deal with *known* problems a lot better than with all the uncertainty that only intensified my fear. Understandably, I did not want to go back to the neurosurgeon who had failed to properly diagnose my problem; so two days later, I was in Houston having the surgery I had needed all along.

My own story turned out well. Thanks to Henry's visit, I had surgery in time. Henry taught me the exercises that helped me regain my strength, the nerve function returned. Several months later, I was able to go on with my specialty training. But for many of my patients over the years, the outcomes have not been as positive; at times, irreversible damage had occurred before they had proper attention for what they had been describing.

Richard Bach said in *Illusions: The Adventures of A Reluctant Messiah*, *"Every problem has a gift for you in its hands."* For me the *problems* were certainly clear at the time. The *gifts* have emerged in many ways since 1979. One of the most meaningful gifts from my herniated disk problems has been the gift of *hearing* patients more clearly and trusting that if I listen carefully, they will tell me what I need to know to help them. Another *gift* was that I learned very early in my medical career just how crucial exercise, healthy food, and a positive mindset are to enhancing the healing process.

"Won't *someone please listen to me?* I *know* I am right. *Something* is wrong. It's *not* all in my head!!!" These are the silent and the spoken screams (sometimes as whispers) that I have heard from women around the country for years, and that have often gone through my own mind in times of health crises. It is *time* for women to be heard. It is also time for men to be heard because these problems have an impact on them as well. As Helen, a business executive in her fifties, said to me:

> I think women are getting short-changed in all this lack of information about hormones and how they can affect our minds and our well-being; and it affects interpersonal relationships, business relationships, and I think a lot of us are suffering.

So for all of you who have not been listened to or answered and for the men in your lives, I have dedicated myself to making your voices heard. This book is that voice. It is also a guide for those who have not yet heard their own inner cries or who have heard them and not found avenues of help. I would like to emphasize at the outset that I think women have incredible *body wisdom*.

Most women are attuned to their body rhythms and sensations in a positive way; indeed, in my opinion, this is one of women's gifts that enhances our survival. Women also seem to have a very good *intuitive sense* about body changes and what might be wrong. This is what I mean by "body wisdom." In working with male patients, I find very few who have this body wisdom. Most men have been taught *not* to pay attention to their bodies and to "gut through" the pain. For men, this "no pain, no gain" attitude often works to the *detriment* of their health. As patients and in my workshops, most women I have encountered are wonderful observers of their bodies and are intellectually inquisitive, asking well thought-out and thought-provoking questions about their health. I find that most women *want* to learn and understand how all these pieces of the puzzle fit together in their well-being and are generally motivated to make positive changes when they are empowered with knowledge and ideas about *what* changes can be made, and *how* to make them.

We health professionals *must* listen to women's body wisdom, learn from it, respect it, and incorporate it into our approaches for healing. I have a deep respect for all that my patients have taught me over the years. All of us, male and female health professionals, can grow in wisdom and understanding about health and illness if we take a moment to *really* listen to what our patients tell us. This is where the art and science of medicine began thousands of years ago. It is the root to which we *must* return if we are to truly *reform* healthcare. Fundamentally, we must come *back to the basics* of the human interaction of healer and person coming for help in the healing process. Listen to the words of Sir Francis Peabody *in 1926*:

> The application of the principles of science to the diagnosis and treatment of disease is only one limited aspect of medical practice. The practice of medicine in its broadest sense includes the whole relationship with the physician and the patient. It is an art, based to an increasing extent on the medical sciences, but comprising much that still remains outside the realm of science.

Isn't this what we are also asking for in 1995? Dr. Peabody's further words, from a speech to the graduating class at Harvard Medical School in 1931, are as relevant today as they were in 1931 and should be indelibly etched in the minds of all who would call themselves "physician": "The secret of the care of the patient lies in *caring* for the patient."

Robert T. Manning, M.D., the founding dean of my medical school and an important role model for me as a medical student as I observed him to be one of the true practitioners of the *art* and *science* of medicine, reiterated to us over and over: *"Listen to your patients, and they will tell you what is wrong."* Thank you, Dr. Manning, for your wisdom, your commitment to patients as people, and your dedication as a teacher. Your words have guided me well in my own journey as a physician. And thank you to the women, and men, who have given me the great priviledge of learning from you by listening to your experiences. You have taught me much that goes beyond the textbooks of medicine. It is time that your words be given a form in which they can touch and help others.

So, let's turn to the voices of women who must be heard, and *heeded*, for us to better meet the intricate health needs for women of all ages. I hope you will find encouragement to trust your perceptions and body wisdom as you read these pages. Remember, no book can take the place of your personal physician in determining your individual health program. I hope you will find answers that may have eluded you before, and to guide you as you work to improve all levels of your health.

Screaming to Be Heard! Listening to Women's Voices

Women are not entirely wrong when they reject the rules of life prescribed for the world, for they were established by men only, without their consent.

MICHEL EYQUEM DE MONTAIGNE, *1588*

Speaking Out: A Woman Physician's Experience

Did you notice that the quotation above was written in 1588? M. de Montaigne's astute observation has continued to be applicable in a variety of settings more than *four hundred* years later as we approach the year 2000. His insights can also be applied to the situation we have faced in women's healthcare. I have spent my medical career as a voice for women's health, long before the current focus finally hit the press. It is hard work to be a pioneer. I have fought many battles for women's health and have experienced the kind of ostracism and "blackballing" by some colleagues in much the same way women have encountered suppression in other fields of endeavor. I am glad to see that desperately needed attention is finally beginning to be paid to women's *unique* health needs.

The magazines and newspapers now carry banner headlines, and many more articles on health topics for women. *Women's health* is a "hot" topic; it's sexy; it sells; it is a "market niche;" it is used in the title of everything from A to Z. But even with all this media hype and long-overdue *apparent* attention to the crucial health needs of women, are things *really* changing for the average woman patient headed to her doctor's office seeking help? As a woman physician, as a woman who has been a *patient* more than

I would have wished, as a women's health advocate for many years before this present focus, and as a clinical researcher who has tried for more than a decade to get attention and funds directed toward women-specific research projects, I would honestly have to say that at this point, *nothing much has changed for the average woman in this country.*

In the words of one young woman who recently came to see me for migraine headaches and mood changes before her menstrual period:

> What bothers me is that I am thirty-six years old and with all the medical doctors I have seen, only one *psychologist* (a nonmedical person who was also a woman), who saw me for four sessions for depression recognized that I may have a hormonal imbalance. It surprises me and makes me angry that I have possibly had this problem for *twenty-three years.* I always told my physicians my headaches happened right before my period, but they dismissed my ideas. Where is the physician who will *listen* to my observations about my body?

And this is not unusual. I hear this same story every day from women of all ages, from all parts of the country. You will hear their voices and read their stories throughout this book. Oddly enough, it doesn't seem to make much difference whether the physician is male or female. Women physicians are taught by the same educational model that men are. There simply is *not* the information and awareness of *just how different* male and female bodies really are! The medical establishment is so dominated by men's thinking and male physiology that women's *different* needs are rarely even in the conscious awareness of physicians, much less adequately addressed even by caring physicians. After seminars I have given on women's health, I have had male physicians come up to me and say, "What you are saying makes so much sense. Why hasn't anyone talked about these connections before? Why hasn't this been in the medical literature? It certainly fits with *what my patients tell me*, but I have not known how to put it all together."

The sad part is that women will guide us in being effective physicians *if we will listen to what they say and think about what is happening to them.* For the woman quoted above, her migraines did indeed have a major hormonal trigger each month. With treatment to address the hormonal factor, her recurring *premenstrual* migraines have been eliminated. She is still susceptible to weather and food triggers for her migraines, but she described feeling an *enormous* sense of relief that a significant dimension of her migraine problem had been resolved by stabilizing the hormonal changes. This was *a factor she herself had been asking about for many years.*

Women's wisdom about their bodies and their experiences, *your* body wisdom and *your* experiences, for example, are simply *not listened to.* All of us as women often encounter a discounting and devaluing of our wisdom about our bodies and our health needs when we walk in the door of most medical offices.

Women's Traditional Healing Wisdom: Devalued and Ignored

What do I mean by women's *healing wisdom*? Let me reiterate what I said in the Introduction:

Most women are attuned to their body rhythms and body sensations in a positive way; indeed, in my opinion, this is one of women's gifts which enhances our survival. Women also seem to have a very good **intuitive sense** about body changes and what might be wrong. This is what I mean by **"healing wisdom."** Most women I have encountered are wonderful observers of their bodies and are intellectually inquisitive, asking well-thought out and thought-provoking questions about their health. I find that most women *want* to learn and understand how all these pieces of the puzzle fit together in their well-being, and are generally motivated to make positive changes when they are empowered with knowledge and ideas about **what changes** can be made and *how* to make these changes.

Without research specifically taking into account women's body chemistry, however, we cannot say *what* changes to make or *how* to make them. If scientific advances were able to put a man on the moon *in 1969*, why haven't we been able to determine whether we can give a woman half an aspirin a day to prevent strokes or whether medication should be adjusted according to the menstrual cycle? I have been making medication adjustments based on the menstrual cycle phase for my patients for about fifteen years, but this was not an approach I was taught in medical school or found in the medical literature. I learned it by *listening* to what my patients were telling me about how they felt, and by observing cyclical patterns to their experiences. *You* know this; *you* experience it. Women's *body* wisdom *knows* the hormonal rhythms; women's *mind* wisdom *knows* there are *connections* to these hormonal shifts. It is a magnificent symphony each month, but sometimes one section may be out of tune with the rest of the orchestra creating discord and disharmony for the rest. Women know this, *feel* it, observe it, ask good questions about it. This is what I mean by women's body wisdom. Why have health professionals not done a better job of paying attention to and heeding what female patients have been telling us for decades?

One answer to this question lies in research based on *males* and male body physiology and the assumption that those findings would apply equally well to female patients. Of course, this assumption ignores a fairly obvious fact: women's body chemistry and hormonal cycles are markedly different from men's. I keep reading about diseases that are 60 percent, 70 percent, or 80 percent female predominant, followed by comments such as, "We don't know *why* there are these gender differences." There is rarely ever mention of studying the most obvious factor that differentiates males and females: the *hormones* that make women *female*! Why have we overlooked or ignored researching something so obvious? It certainly isn't because *women* are unwilling to accept a hormonal connection. We *already know it is there.* Women I talk to would like to know *more about what it is* and how hormonal effects work throughout the body.

This book is about these **overlooked and ignored hormonal connections;** what we *do* know about hormonal effects on brain-body systems and how these hormonal effects interact with the endocrine, immune, metabolic, cardiovascular, respiratory, musculoskeletal, reproductive, urinary, and nervous systems. Every cell of our bodies participates in the flow of our menstrual rhythm. Changes occur in almost all body functions and secretions as the levels of female hormones rise and fall every month. These changes have been measured and objectively documented in *many* factors as the *partial* list on the next page illustrates.

Does this list begin to give you an idea of just how *profound* the relationships are in every part of our body to the changing hormone levels each month? It seems to me there is a wealth of opportunity to study these and learn ways of working *with* women's natural body cycles for optimal health and well-being. As you journey with me in this book to explore the unfolding story of this intricate web of connections, I will tell you what I *know* I know—from medical research, from listening to women's experiences and descriptions, from clinical study of women's hormone levels *when they have the symptoms they describe*, from

MENSTRUAL CYCLE MEASURABLE BODY CHANGES

- body temperature
- bile pigments (to digest fat)
- breast size, texture, skin/nipple color
- cervix changes: size, color, position
- production of neurotransmitters
- thyroid and adrenal hormone production
- red and white blood cell counts
- fluid balance
- skin color, texture, permeability
- respiration functions: CO_2, O_2 arterial
- blood pH
- serum bicarbonate
- citric acid (Vitamin C) content of mucus
- brain wave (EEG) patterns
- heart rate and rhythm
- balance, finemotor coordination
- ESR ("sed rate") measure of inflammation
- pupil size and reactivity
- platelet counts

- basal metabolism rate
- estrogen levels in blood and urine
- progesterone levels in blood and urine
- levels of brain hormones
- blood glucose regulation
- blood levels of adrenalin
- blood protein levels
- body weight
- GSR (galvanic skin resistance)
- pulmonary (lungs) vital capacity
- amounts of blood proteins
- vaginal mucus characteristics
- vaginal cytology (cell types)
- visual, auditory, olfactory acuity
- urine volume, pH, specific gravity
- memory and concentration
- pain threshold
- feeling state and behavior
- concentrations of vitamins A, C, E, and B group
- urine volume, pH, specific gravity
- energy levels and sleep patterns

psychological and sociocultural research, from cross-cultural research findings, and from my own experience as a patient who has been through much of what this book addresses.

I will also tell you honestly what I don't know or what isn't yet known from scientific research. My commitment to you, the reader, is the same commitment I have always given my patients: I will do my best to be honest with you, to give you the best information I am able to find, and to *admit* I don't know and help identify resources for you to get your questions answered. I don't expect you to find the answers to *all* your questions in this one book, but I do hope that you will find answers that you have *not found* addressed in other books.

My commitment is also to say very clearly at the beginning of this book: *I have not made any recommendations or any interpretations* from the medical literature (Western, Eastern, or any other) in this book *that I would not use myself for my own health needs* or recommend to my own family to consider with their physicians. When I am asked, I tell any member of my family the same things I am saying to you in my book. I take my commitments seriously, and I hope this gives you a degree of trust as you explore with me the *overlooked hormonal connections* that *interact at* all levels in women's health: mind/brain, body, soul/spirit and relationships. Let us begin our exploration of where we are with Women's Health in the United States as we rapidly approach the twenty-first century.

By now, you have probably read that the U.S. General Accounting Office (GAO) investigated charges in1990 that research funded by the National Institutes of Health (NIH) have been ignoring research focused on crucial areas specific to women's health needs and that women have been systematically excluded from research protocols investigating new treatment approaches, health promotion strategies, and diagnostic medical testing. The GAO audit revealed that in 1989 *less than 3 percent* of the NIH budget had been spent on total women's health issues, *less than two percent* on obstetrical and gynecological health concerns, and *less than 0.5 percent* on basic research in the area of breast cancer. There has been good progress since 1990. *We have a long way to go.*

Challenges and Controversies in Women's Health

In the four years since the GAO published the results of its audit, a groundswell of individual and group pressure has effectively pushed for rectifying such appalling imbalances in the NIH expenditures for women's health research. Here are some of the many accomplishments resulting from these efforts, primarily by *women* speaking out and casting votes for change:

- Launching of the NIH Women's Health Initiative
- Increased allocation of research dollars to disorders affecting women
- Establishment of the Office of Women's Health at the NIH
- Publication of the results of the Postmenopausal Estrogen and Progestin Intervention (PEPI) trials, the first major U.S. longitudinal double-blind placebo controlled study of menopausal hormone therapy regimens. Although this study used only *one* type of estrogen (native to horses), it did compare synthetic and natural progesterone for the first time in the U.S.

- Formation of new alliances and consumer groups for women's health
- Establishment of new medical journals devoted to women's health
- Increase in newspaper, magazine, TV, and radio articles or shows on women's health topics
- Hospitals and community and professional groups sponsoring women's health programs
- Most importantly, women doing what we have always done: networking with each other, starting self-help support groups, nurturing each other, and making efforts to ask questions and to learn more about our individual and collective needs

There is still more to be done. Fundamental and basic hormonal effects must be addressed in order to better understand crucial needs in healthcare for women. For example, it is well known clinically that the menstrual cycle is an important factor affecting drug metabolism and interactions; yet few systematic studies have been done to determine exactly how best to adjust medication dosages according to the menstrual cycle. These clinical observations of menstrual cycle hormonal effects on medication and disease severity and frequency have been observed in areas as diverse as herpes outbreaks, epileptic seizure activity, allergies, migraine headaches, yeast infections, bipolar affective disorder, and depression.

But we *still* have not studied HOW hormonal changes affect these cyclic changes in various disease flare-ups. The authors of a 1994 study of similar clinical patterns in Chronic Fatigue Syndrome (CFS), Fibromyalgia Syndrome (FMS), and Multiple Chemical Sensitivities (MCS) looked at many characteristics of these clinical problems more common in women. They did correctly identify these disorders as being much more common in women in their forties. Yet, there was *not one word* in the study about, or any methods used to assess, *possible ovarian hormonal factors contributing to these diseases.* Interestingly enough, all three researchers were women, so we can't just sit back and say *men* don't listen! Why is such an obvious potential "trigger factor" being overlooked? Health care professionals must find ways to remove the blind spots in women's health studies. In addition, it seems to me that studying the *differences* between males and females can be *beneficial to both sexes* and reveal important information about factors affecting disease onset and progression.

The relationship of premenopausal hormone changes to a variety of disorders seen more commonly in women, such as depression, fibromyalgia, and migraines has also not been adequately addressed. I have included a chapter on each of these important subjects because each one affects women *much more frequently* than men. The fluctuations and declines in hormone levels are normal physical changes that may have a significant impact on *premenstrual* and *premenopausal* sleep and mood changes.

Mood changes in the years before menopause (from about age thirty to age fifty) have traditionally been *assumed* to be primarily the result of life stresses and psychological transitions, but almost nothing has been done in systematic research to study *hormonal effects on the brain* as a factor causing these problems. We live in a culture that hasn't even been fully convinced that women *have* a brain, much less that it is connected to the body! If you think I am being too harsh, just look at the cartoons, ads, and body images used to sell products and present health information and notice how many headless bodies there are and how many jokes are printed daily about "brainless" or "nutty" women. We must remember, the brain *is* connected to the body, and hormones are one of the most potent chemical messenger systems affecting the brain and all its functions, including, of course, mood, sleep and memory.

In particular, both estrogen and progesterone have profound effects on the serotonin, norepinephrine, dopamine, and endorphin receptor systems that are involved in mood regulation; yet, almost no clinical research has integrated these findings to identify effective treatment regimens for premenopausal women. Because this *crucial information* is so woefully neglected in women's health, it will be a major focus of this book. You will hear the stories of women much like yourself interwoven through the scientific and medical information I discuss. You will also, mark my words, see much more on these issues emerging in clinical research as the cross-fertilization occurs with other countries (Canada, England, Australia, Japan, to name a few) where these concerns have been taken seriously and studied more systematically.

In the past, women have been excluded from health and medical research studies for a variety of reasons, *including the presence of the very hormonal changes that need to be studied*! Here are some of the complex factors that have contributed to the invisibility of women in health research studies:

- The hormonal cycling and complexity of women's physiology were considered "background noise" that complicated study design.
- The male body has been considered the "norm." What was learned about men was *assumed* to apply equally well to women.
- Research done on males without hormonal cycling was deemed to be *more reliable*. The bias against excluding women in research studies had even extended to a preference for male laboratory rats!
- Men dominated the research funding committees, medical school and university research settings, and they determined where the dollars went and for what types of studies.
- Most disorders that were known to be more common in women were *assumed* to be primarily psychological in origin and not as important to study as the "real" diseases more common in men.
- Women in general, until the past two decades, have been almost invisible, apart from their reproductive functions, in our culture as a whole.

Women's invisibility in health and medical research extends far beyond what I have just described. For example:

> The Baltimore Longitudinal Study of Aging was started 1958 in 1958 but **excluded women until 1978.** The last major report was published in 1984 and was titled *Normal Human Aging*, but this report contained *no data on women*.

It appears that, in this research, women weren't even considered "human!"

Risks You Are Not Told

Bernadine Healy, M.D., the first woman to be appointed director of the NIH said,

It is now time for a general awakening. Women have unique medical problems. They have greater morbidity [medical term for suffering, disability] than men and are affected by more chronic debilitating illness. Although women live longer than men—i.e., as much as seven years on average—the quality of life of those years is exceptionally burdened by cancer, particularly of the lung, breast, and colon; by

heart disease and stroke; osteoporosis, depression, and social isolation; Alzheimer's disease and general frailty. These conditions, which
tend to afflict women in the last third of their lives, are not the
inevitable ravages of age but, in many cases, are highly preventable
and eminently treatable. We must awaken fully to these facts and
address the diseases of women as different from the diseases of men
but of equal importance.

To illustrate Dr. Healy's point about the quality-of-life concerns for elderly women, osteoporosis alone is a major factor in
the increased cost of health care and the rising need for nursing
home care for elderly women. It is striking that **over 75 percent of
nursing home residents over sixty-five are female**. The even more
tragic aspect of this statistic is that women in this age group who
end up so debilitated that they are forced to be in nursing homes
are suffering from diseases that *are largely preventable* through
early education about risk factors and emphasis on healthy
lifestyle changes.

What contributes to women not getting the information and
education they need on these potentially preventable later-life
diseases? One factor is clear: The media imbalance in focusing predominately on breast cancer has significantly distorted the *real*
health issues that affect you as you grow older and adversely affect
your quality of life: the disabling and potentially deadly conditions
of osteoporosis and heart disease. Osteoporosis has become a
national health epidemic, with $8 to $10 billion spent annually on
health care for osteoporotic-related fractures and subsequent long-
term disability. And these figures *do not include* the dollar and
human cost of pain and suffering or the devastating effects on
quality of life. A hip fracture is definitely a serious health problem,
not as simple as ads about "total hip replacement" as the solution
would have you believe. After a hip fracture, about *20 percent of
women die from complications within three months*, and 50 percent *never* walk independently again. Pretty scary, I think. I am
concerned that women do not get an accurate picture of the consequences of bone loss and osteoporosis complications, especially
since greater emphasis on preventive approaches to osteoporosis in
the decades of the 20s, 30s and 40s, could dramatically reduce the
frailty and debilitation seen in older women.

The issues of older women and bone loss represent only the tip
of the iceberg of the *potential* osteoporosis *epidemic* in this country. We aren't even really addressing the millions of young women
who are starving themselves to be thin to reach some "magazine

ideal" for their bodies. In the process, they are losing bone at the very time in their lives (teens, twenties, and thirties) when they should be *building bone* toward peak bone density. These women do not even *arrive at menopause* with optimal bone density. Often, however, they *appear* healthy on the <u>outside</u> and don't even know that "silent termites" are eroding their bone from the inside. We think these young women look "great," "healthy," "vibrant" because they are *thin*. The "thin look" is what we have been *conditioned* to think is normal. But women need about 20 to 25 percent body fat in order to have normal menstruation, fertility, bone growth, hair and nail growth, and other measures of good health. I assure you, the models you see in most of the magazines have *less than* the 20 percent healthy body fat level. Have *you* had your body composition checked recently?

Alcohol is another area of challenge in women's health. Alcohol abuse and alcoholism *hit women harder than men* in all dimensions: physically on the body and brain, psychologically, financially, and sociologically. I include it as another one of the risks you don't hear much about relative to other topics in the popular press. A 1990 study in the *New England Journal of Medicine* by a team of Italian and American researchers revealed that women had smaller quantities of the protective enzyme alcohol dehydrogenase, which breaks down alcohol in the stomach, and that as a result women absorb about 30 percent more alcohol into their bloodstream than men do. The researchers also made another startling discovery: Alcoholic men have about half as much alcohol dehydrogenase as healthy males do, but *alcoholic women* show *almost no enzyme activity*. The researchers concluded that alcoholic women appear to lose all gastric protection in the absorption of alcohol; this is one of several reasons alcohol hits women harder and sooner than men.

I hear from women around the country that they are terrified of breast cancer. I understand this fear. Did you know, however, that cigarette smoking *now* represents one of the *worst* threats to women's health? Yet, in 1989, six *new* brands of cigarettes were *target marketed to women*. In 1991 alone, 51,000 women died of lung cancer, and 191,000 new lung cancer cases were diagnosed in women. In 1965, there were 14,000 tobacco-related deaths in women; by 1995, there are projected to be *240,000 tobacco-related deaths in women, almost SIX times the number of breast cancer deaths.*

Tobacco use is a hidden epidemic killing women. In 1986, lung cancer became the leading cancer death in women, *exceeding* *breast cancer*, and remains the leading cause of cancer death in 1995. The dramatic rise in lung cancer in women is *directly attributable to the rise in smoking* in women since World War II. But *90 percent* of women still think their leading cause of cancer death is breast cancer. Other disease risks associated with smoking include heart disease, early menopause, osteoporosis, emphysema, reduced fertility, miscarriages, low-birth-weight babies, and possibly ovarian and breast cancer. Adolescent and young adult women are beginning to smoke in alarming numbers. Those of you who are mothers, take note of this: **The fastest-growing group of smokers in the United States are girls under age *eleven*.**

Why don't you know this? The bottom line is money. **All** the women's magazines except *Good Housekeeping* and the new *Ms.* (which accepts no advertising at all) in the United States are heavily supported by advertising from the tobacco companies. Women's magazines, whose bottom lines would be jeopardized by offending their large advertisers, *do not run stories on the health consequences of cigarette smoking*. A recent study published in the *Journal of The American Medical Association* objectively documented the correlation that had been long suspected: The *greater* the percentage of advertising revenue from tobacco companies, the *less likely* a magazine was to publish any information on the health effects of tobacco use. Go back and look at your typical women's magazines. How many articles about lung cancer in women do you find? How many full-page color ads do you see showing pretty, smiling, *thin* young women smoking?

Cigarette smoking has been shown to cause earlier menopause and bone loss both in female smokers *and in <u>nonsmoking</u> women whose spouses are smokers*; yet, the number of women smokers is *increasing*, not decreasing. Fewer women than men quit smoking. Reason? Women value their appearance more highly than their health, thinking, "If I quit smoking, I'll gain weight."

The bottom line is that tobacco companies sell glamour, glitz, thinness, and an image of good health in advertisements that specifically target young women to buy a product that will enslave and potentially kill them. When are we women going to have our voices heard and heeded? Just as we have been outraged over the inadequate research and funding for breast cancer, we must raise our voices against this larger threat to the health of the next generation of women, our collective daughters. Cigarette smoking has also been found to impair fertility, although the components of cigarette smoke that are toxic to ovarian follicles are unknown. Cigarette smoking has also been implicated as a factor that increases the risk of breast cancer, perhaps by increasing cell mutations. If this turns out to be as important a link as many physicians and researchers suspect, women will have been sold a literally **lethal** bill of goods. Yes, "you've come a long way, baby." But is *more disease* what you *intended* or *wanted*? Smoking-related costs and deaths affect us all, whether we smoke or not, whether we have daughters or not. We must all have the courage to speak out to stop the glamorization of cigarette smoking and help our young people, especially vulnerable adolescent girls, make the choice NOT to start smoking.

Behind the Headlines: Alarming Facts You Don't Hear

Prevention of osteoporosis is a compelling reason for prescribing estrogen to postmenopausal women; yet, many of these women are reluctant to take estrogen because of the distorted picture in the media about the risk of breast and uterine cancer. In an article entitled "Endometrial Cancer From Estrogen Replacement Therapy (ERT): An Unfounded Fear," distinguished menopause researcher Dr. R. Don Gambrell reported that the absolute risk of endometrial (uterine) cancer is quite small, occurring in one in every thousand women over age fifty each year. This type of cancer is easily detected, very treatable, and less aggressive in women using hormones than in women who are not on hormone therapy. Dr. Gambrell also stated that *estrogen itself is not carcinogenic.* In patients diagnosed with endometrial cancer while on estrogen therapy, the *five-year survival rate is* 95 percent, a significantly *better* survival rate than that of women diagnosed with endometrial cancer and who are *not* on estrogen therapy. Many specialists think that the type of cancer that occurs in women who don't take hormones is a more aggressive form of cancer than in those who do take hormones. You don't see *this* information in the magazine and newspaper articles. As a physician, and as a woman consumer, it disturbs me that the available information is not more balanced and current. In Chapter 14, I will talk more about these issues as they relate to *what* information you get about breast cancer and *how* this information is presented. The same types of misinformation are perpetuated in article after article.

Eating disorders are other behind-the-scenes problems that affect women in enormous numbers, but rarely generate the same degree of media interest as topics like breast cancer. The cultural "thinness mania," beginning with Twiggy in the 1960s and continuing with the 1993 "waif" look, has created a female obsession with weight, dieting, and being thin no matter what the price to one's health. The ads bombard us constantly with headlines and images: Change your body. Change your self. Fix your flaws. Blast those jiggly hips and thighs. Get that tummy FLAT. Have a "tummy tuck" (major surgery and painful recovery, but they don't mention *that* in the ads). Become new and sexy, more attractive and exciting to your man: spray, powder, paint, nip, and tuck your body until you reach PERFECTION. No matter what the cost.

The idealized female body shown in our magazines is thin, bony, slouched, lean, and usually devoid of the normal female curves. These images have been a major factor in the creation of a multibillion-dollar diet industry in the U.S. largely aimed at YOU—the women. These ads and images play on our cultural obsession with thinness to ensure continued sales of products. It is an entrepreneur's dream: sell the same products over and over to the same group of people. The reason it tends to be the same group of people is that 95 percent of people who go on repeated quick-weight-loss diets end up *regaining* the weight they lost, and usually another added five or ten pounds!

Chronic "yo-yo" dieting has a major adverse effect on your health; going on and off diets stresses the heart, brain, bones, and other organs. Excessive thinness is associated with increased cancer risk, early menopause, osteoporosis, ulcers, anemia, and emphysema. There has been little research done on the connection between underweight and illness. The preliminary evidence suggests that it is actually healthier to be a little overweight than to be chronically dieting, going on and off fasts and other quick-fix approaches. Susan Powter has it right: *Stop the Insanity!* Chronic dieting can be lethal.

Why Women Aren't Heard

Additional problems in the area of women's health include the media's substantial role in perpetuating other stereotypes that adversely effect women. Think of the many negative labels applied to women: *anxious, overworried about their health, complainers, difficult patients, crocks, neurotic, emotionally-starved, empty-*

nesters, ditherers, bitchy. As a culture, we laugh at the cartoons about PMS, and we do not take seriously the women who struggle with the problematic symptoms of PMS that can at times be severe enough to adversely affect work, family, and social relationships. Feminists complain that physicians try to make PMS a psychiatric disorder. Women who *have* PMS complain that physicians aren't listening. Many of us physicians who have worked extensively with PMS patients are frustrated that the culture trivializes and discounts the very real physical and psychological symptoms of PMS to such a degree that *even WE physician advocates don't get listened to* when we try to speak up on behalf of our patients.

Women with breast cancer have been treated as *breasts* rather than persons. One woman wrote an eloquent piece about her experience in a cancer center, describing her depersonalized treatment to feeling like "a piece of baggage on an airline baggage carousel." Studies clearly show that a patient who speaks up and is assertive about her care and is involved in decision making about her treatment has a better survival rate and prognosis. But when women *do* speak up about their health care desires and needs, they tell me over and over they are then labeled "difficult, demanding, and bitchy" by both *nurses* (still mostly female) and doctors (still mostly male). How is a woman to figure out what to do?

Menopausal women are given one "recipe" for hormones, whether they feel well on it or not. We don't approach any other areas of healthcare that way. Can you imagine giving every patient with an infection the same antibiotic? Do you think that all diabetics are prescribed the same dose and type of insulin? Of course not. So why have menopausal women been relegated to a "cookbook" approach? One woman described it succinctly on her initial consultation form: "My doctor gives everybody the *same thing*: 0.625 and 2.5 every day are his current buzzwords." Is it that older (i.e., menopausal) women just aren't valued enough to take the time to work out an individualized approach? Is it that menopausal women are viewed as *complainers*, so they are just give the standard approach and sent home as quickly as possible? I think these are part of the issues leading to the *standardized* prescriptions. Here's an exercise I would like you to do NOW, as you are reading this:

TASK: Quickly write down the first three words that come immediately to mind with the phrase "An older man is _____." Just spontaneously fill in the blank with whatever words pop into mind. What did you come up with? Now do the same thing with this phrase: "An older woman is _____."

Do you see any pattern to your responses? When I ask these two questions in my seminars, the words that most frequently come to mind in the audience for describing older men are "distinguished," "successful," "powerful," "attractive." I rarely hear a negative word used to characterize older *men*. The common audience responses for the statement about older women are words like "dowdy," "old," "tired," "fat," "alone," "invisible," "poor," "over the hill," "unattractive." These stereotypes of older women are so deeply ingrained in our minds that we don't even consciously realize how *differently* we view aging men and women. We can't help but *feel* those images, and incorporate these ideas into our sense of self. The cumulative impact for women, however, adds up to an even lower sense of self-worth as we grow older, since we have been part of the culture for too long to easily shrug off such belittling messages.

I do not agree with such descriptions of older women, but such stereotypes are alive and thriving. We need to know they are present in our culture in order to understand why our questions and concerns are frequently overlooked or ignored. Programs in midlife women's health must address these adverse impacts on our self esteem and sense of self worth. That is another challenge for us as we forge a new, healthy, vital, "full-of-zest" image of ourselves growing older.

SHOCKING FACTS IN WOMEN'S HEALTH

Risks You Are Not Told:
Heart disease is an equal-opportunity killer. The number one cause of death in women over forty—yet it is generally assumed to be a disease of <u>men</u>. Prior to the Nurse's Health Study, women have been *excluded* from *every major study of heart disease* prevention, diagnosis, and treatment.

Risks You Are Not Told:
Women who are seen in the Emergency Room for chest pain and palpitations are far more commonly given a diagnosis of "anxiety" and sent home with a prescription for a tranquilizer rather than having a full evaluation for heart disease. Men with similar symptoms are more likely to be kept overnight to rule out a heart attack.

Risks You Are Not Told:
Between the ages of forty to sixty-five, almost 500,000 women die each year from cardiovascular disorders, versus 60,000 deaths annually from *all reproductive cancers*: breast, uterine, cervix, ovarian, and vaginal. But women and their physicians often don't know to start screening for heart disease risk factors in women in their forties.

Risks You Are Not Told:
A 1991 study published in the *New England Journal of Medicine* provided further evidence of sex bias in the management of coronary artery disease: Women were significantly less likely to have prescribed coronary angiography, angioplasty, or bypass surgery when admitted with a diagnosis of myocardial infarction, angina, chronic ischemic heart disease, or chest pain. Men are routinely offered these options.

Risks You Are Not Told:
Postmenopause estrogen therapy (ET) dramatically reduces (more than 50 percent in recent studies) risk of heart disease and osteoporosis, yet *less than 15 percent* of postmenopausal women take estrogen, in part because of an exaggerated fear of breast cancer in media reports and to lack of adequate information and screening for *individual* health risks.

Risks You Are Not Told:
Despite the fact that a *natural human form of estradiol has been FDA-approved in the U.S. since 1976,* women in this country are usually given only one recipe for hormone therapy (I call it the "cookbook approach" or the "Premarin-Provera" song). Rarely are other options offered to women, even if they have adverse reactions and unwanted side effects with the standard therapies.

Risks You Are Not Told:
In 1970, there were nine U.S. companies developing new forms of birth control. In 1990, there was one.

Risks You Are Not Told:
The United States is 20 years behind Europe in our options for natural hormone therapies for menopause. In other developed nations, many different forms of native human estradiol, progesterone, and testosterone are routinely available.

How many of these facts and health risks did you already know? I suspect not many, since these don't often make the headlines. The more you look at coverage of women's health, the more you see the imbalance in focus on topics which are more likely to have an emotional "hook" that gets you to *buy the magazine.* The distortion in risk has an impact on what choices women make in lifestyle changes as well as other interventions to reduce disease risk.

My intent is not to make this a political book. I raise these issues for three primary reasons:

1. to help you see the undercurrents that enhance or distort the health information you receive,
2. to paint an overall picture for you to critically evaluate, and
3. to emphasize the importance of YOU being active in getting information YOU need to make YOUR OWN decisions. When you become an informed consumer, working with your physician to assess your various health risk factors individually you can select the options which best meet your individual needs.

Setting the Stage for Change

The Women's Health Initiative, launched by Dr. Bernadine Healy and NIH, is long overdue and much welcomed by physicians, health professionals, and researchers in many fields, as well as by patients. The proposed research studies will focus on areas such as effects of hormone treatment in breast cancer, the role of diet in contributing to cancer, and the effectiveness of estrogen in preventing bone fractures. Major studies of medications are being implemented to specifically include women and to address public outcry over the lack of such information. But even these studies aren't optimal. Only one type of animal estrogen is being used in most of these studies, and it isn't the best source of native *human* estrogen, *17-beta estradiol*. We still have a long way to go. We need to keep the pressure on. It helps that women's interest groups have taken up the banner and are raising the public consciousness and politicians awareness.

We as women also need to challenge medical schools to see that they are in a primary position to elevate awareness of gender concerns in the new generation of physicians. I am a strong advocate of having Continuing Medical Education (CME) programs better designed to address the male-female differences in disease recognition and treatment. I have designed a number of CME courses with this integrated approach. Pharmaceutical companies must demonstrate their involvement in increasing the knowledge of male-female body/mind differences through research and support of educational programs for all health professionals as well as consumers. It is aggravating to me that some of the same people who criticize physicians and "those bad drug companies" for such jointly sponsored programs are often the same people who have a vested interest in *their own* products: vitamins, herbs, self-improvement tapes—you name it. People have sometimes asked why I have agreed to be on national speaker's programs which have educational grants from pharmaceutical companies. To me, the answers are straightforward and important:

- I want to advance the knowledge base in women's health issues by speaking to as many groups as possible.
- I believe it is part of the social responsibility of for-profit companies to invest some of their profits back into the educational process.

- I will be speaking the crucial messages taught me by my patients and my clinical experience, based on sound principles of normal physiobiology, *regardless of who is providing financial support*. If a company or organization does not agree with my position and my clinical program content, they don't have to invite me as a speaker.
- I am alarmed by the fact that women are not told about available options, such as natural hormones. If there are products on the market deemed safe by the FDA, and they are ones I would use myself or recommend for my family and patients, wouldn't you want me to also be telling you about such options to consider in *your* decision-making?

I don't have many illusions about what has motivated the current surge of interest in women's health when many of us have been "screaming to be heard" for many, many years. Women's collective *economic* clout is finally too great to ignore any longer. And it gets the attention of businesses in all sectors. Even "women's health" has become a "hot topic," getting more attention in magazines because it sells! Have you noticed how many new "women's health" newsletters have popped up in the last couple of years? Many of these contain the same information recycled in a new graphics design. There is very little that I have read in any of these "new" newsletters that is truly *cutting edge* information for women. You are buying magazines and books (yes, even mine) because you are hungry for the information and answers.

Am I glad to see *more* such articles, newsletters, and shows on these topics? You bet I am. I also want to see information given that is sound and up-to-date, not just perpetuating old myths and old polarizations. I would say to all of us: Be aware of underlying motives that may bias the selection of information presented, and evaluate carefully what you hear in the news, in magazines, in health education programs, in conversations with friends, or wherever. Remember, no one authority has all the answers, and each of us is an individual with different needs.

Setting the stage for, and implementing, change will continue to be our task in the interest of future generations of women. We can work to see that pressures are intensified in the search for answers by encouraging research and educational activities, and by helping to develop sources of funds to create more health care options and choices for all of us. We must become "activated" patients, in a *partnership* with our health professionals, to improve communication, increase awareness of the special needs of women's bodies, and further enhance awareness of gender differences and gender concerns as they impact on prevention and health care. We can, and should, "vote with our feet" by changing physicians and other health professionals when we feel we are not being listened to adequately.

Another resource is the increasing number of women in the health professions in all fields. We must be the ones to lead this agenda into the twenty-first century. We can be, and should be, in the forefront of the women's health agenda efforts. Health **costs** can be reduced and health **care** improved by attention to the significant differences between the needs and body chemistry of men and women. You will find in this book some unrecognized connections and issues that are crucial to our understanding of how women's bodies work. You have known or suspected some of these hormonal connections because you live them. Some will seem so obvious you will wonder why they haven't been addressed before. Some will make you cry; some will make you angry. "I *knew* it was real," women say in my office. "At least I don't feel like I'm crazy. There's something going on that makes sense." "Finally, someone is telling it like it is and putting it together." For example, I have drawn a number of diagrams throughout the book to show hormonal connections that seem *basic* to me. I have never seen these connections laid out like this before. I continue to be astounded by the apparent blind spots about the role of female hormones in so many different body-brain functions.

I have provided a lot of medical information in the chapters ahead. Use this information to become a powerful advocate for your own health and well-being. Write me with your comments, your feedback, your experiences in health care settings, and your ideas or suggestions for how we can all work together to reach our goals to improve the delivery of women's healthcare: for ourselves, for our collective aspirations for our daughters' and granddaughters' generations. While I may not be able to respond personally to each of you, I can assure you that your voice WILL be heard, taken seriously, and incorporated into future programs, courses, services, and research in women's health. Let's make the slogan "You've come a long way, baby" mean something HEALTHY!

CHAPTER 2

Making "Holistic" Medicine Whole

In recent years, there has been a dramatic increase in the variety of alternative medicine therapies in use by individuals, hospitals, physicians, and other health professionals in many fields. I am excited to see this changing trend and have been an advocate for integrating alternative approaches Western (allopathic) medicine. I am such a proponent for the inclusion of these therapies in our usual medical approaches that I designed an annual CME course for physicians to learn more about complementary or alternative medicine and use these therapies with their patients. Although *alternative medicine* is the term in general use today, I prefer the term *complementary medicine* because I think these therapies are necessary for many patients and indeed do "complement" the techniques used in Western medicine.

I have used many of the complementary medicine modalities for my own healing from various surgeries. I know with certainty that I would not have the mobility and range of motion I have today if I had not incorporated massage therapy, neuromuscular therapy, myofascial release, and hydrotherapy into my own rehabilitation. I have also personally used biofeedback, hypnotherapy, visualization-guided imagery, aromatherapy, therapeutic hot mud packs (prescribed by an Italian physician), physical therapy, chiropractic, acupuncture, and herbal therapies for reducing chronic pain and enhancing relaxation.

I have also needed the best of Western medicine, involving complex imaging to diagnose my back and neck problems, precision neurosurgical approaches using "high-tech" operating microscopes to remove herniated cervical discs, and medications to reduce pain. I know at many levels, intellectually and from personal experience, how important it is for patients to have an *integration* of these therapies in order to get well and become healthy again.

As you read this book and hear me talk about the new scientific advances and hormone therapies in women's health, remember this: *First and foremost*, my belief system emphasizes wellness and natural options as the foundation, with medical (surgery, medications, etc.) approaches to be added when needed. I know firsthand, however, how important **both** are to providing *complete health care*. I am convinced that the key to reducing future health care costs, maximizing patient recovery, and improving well-being will come from the blend of traditional Western and complementary therapeutic approaches. As you read this book and hear me talk about the new scientific advances and hormone therapies in women's health, remember this: In the best sense of the word, such an integrated approach can be called *wholistic* medicine. The term "holistic" (wholistic) medicine as used today, however, tends to have a different meaning: "holistic" has come to refer primarily to therapies perceived as "natural," and usually means any "non-Western medical" approach to healing, such as herbal medicine, homeopathy, naturopathy, chiropractic, Chinese medicine, acupuncture, bodywork, energywork, and others.

I would like share with you what *wholistic medicine* means to me as a practicing physician: **To make "holistic" medicine truly *whole* or *complete*, it must mean "a <u>combination</u> of medical AND complementary modalities for healing that takes into account the WHOLE individual and the individual's physical-emotional-spiritual-social needs in designing a plan for enhancing health, creating an environment for healing, and treating illness."**

Even though we have seen a surge in interest in complementary medicine, the above definition has been my philosophy and approach to health care since *before* I started medical school, and I have continued to learn and grow in my own understanding of the many approaches which can help people in "dis—ease." The way I view it, *wholistic* health care is not so much *a technique* as it is *an attitude*. It is an attitude of seeing each individual as a unique blend of physical, psychological, and social needs, then designing a tapestry of techniques and interventions that will best address the particular needs of that person.

You may have a definition of "holistic" medicine similar to mine and wish it were more available as a model of health care delivery. Consumers who use complementary therapies usually have to pay out of pocket, because these services are not generally covered by health insurance plans. I hope we will see a time in the near future when the benefits of complementary therapies are well established from the point of view of both clinical effectiveness and economically lower cost than is our present fragmented system. As a teacher for physicians and other health professionals, I strongly believe that we are making progress toward an integrated approach. I hear more and more physicians genuinely interested in learning about *complementary therapies* and incorporating these modalities for their patients *and for themselves*.

At the same time, it is distressing that I hear *more condemnation* of Western physicians among the alternative practitioners, who now appear as closed-minded to Western approaches as allopathic physicians had previously been to the alternatives. *Holistic* medicine *cannot* be **whole** if its practitioners refuse to accept what allopathic Western medicine has to offer, anymore than we allopathic physicians can be *whole* in our approaches if we fail to include nutrition, exercise, bodywork, biofeedback, acupuncture, chiropractic, and a host of other *complementary* options. All of us, in the best interests of our patients and clients, need to *stop* the turf battles and *start* collaborating.

Women in particular seek a total approach to their healthcare, integrating techniques from traditional Western medicine with techniques from traditions of Eastern, Native American, and other ancient healing approaches. Women's wisdom down through the ages provides us with an understanding of the ways women had an intuitive knowledge of the value of all these approaches to healing. In the Greek mythology, the two daughters of Aesculepius (god of healing), Panacea and Hygiea, were the goddesses of different realms of healing: Hygiea's domain was health practices (now known as *hygiene*) and Panacea's role was to apply the "healing balm" of kindness and compassion.

The word *panacea* has now come to imply a relatively meaningless cure-all, something of little *real* value in technological medicine. But in its ancient meaning, you can see how crucial the healing balm of kindness and compassion is whenever there is suffering and a need for healing. In the ancient Greek view, the domains of both Hygiea and Panacea were important to the total healing process. This is the balance we again seek to achieve today.

Such ideas were important to early American women physicians. Elizabeth Blackwell, the first woman ever to earn a formal medical (M.D.) degree, had a profound influence on health care delivery for women in the nineteenth century. Dr. Blackwell was a strong proponent of proper use of the medicines available in her time (the late 1800s), along with healthy food, exercise such as walking, fresh air, and sunshine, good hygiene, sanitary practices in hospitals and doctors offices, and other modalities we would today call wellness approaches. At the time she pushed for sanitary practices in hospitals, surgeons still did not know the value of hand washing between surgeries to cut down the infection rate. At Dr. Blackwell's hospital for women, where she insisted upon such procedures of good hygiene and washing, the infection and death rates following childbirth were a minuscule percentage of the rates at the more prestigious New York hospitals run by her male medical colleagues who did not believe hand washing was necessary. Women physicians have been in the forefront of encouraging the use of traditional therapies and wellness lifestyles, and women patients seem genuinely more responsive to and interested in these complementary approaches.

I have seen an ominous trend in the last several years as I speak to groups of women around the country. I have seen an emerging antagonism toward *all* Western medicine physicians and Western medicinals (pharmaceuticals). At every seminar I present, I hear women talk about how "good" the alternative therapists and herbal remedies are and how "bad" doctors and "drugs" are. Recent medical research has helped to clarify many of the health risks specifically threatening women's well-being and longevity, and to develop effective therapies and medications with fewer side effects. At the same time, however, women are turning away from Western science and medicines in droves. I feel strongly that **none of us can afford this "either-or" polarized model of thinking.**

I recognize all too well, and with sadness, just how much my own profession has failed to address the needs of women, but I believe women around the country are now in danger of throwing out the baby with the bathwater when they reject what Western medicine has to offer. Women have rightly asked for more research into the health problems experienced by women. Yet, when that research shows that hormone therapy after menopause reduces the risks of certain diseases, many of the voices who cried out for more research now turn around and accuse physicians of *medicalizing* the natural menopause transition. I have been shocked and saddened by such views, and the anger with which they are spoken.

A mistaken idea often espoused by alternative therapists is that it is only medical drugs that are dangerous and cause unwanted side effects. *Iatrogenic illness*, meaning that illness caused or aggravated by treatment procedures or medicines, has been with humankind ever since the first medicine man/woman gave someone an overdose of ground herbs. Curare is a *plant*-derived nerve toxin: It is therapeutic in small amounts, yet causes death by paralysis of the respiratory muscles if given in large enough amounts. You can become toxic on too many vitamin supplements, as well as by taking too much of a particular prescription drug. When I give a seminar, women tell me that herbal medicine is "more natural" and *therefore safer*. Herbs aren't *necessarily* "gentler" or "safer" than pharmaceutical products, although they *may* be in some situations. For example, I have seen quite a number of patients, as well as myself, who have had allergic reactions or toxicity symptoms to some herbal products, contrary to the reassurances of herbalists who have said herbs are "balanced" and don't cause allergic reactions. I also have patients who have had adverse reactions to Western pharmaceuticals. The street runs both ways. Whenever you are taking "medicinals," *no matter what the source*, there is the potential for benefit as well as the possibility of an undesirable reaction.

Yet many times, the same person who objects to taking a purified estrogen because it is made in a laboratory will take a herbal product *with no ingredient list* or, as a recent patient said to me "Here is the list of herbs in this tonic, but *I don't have any idea what the words mean or what they do*." I have a hard time understanding the logic of this. I do not think women's health needs are well served by taking an "either-or" stance. When women turn to alternative therapists as their primary or only provider of health services, and seek the road to wellness *only* through herbal remedies, vitamin supplements, colonics, and other practices which may or may not have appropriate application for a given person, they may miss important and treatable medical problems. A common problem I see is the loss of energy and fatigue that occurs early in the course of thyroid decline, which may be missed if you just take extra vitamins and don't have the appropriate thyroid tests done. Too often, particularly in women's health care, both physicians and alternative therapists apply *only their specialty*, regardless of whether this resolves the problem. To put it another way, both groups get too involved with treating a *symptom* rather than the *person* and seeking the underlying cause(s) of the problem.

Keep in mind as you design your health plan: **Balance is the key.** The body is an exquisitely sensitive, precious machine, and it needs the proper balance in order to function optimally. That balance will be achieved in different ways, and with different techniques, for different individuals, using the tools of modern medicine ALONG WITH the tools of complementary therapeutics. Each one of us is an individual with different needs. The key is to integrate and blend the therapeutic approaches right for you.

Perhaps several case vignettes of actual patients of mine will best illustrate these points and help to set the philosophy from which I write this book and approach the variety of common problems which affect women in greater numbers than men.

Ms. M is a young woman in her early thirties who was referred to me by another physician who said, "She is having significant problems with anxiety and mood swings, and I have her on these various medications, but she doesn't seem to be getting better. She is having a hard time keeping her appointments with me, and I am really not sure what to do to help her. Would you see her and see what you think should be done?"

In doing a systematic medical and psychiatric evaluation of this young woman, I found an unrecognized medical problem (severe changes in her blood sugar levels and abnormally high levels of body insulin production) that had a major impact on her mood swings. Her symptoms were much worse just prior to her menses because of the rise in progesterone that also affected her blood sugar regulation. She also had an unexpected "anxious agitation" reaction from the tranquilizers she had been receiving from several physicians. An additional factor causing her anxiety and agitation was the "withdrawal syndrome" each month that occurred when she stopped the large doses of natural progesterone she was using for PMS.

I tapered her off these medications gradually over several months. I later suggested a small dose of a more appropriate anxiety-reducing medicine for her problem of adrenalin overactivity and treated her with a small amount of supplemental estrogen to correct her hormonal imbalance. Her meal plan was designed to stablize the blood glucose highs and lows, and she was started on a basic vitamin program with added calcium and magnesium. I used techniques of self-hypnosis, with relaxation-visualization training to help her with her stress reduction and performance anxiety. I referred her to a massage therapist, and to a chiropractor to help diminish the muscle tension and spasm she experienced from the stress in her life. I recommended she seek training in the Alexander technique as well to improve her concert performance.

This woman also needed more intensive psychotherapy to work through problems from her childhood, and as she worked through these issues she did not need large doses of tranquilizers which had previously been prescribed. She is now doing very well, is taking far less medication, and has made enormous strides on her road to well-being by understanding how she needs to eat, using effective relaxation techniques, working with various body therapies to address chronic neck and back problems, and having therapy sessions focused on her particular concerns for psychological health and spiritual growth. She has blossomed as a concert musician, confident in her abilities as a soloist, as well as her newer roles as wife and mother.

What can we learn from this? The message is to *listen carefully*, look for *patterns* of symptoms (such as the premenstrual worsening of her mood changes, blood sugar swings, back and neck pain) and then systematically identify tools to improve overall health, comfort, and sense of control over life's choices. Another lesson, which was reinforced for me as I worked with this woman, is that women often need *much less* medication than the standard doses recommended (based on clinical drug studies done primarily on *men*). If you are not getting better with dose *increases*, talk to your physician about *decreasing* the dose of your medication to see if that will provide relief of troublesome symptoms. The gender differences in response to medication are quite striking, and have not been addressed adequately in good research. I will talk more about these aspects in future chapters.

Mrs. B. was sent to me by a psychic healer who intuitively "saw" a medical problem that doctors had not been able to diagnose. This woman had a back problem and had seen a chiropractor who recommended adjustment treatments and a long list of vitamin supplements. The manipulation helped ease the muscle spasm, but when this patient began on a lemon juice–maple syrup "cleansing fast" for a week or so (recommended by a naturopathic practitioner), the large doses of vitamins gradually began to create other problems. The imbalanced fasting formula, with such a high level of simple sugar carbohydrate and **no** protein, caused the excessive vitamins and minerals to become even more toxic.

Over the next three months, the patient developed bizarre "burning, electric shock-like sensations up and down my spine and body," along with occasional numbness and tingling, marked mood changes, and generalized muscle weakness. She was seen then by a neurologist, but her unusual emotional expressions and behavior made him think she was "psychotic." Since I worked in both internal medicine and psychiatry, I was asked to see her for a consultation. After getting the history I have just described, I asked her family to bring in *all* of the supplements she had been taking. It turned out to be a *grocery bag full of various vitamins and herbal products*. When I reviewed all of the overlap and duplication among the different products, and put the pieces of the puzzle together, it became clear that she had multiple vitamin and mineral toxicities from over-supplementation. These problems were then made worse by the syrup-lemon juice "cleansing" fasts that further upset body balance. *She had not been on any allopathic or Western medications*, and yet she clearly had toxicity symptoms. She was also a cigarette smoker, so, of course, the nicotine only aggravated her other problems.

To regain normal nerve and muscle function, along with better mood stability, her body needed to be "de-toxified" from these excesses. The situation for this women was complicated enough that she required hospital admission in order to sort out the problems and do the necessary evaluations. The excessive supplements were stopped, and the dietitian worked with her on a healthy meal plan. Hypnotherapy was used to help with relaxation so she could stop the smoking which she said "calmed her nerves." She had a partially ruptured lumbar disk that intermittently caused some of the tingling sensations in her legs when she got into certain body positions. I prescribed physical therapy so she could learn good body posture, exercises to strengthen her back, and how to lift correctly. Since this woman's only daughter was about to leave home for college, I felt that some of her mood symptoms were related to feelings of loss that could best be helped with supportive psychotherapy.

What can we learn from what happened with this patient? One message is that multiple practitioners can unknowingly create problems by adding therapies that don't blend well with something another therapist has recommended. When you are seeing several health care providers, make sure that you tell each person what you are doing or taking under the care of someone else. For Mrs. B., the chiropractor had not recognized the toxicity from too much vitamin supplementation, and that his patient needed proper medical diagnosis about the unrecognized lumbar disk problem before she should start on a course of manipulation. Later, when she did see a neurologist, this physician did not take seriously her complaints of back pain because her behavior and emotionality, as well as the multiplicity her unusual symptoms, made it difficult for him to see a neurological problem; he decided she was "psychotic."

It does often happen that when a *female* patient (compared to a male patient) has symptoms that are unusual or puzzling, the *female* patient much more commonly will be told "there is nothing wrong," or she is written off as "neurotic" or "psychotic," and the actual medical issues do not get promptly identified and treated appropriately. Neither Mrs. B or her family had communicated to anyone information about the juice–syrup fasting or the complete list of supplements she had been taking. No one can put a puzzle together if major pieces are missing! The subsequent integration of medicine, psychiatry, physical therapy, dietary therapy, hypnotherapy, and emotional support was crucial to provide the various modalities she needed for solving the puzzle of interconnected medical and behavioral problems. The point here is that vitamins, although natural, can be toxic in large amounts and can cause changes in mood and behavior along with unusual "nervous" symptoms which can be confused with a medical or psychiatric disorder.

The cases of Ms. M. and Ms. B. illustrate the success of an integrated mind–body comprehensive approach, with traditional medical care an important dimension of their initial assessment and treatment. Even though I am interested in many of the complementary therapies, one physician cannot provide all the therapeutic modalities that are needed to help solve all the problems. It requires the efforts of a team of people, each adding expertise to put together the pieces to create an integrated "whole." These patient cases further illustrate the dangers of taking only one part of the continuum of available treatment approaches. On either end of the continuum, an imbalance may occur, causing the patient to become clinically worse. Modern medicine may take an "overkill" approach at times, but so may chiropractors, advocates of megavitamin supplementation, herbalists, and other alternative therapists who encourage people to avoid what traditional Western medicine has to offer. At either extreme, such a stance is potentially dangerous. In like manner, physicians must be knowledgeable about and consider the value of complementary therapeutic modalities that may benefit patients, and seek to include these in medical therapeutic regimens.

You must always remember that health problems are *highly individualized*. Similar symptoms in two different people can mean entirely different things. A therapy of any kind that brings rapid relief to one person may be of no help to another and may cause serious side effects in a third. I think it is critically important that all health problems be initially evaluated by a competent, concerned physician, one whom you feel listens to you, has your best interests at heart, and who encourages you to add other appropriate and compatible therapeutic approaches to your overall health plan.

If you do not now have such a physician, you have every right as a patient to seek one. Such a physician should ideally work *collaboratively* with other therapists and therapeutic options as needed to assist the individual patient reach her optimum level of wellness. It is also important for YOU to tell your physician what supplements you are taking and what other therapies you are using. I think it also is very helpful when alternative medicine practitioners communicate with you and your physician when they see something unusual.

I remember one situation that really illustrates this latter point well. One of the massage therapists working with me in my medical practice told me she was worried about a woman who had just started bruising excessively during a massage session. I checked on the patient and discovered she was taking Coumadin (a blood "thinner" to help prevent clots); she had misunderstood her directions and was taking *double* the prescribed dose. She was now bleeding under the skin, which caused the bruises, and she needed immediate vitamin K injections as well as to decrease her Coumadin. Even though she did not know the cause of the bruising, the massage therapist's astute observations, which she promptly communicated to me, helped prevent this patient from having a potentially serious hemorrhage.

This story also illustrates one of the very positive aspects of modern medicine: the ability, using various laboratory and other diagnostic means, to determine more precisely what is needed for a given patient, such as fine-tuning the amount of anticoagulant or measuring blood sugar levels to determine the amount of insulin to give a diabetic. This is a valuable aspect of modern health care that alternative practitioners would do well to recognize and utilize. On the other hand, there may be many herbal options for common ailments that are safer and more effective than taking repeated courses of antibiotics, which themselves carry a risk of contributing to recurrent yeast infections in women and the problem of developing resistant bacteria. Modern antibiotics are also usually quite expensive.

The primary disadvantage to herbal remedies, in my opinion, is that often you are not able to determine the actual amount of the active ingredients you are getting or what is actually in the preparation. If, for instance, a natural prescription says to take 6 bay leaves every day, how much of the desired ingredient is in that leaf, and what size leaf is used? An advantage of Western medicine is that one knows exactly how much 5 mg of a compound is. The dosage can be adjusted up or down with greater precision and accuracy than a random selection of 6 leaves. On the other hand, physicians may be too heavy-handed in the amounts of allopathic Western medicines they prescribe, especially for women patients.

Doses of many medications for women often need to be started at much lower levels than are used for men. I have a number of women who have benefited from Prozac for premenstrual symptoms *but may need only 2 mg instead of the usual 20 mg dose described as the starting amount.* If the differences in women's body size and physiology are not taken into account, the likelihood of adverse side effects increases dramatically. No matter what therapy is being prescribed, all of us involved in the health field and in helping others become well should keep in mind the important premise of ALL healing traditions: "DO NO HARM."

I think the overall keys to providing the best health care for women are the recognition of *gender* differences and the recognition that *each individual* person will have *different needs.* I think each school of thought has much to teach the others. To provide optimal care for women of today, we must be open to all options. Our goal should be to find the particular blend of physical, medical, psychological, and spiritual approaches for the individual woman to help her best regain balance and achieve harmony and good health. Two critical elements are necessary: the healing *relationship* with the health professional, and the involvement of the woman's capacity for developing *self-healing* skills. I believe in the idea that the most important healing comes from within, tapping into the power of our minds in taking an active role in our individual wellness.

When we combine our *internal* healing power with the appropriate *external* modalities available to us, the integration enhances our ability to achieve the best state of health we can. Even if you have a disease, such as diabetes, you may still move to a greater state of *wellness* by eating healthy meals, exercising regularly, practicing relaxation skills, having massage therapy to improve circulation, and maintaining a positive outlook on life. It's a different way of looking at things: someone who has no disease or illness may still be *unwell*; another person who practices the integration of internal and external healing options may be much more *well* even in the face of significant disease.

If we CHOOSE to use it, engaging our minds to activate the healing ability *within* us is the most powerful medicine that exists for all of us. My emphasis throughout this book is creating a "health partnership" between you and your physicians, and assisting you to feel in control of your choices and options. Without YOU, the patient, having an active commitment to and involvement in YOUR own health care, the healing process breaks down. YOU are the most crucial member of any health care team! My desire is to help you learn the information and skills to take responsibility for your own well-being, and then help you find the necessary resources to reach your goals. I hope this book will give you many ideas, new insights, and options to better understand the wonderful miracle of your body and the means to help you achieve your best level of health, wherever you are on life's journey. ***Be A Well, Educated Woman!***

CHAPTER 3

Hormones: A Guide to Body Cycles

What Are Hormones?

HORMONES. Today, whenever I mention the word *hormones*, women have almost instantaneously an intense reaction, either very positive or very negative, but not much in-between:

"I don't want strange chemicals in my body."

"All doctors ever do is prescribe hormone pills."

"Those are drugs. I don't take drugs; I want to be natural."

"I know it's my hormones out of whack that's making me feel so bad, but my doctors won't listen. Why won't anybody give me hormones?"

"I felt like being on hormones has lifted the fogginess off my brain and I have more energy now."

This polarization of opinions crops up everywhere these days. Betty Friedan, in a speech at Omega Institute in the fall of 1994, called hormones, specifically estrogen therapy, a *hoax* perpetrated on women by the medical industry. Dr. Trudy Bush of Johns Hopkins said in several 1994 publications that the majority of women after menopause would benefit from estrogen therapy. Both speakers are women, yet 180 degrees apart in their views.

Why such emotional intensity and polarization over "hormones"? I hear these statements and the anger about the use of hormone therapy from many women, and it reminds me of the intensity of the debates between the "Prolifers" and the "Prochoicers" over abortion. Why is this? What are these things called *hormones*? What do they do? Why are they important? How do we tell when a woman (or a man, for that matter) needs hormones? This chapter will help clarify these questions; in later chapters, we will look more closely at factors I think contribute to the polarity in views and the intense emotionalism on these issues. I will also provide you with the latest research and clinical information that helps to show unrecognized hormonal connections affecting many conditions that are more common in women.

The word hormone means "a product of a living cell that circulates in body fluids or sap (in plants) and produces a specific effect on the activity of cells remote from its point of origin; or a synthetic substance that acts like a hormone" (*Webster's Tenth Dictionary*). I think of hormones as "chemical communicators" or "connectors" that carry messages to and from all organs of the body and serve to connect one organ's function with another organ's function to keep the body balanced and functioning optimally. Without our hormones to keep the connections and messages flowing smoothly and our organs functioning in an integrated manner, we would eventually die. It's that simple. The secretion and interaction of hormones throughout our bodies every day is a highly complex and ongoing process.

For many years, I have used the visual image of a "key in a lock" to describe the way brain chemicals fit at special receptor sites in the brain, and the way hormones bind at their specific receptor sites to trigger their action on the target cells. Each hormone, neurotransmitter, neuropeptide, or other chemical messenger is a unique "key," and each has a "lock" (receptor site) into which it fits (see diagram). The receptor sites may be located on cell surfaces (membrane receptors) or inside cells (cytoplasm or nucleus receptors). Each hormone provides a specific set of directions or messages to the target cells to enable the cells to perform certain functions.

The cells of the body are like manufacturing plants, making the many chemicals the body needs to function. Hormones have a variety of functions, some similar to those of assembly-line supervisors directing the manufacturing processes, and some similar to those of team facilitators acting as catalysts for chemical processes to occur in the cell. Hormone actions may be rapid if they trigger immediate chemical release via effects on membrane receptors or slower if acting at the cell nucleus receptors to influence the DNA and direct the manufacture of specific enzymes and proteins. The molecules of each hormone fit exactly into the proper receptor site; changes in the molecule configuration produce different notches on the molecule key, which means that a different configuration may not work as well at that receptor. This effect of molecular change is evident from the way in which the various types of estrogen molecules produce different results at the estrogen receptors throughout the brain and body. We also see this difference in response with many other hormones and their synthetic "look-alikes." If the hormone molecules don't bind just the right way and "click into the lock," it's like a key getting stuck in a lock. The door doesn't open easily; the cell doesn't function properly, and you may experience the body effects of missing that particular hormone.

As a specific example of the importance of molecule structure, consider the primary human estrogen, 17-beta estradiol, and the primary horse estrogen, equilin (one of the components of Premarin). Both types of estrogen have four connecting rings as the basic shape of the molecule. But equilin has some important differences in the makeup of one of the rings, which makes it a slightly different key. Consequently, it does not fit the estrogen receptor exactly (like a key getting stuck); it sometimes keeps the human estradiol key from fitting into the receptor, which means the effects can be different from those of native human estrogen. The length of time it attaches to the receptor varies compared with human estrogen; and the process for the body to metabolize equilin is different. Because the equilin metabolite is not a normal one for the human body to process, the enzymes needed to break it down aren't necessarily readily in place, so excretion takes longer. All this because of a few changes in one ring! The body is quite amazing in its ability to recognize its exact molecular keys.

Hormones are very potent molecules, and it usually takes minuscule amounts, sometimes as little as a billionth of a gram, to exert their effects on cells of the target organs. After initiating actions at the target organs, hormones are broken down and "inactivated" by the target cells themselves or carried by the blood to the liver to be metabolized. The metabolized hormones are used again by the body's synthesis processes to make new hormone molecules, or the metabolic by-products are excreted in the urine (tests can measure hormone breakdown substances in urine) or feces. For example, Premarin produces two of the human types of estrogen (estradiol and estrone) in a smaller amounts, along with the higher amounts of horse equilin estrogens. All that's needed to activate the human body's estrogen receptors is the estradiol (and possibly estrone, although this is not yet clear), but the remaining equilin hormones still have to be processed by the liver for excretion in the urine.

Equilin isn't necessarily "bad," but it does place an unusual extra demand on the body that isn't needed for estrogen's beneficial effects. For some women, this appears to be the reason that they still have symptoms of estrogen loss, even when taking the conjugated equine estrogens (Premarin); that is, the keys are not opening the receptor locks quite as well, or perhaps the mixed estrogen tablets aren't providing quite enough of the human forms (estradiol and estrone) that woman may need. This may be why the dose is often increased, that then means even more equilin for the body to have to process. I will talk more about the many effects of some of these differences in the chapters ahead, but I wanted you to begin to realize the crucial importance of the *fit* of hormone molecules into their receptor sites throughout the body.

Some of the major hormones, where they are produced, and what they do, are described in the diagrams and charts below. As you read them, think about the brain as the orchestra conductor who provides direction to the various "instruments" (hormones) to produce the "symphony" of our body rhythms and functions. Hormones affect the brain, and the brain affects hormone production and interactions. The brain and the body *really are* intimately connected!

Diagram 3.1—HORMONES AND RECEPTORS:
A LOOK AT HOW THEY WORK

The hormone molecule "key" fits into its own receptor site "lock" at the target cells for that hormone. Molecules with different configurations may also occupy the "lock" but may or may not trigger the normal action like the own body's molecules do. Sometimes other molecules may block the body's own hormones from working properly.

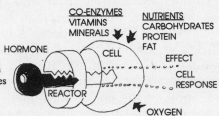

MEMBRANE RECEPTOR MODE OF ACTION
The hormone "key" fits into the receptor "lock" located on the membrane surface of the cell. This binding triggers adenylate cyclase, the enzyme in the cell, to increase production of cyclic AMP. cAMP then acts as a "second messenger" to link the hormone at the cell surface with the inside of the cell where the metabolic actions (triggered by the hormone) take place. cAMP is one of a number of such "second messengers" in the body.

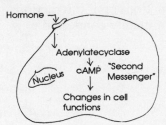

NUCLEAR RECEPTOR MODE OF ACTION
Here the hormone "key" is small and soluble enough (like estradiol) to be able to pass through the cell membrane, to fit into the receptor "lock" in the nucleus of the cell. It sets off its effects on cell metabolism by interacting with DNA in the nucleus, which directs the making of RNA from DNA. RNA moves into the cytoplasm outside the nucleus and directs the cell's "metabolic machinery" to make proteins and enzymes for the cell's functions.

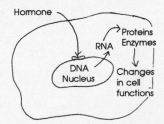

Diagram 3.2—THE ENDOCRINE SYSTEM: A LOOK AT KEY HORMONES AND WHAT THEY DO

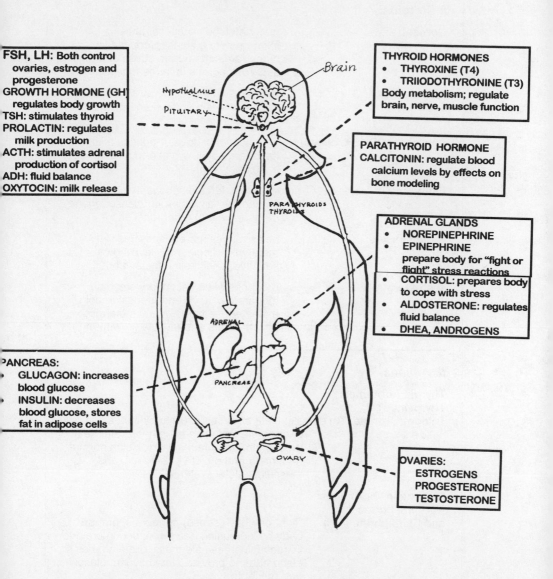

FSH, LH: Both control ovaries, estrogen and progesterone
GROWTH HORMONE (GH) regulates body growth
TSH: stimulates thyroid
PROLACTIN: regulates milk production
ACTH: stimulates adrenal production of cortisol
ADH: fluid balance
OXYTOCIN: milk release

THYROID HORMONES
- THYROXINE (T4)
- TRIIODOTHYRONINE (T3)
Body metabolism; regulate brain, nerve, muscle function

PARATHYROID HORMONE
CALCITONIN: regulate blood calcium levels by effects on bone modeling

ADRENAL GLANDS
- NOREPINEPHRINE
- EPINEPHRINE
  prepare body for "fight or flight" stress reactions
- CORTISOL: prepares body to cope with stress
- ALDOSTERONE: regulates fluid balance
- DHEA, ANDROGENS

PANCREAS:
- GLUCAGON: increases blood glucose
- INSULIN: decreases blood glucose, stores fat in adipose cells

OVARIES:
ESTROGENS
PROGESTERONE
TESTOSTERONE

Brain
Hypothalamus
Pituitary
Parathyroids
Thyroid
Adrenal
Pancreas
Ovary

CLASSES OF HORMONES AND WHAT THEY DO

Primary Actions

I. Steroids

Cortisol . . . . many metabolic actions, anti-inflammatory actions, produced in higher amounts during stress and may suppress normal immune function

Aldosterone . . . . regulates fluid balance by stimulating kidney to retain sodium and water, excretes potassium

Androgens (DHEA, others) . . enhances sex drive, produces mild male features in women (e.g. facial hair, male body shape)

Estrogens (three) . . . . produces female secondary sex characteristics; key role: menstruation, pregnancy; 400 other functions

Progesterone . . . . helps maintain pregnancy, many metabolic effects, high levels give sedative, analgesic effects at brain

Testosterone . . . . produces male secondary sex patterns; triggers sex drive and arousal in both males and females, many metabolic effects (bone and muscle growth, etc.)

II. Amines

Thyroid hormones:
Thyroxine (T4),
Triiodothyronine (T3) . . . stimulate body metabolism by increasing cell energy release; increasing heart rate, heat production, and brain activity. Helps normal regulation and growth of nervous, and musculoskeletal systems

"Adrenalin" hormones:
Norepinephrine (NE)
and Epinephrine (EPI) . . "fight or flight" (stress) hormones, prepare body by increasing heart rate; act on brain to lift mood, increase alertness; dilate arteries to key organs to provide more oxygen, glucose, and nutrients

III. Peptides and Proteins

Insulin . . . . *lowers* blood sugar (moves glucose into cells), stimulates fat storage and protein synthesis

Glucagon . . . . *raises* blood glucose (glycogen breakdown and glucose release from liver, gluconeogenesis)

Somatostatin . . . . mild effect to raise blood glucose

Parathyroid Hormone (PTH) . . . major role: increase blood calcium levels by stimulating bone breakdown, calcium release

Calcitonin . . . . involved in regulating blood calcium levels by inhibiting bone breakdown, calcium release

Thymosin (thymus gland) . . . . . major role in development of immune system

ACTH . . . . Adrenocorticotropin Hormone; stimulates part of the adrenal gland to make cortisol

FSH . . . . stimulates ovaries, activates and promotes follicle growth to produce estrogen

LH . . . . triggers ovulation, formation of the corpus luteum, secretion of progesterone, estrogen

Growth Hormone (GH) . . . . oversees entire process of normal body growth

TSH . . . . stimulates the thyroid gland to release T3, T4

Prolactin . . . . stimulates breast enlargement during pregnancy and milk production after delivery

Anti-Diuretic Hormone (ADH) . . prevents dehydration by stimulating kidneys to increase reabsorption and retain water

Oxytocin . . . . stimulates uterine contractions during labor, helps trigger milk release after delivery.

Melatonin (pineal gland) . . . . regulation of sleep cycles, body rhythms

Brain–Body Hormonal Communication Pathways

The brain and body are interconnected by an incredible array of chemical and electrical circuits, each one interacting with and affecting others. The brain has a multitude of ways to direct the orchestra of the body to respond to what it (the brain) perceives, whether from inside the body physically, inside the mind's thoughts and feelings, or outside the body. In women's bodies, the entire process is even more complex: the menstrual cycle rhythm of changes causes the brain-body systems to continuously adapt to the changing hormonal environment. Unlike the male body, which maintains a fairly steady production (*tonic* pattern) of testosterone all month, the female body has a *cyclic* pattern.

The major underlying influence of these crucial female hormonal rhythms has never been fully appreciated for the diverse effects on *all* parts of the female body, not just reproduction. The diagram that follows shows some of the ways that *stressors* (stimuli) of all kinds require the body processes to change and adapt. Hormonal change is another one of those stressors that mean that the body systems must constantly be changing and adapting.

When the body systems are overstressed, a variety of phenomena may occur. Sometimes we call these changes *symptoms* if they feel unpleasant to us. These changes themselves may become additional stressors on the body and contribute to more stress overload and possible illness. The interconnections and the ways in which hormonal production may in turn be altered by stress on the body are often overlooked when women seek medical care. The two-way nature of these pathways is a critical connection throughout all facets of women's health that has generally been the frequently overlooked "missing link."

Diagram 3.3—STRESS

SITUATIONAL
*finances
*work
*relationships
*community

PSYCHOLOGICAL
*fears
*worries
*view of self
*mid-life angst

PHYSICAL
*hormones
*diet
*illness
*alcohol,drugs

ENVIRONMENTAL
*pollutants
*allergens
*weather

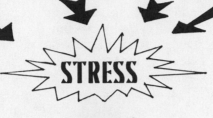

STRESS

DISRUPTS BODY BALANCE (HOMEOSTASIS), WHICH CAN LEAD TO

PSYCHOLOGICAL SYMPTOMS
-Anxiety
-Sleep Problems
-Depression
-Anger Outbursts

PHYSICAL ILLNESSES
-Fibromyalgia
-Chronic Fatigue
-Infections (Viral, Bacterial)
-Allergies
-Autoimmune diseases (Lupus, others)
-Cancer

ADRENALIN OVER-ACTIVITY
-Headaches
-Colitis
- Arteriosclerosis
-High Blood Pressure
-"Panic Attacks"
-Eczema
-Ulcers

The Menstrual Cycle RHYTHM of Changes

Most women learn about menstruation initially from mothers or girlfriends. The first more scientific explanation we receive is often in health class, about the sixth or seventh grade. We then live it each month and don't really think about which hormone is doing what at any given time. In case you've forgotten your health class, I'd like to give you a quick rundown on what happens in the normal menstrual cycle. My description is based on the average cycle length of 28 days, but keep in mind that variations in length from 25 to 35 days may be perfectly normal.

We arbitrarily mark the cycle by labeling the first day of bleeding DAY ONE (M). We could define any day as Day One, but it helps to have such a clear-cut marker as bleeding to use as a starting point. Bleeding is really the finishing of the previous cycle with the shedding of the lining of the uterus (womb) that is not needed if there is no fertilized egg to nourish. As the uterine lining is being shed, the body is preparing for the next cycle. The follicle ("little sac") in the ovary that will become the egg is already being "recruited" by the hormonal changes. Progesterone and estrogen both dropped sharply in the waning days of the previous cycle, and these two hormones are now at their lowest point of the cycle as bleeding begins (DAY ONE of next cycle).

From Day One until ovulation, estrogen levels are rising as growth of several follicles is being stimulated by FSH (follicle stimulating hormone). Once estrogen reaches a certain amount, all but one of the follicles shrink; this one is the egg released at ovulation. For the entire first half of the cycle progesterone levels remain extremely low, usually less than 1.

This first half of the cycle is dominated by estrogen and is called the *Follicular Phase* (refers to the egg development in the ovary) or *Proliferative Phase* (refers to the process of growth of the endometrial lining of the uterus). Estrogen levels average about 200 pg/ml across the first two weeks of the cycle, with the estrogen low point being DAY ONE and its high point being OVULATION, usually about Day 14. Peak estrogen levels at midcycle are in the range of 350 to 500 pg/ml. The first few days of the cycle, estrogen levels are about 60–90 pg/ml until the decline in estrogen in the pre(peri)menopause years.

Thus, keep in mind that in the first two weeks each cycle until ovulation occurs, estrogen levels are *high*, and progesterone levels are *low* (in fact, there's very little progesterone present for these two weeks). This is typically the phase of the cycle during which women experience a sense of well-being, optimal energy level, normal sleep, and an "up" mood. Estrogen has more of an activating effect on brain centers and enhances energy and mood. In Chapter 4, I will show you some of the many ways estrogen acts on the brain that are similar to the actions of present *antidepressant* medications.

FSH is the brain hormone that stimulates the growth of the follicle. FSH begins to rise in the cycle when the brain senses the drop in estrogen at menses; FSH stimulates the ovary to produce the next egg. FSH and LH (luteinizing hormone), are the two primary brain hormones that govern the egg maturation and release for the menstrual cycle. I won't focus on FSH and LH because I want you to have an overview about the estrogen and progesterone patterns and effects. In the perimenopausal years, as estrogen production from the ovary *declines*, the brain produces more FSH and LH trying to increase hormone production by the ovary. So you will see high levels of FSH and LH prior to and after menopause because estrogen levels are then low.

In the first 10 days of each new cycle, rising estradiol levels stimulate the release of LH from the brain. When estradiol reaches its peak level (about 400–500 pg/ml) at mid-cycle, LH triggers the follicle to be released as an egg, called *ovulation*. Some women can feel ovulation as a brief, sharp pain in the area of the ovary (called "mittelschmerz"); other women do not feel any physical sensations at ovulation. The rapid drop in estradiol as the egg is released may trigger onset of a migraine in some women; it may also contribute to brief disruption in sleep. For some women, it may trigger a brief mood swings as the brain chemicals are changing in response to the drop in circulating estrogen. I will talk more about these important connections in upcoming chapters.

The egg develops into the *corpus luteum,* (from Latin for "yellow body" due to its characteristic appearance). This half of the cycle is called *luteal phase* (if referring to the ovary changes) or *secretory phase* (if referring to the further thickening of the uterine lining to prepare for fertilization and implantation of the egg). This phase of the cycle is dominated by the hormone progesterone, which is produced by the corpus luteum. Progesterone is the "pro-*gestation*" hormone whose primary role is to prepare the body to sustain and nourish a pregnancy. It is the *dominant* hormone of the second half of the cycle, with blood levels higher than the level of estrogen.

Circulating levels of progesterone reach a peak by about DAY 20 to 22, the midpoint of the second half of the cycle (or about week three from last onset of bleeding). If the egg is fertilized, progesterone levels stay high until the placenta takes over producing the progesterone for pregnancy. If there is no fertilization of the egg, the corpus luteum begins to disintegrate, and progesterone levels drop sharply, triggering the onset of bleeding. Estrogen also drops at this time of the cycle, but it is the decrease in progesterone that causes bleeding to occur. Shedding the uterine lining is part of the process of preparing the body to begin a new cycle.

Estrogen levels also rise again from ovulation until about Day 20, and reach the peak for the second half of the cycle at the same time progesterone is peaking, but the level of estrogen in the LUTEAL phase is less than it was in the FOLLICULAR phase of the cycle. Average luteal phase estradiol levels are about 150–300 pg/ml.

Since progesterone prepares the body for pregnancy, it makes sense that some of the changes you notice—water retention, increased appetite, breast enlargement—are triggered by the metabolic effects of progesterone, since these are needed changes to help the body provide for a growing fetus. Hormones, such as insulin, that control blood glucose levels are affected by progesterone, and this contributes to some of "sweet cravings" women describe in the premenstrual week. The metabolic rate is also increased. Tufts University researchers show a 12 percent increase in appetite and metabolic rate under the influence of progesterone. You're not imaging it, you *do* notice feelings of hunger more in this half of the cycle for very real, physiological reasons based on the higher levels of progesterone at this phase of the cycle.

Another effect of progesterone is to slow down the movement of food through the gastrointestinal (GI) tract by decreasing the muscular waves (peristalsis) that move material through the entire digestive system. This is one reason you feel full or bloated at this phase of the cycle. Another lifestyle factor that intensifies the natural effects of progesterone is our low-fiber diet. In stone age cultures, humans may have eaten a 100 grams of fiber a day or more. It was an evolutionary advantage to survival in having the hormonal effect in women slow down the GI tract so that more nutrients could be absorbed from the food into the blood stream. With a high-fiber diet (which causes "rapid transit" through the GI tract) and in times when food was scarce, the hormonal effect of progesterone further helped a woman's body sustain a pregnancy.

In our culture with the typical American high protein, high fat diet, women may only get 10 grams of fiber a day! Slowing down the gastrointestinal tract when you're eating a low-fiber diet has some very unpleasant side effects...*constipation*. Women in the luteal phase frequently describe feeling lethargic, constipated, bloated, headachy, and irritable.

Progesterone has a tranquilizing effect on the brain, much like our current antianxiety medications. For some women, progesterone has such a calming effect, it acts more like a sedative. For some women, the "slowing down" effect of progesterone feels "wonderful," "soothing," "relaxed," "more centered," for others, it feels like "depression." These women say, "I don't have any get up and go." "I withdraw." "I can't get out of bed." "I don't have any energy." You can see how a hormone having a calming, tranquilizing effect is an evolutionary advantage in the early stages of pregnancy; it would facilitate diminished activity at a time when the egg is being implanted and facilitate early embryo development. In pregnancy, progesterone levels decrease sharply at the sixth to eighth week and do not rise again until about the thirty-fourth week of gestation to prepare the body for delivery. If you have been pregnant, think about how you felt the last six weeks of pregnancy compared with the middle months of pregnancy, and you can once again recognize some of the physical and psychological differences in the hormones estrogen and progesterone.

The hormonal ebb and flow that occurs in this cyclical manner has widespread effects on the brain-body processes, as well as on our psyche. When you understand the specific effects and roles of each of the primary female hormones, you can see how beautifully orchestrated the female endocrine system is for its role in bringing new life into being and keeping the species alive. These hormonal actions make sense for the tasks they govern in the body.

The problem today is that in our culture, food is no longer scarce; for most people, it is overly available. We don't eat as much fiber in fruits, whole grains, and vegetables; we have too much sugar, caffeine, and alcohol easily at hand: we're not getting pregnant as often, and we are trying to do multiple tasks, with a marked increase in overall stress levels. Consequently, some of the natural hormonal metabolic effects are now experienced as *negative, unwanted physical-psychological "symptoms"* because of our changing, unnatural lifestyles and diet. I think this is one of a number of reasons that we see so many more women experiencing PMS in today's culture compared to women at the turn of the century when diets had lower overall fat, sugar, salt, alcohol, and caffeine and far higher intake of fruits, whole grains, and vegetables.

All these underlying physiological changes have a bearing on how we respond to the external world and the impact of external stresses on our brain–body pathways. Please don't think that I'm saying we are at the mercy of our hormones. I am concerned that we need to appreciate the physiological changes. We desperately need more gender-specific research on these issues so that we can learn to constructively manage our complicated lives along with our bodies that are more complex than the male body. I don't think that the hormonal cycles mean that we should do anything less than whatever it is we would like to do with our lives. But we need to know about the hormonal cycles, and we need better medical and health research that's will help our therapeutic approaches take into account the unique and *natural* needs of the female body.

Diagram 3.4
THE MENSTRUAL CYCLE HORMONE RHYTHM

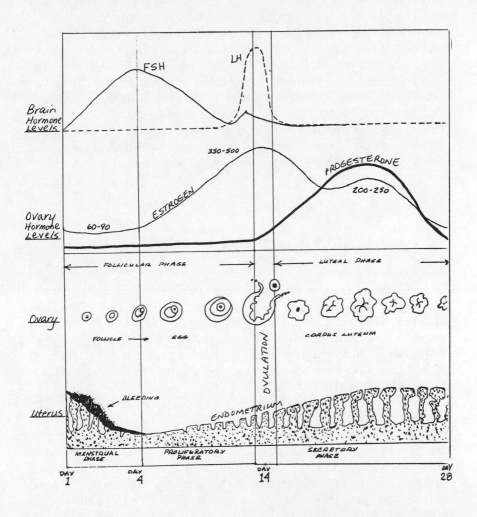

What Happens When Estrogen Declines

At birth, a newborn girl's ovaries contain about 500,000 follicles, which are the source of her future eggs. One egg will be released at ovulation approximately each menstrual cycle. By puberty, the number of follicles has decreased to 300,000 and by age 38 to 40, the average woman has only 5,000 to 10,000 follicles remaining.

The follicles and maturing eggs produce estrogen; when the ovaries run out of follicles (and therefore out of eggs), they also run out of the supply of estrogen. The brain senses the decrease in estrogen, and produces more FSH and LH to try to stimulate the ovaries to produce more hormones. FSH no longer can do its job because there are no more follicles to develop into hormone-producing eggs. This is the end of a woman's *reproductive* stage, known as **menopause**. The journey from puberty to menopause has many developmental stages along the way. Here are some of the highlights of those stages as they relate to hormone cycles.

Early Puberty and Adolescence

Girls in the United States typically enter puberty anytime between about nine and fourteen years of age. Breast development begins to appear first, followed by the appearance of pubic hair. Menstruation usually doesn't occur until the breasts are well-developed and a critical body weight of about 110 pounds is reached. This generally follows soon after the peak of the girl's adolescent growth spurt, at about age twelve. The average age at the onset of menstruation is about twelve and a half to thirteen, although it may take several years for the menstrual cycle to stabilize into a regular pattern.

During these years, a young woman's ovaries are beginning to develop their individual cycle rhythm. It can be a time of erratic periods, feelings of uncertainty about what's happening to the body, mood shifts, new physical sensations, and unpredictable menstrual flows. Some young women experience only mild cramps, or no cramps at all, with bleeding; while others have severe and sustained cramping. Some can tell physically when ovulation occurs; others have no conscious awareness of it. Fertility (the ability to conceive and bear children) occurs when ovulation begins. The problem for many adolescent girls is that since ovulation may be erratic in the first year or two of menstruation, it may be difficult to know when they are fertile. This is often one reason girls in this age group are surprised when they accidentally become pregnant. It is also an excellent reason for girls who are sexually active at this time to be certain to use some form of contraception.

Throughout history many cultures have had ceremonies (rites of passage) for young girls to mark this transition into womanhood. In our culture, this has not been a usual practice, and many young girls are embarrassed by the onset of menstruation. In our culture, language about menstruation tends to be negative: "on the rag," "the curse," and other demeaning terms don't help girls feel proud about becoming a woman. Celebration ceremonies could serve to provide positive images and role models for girls as they become young women.

Reproductive Years: The Twenties and Thirties

During her twenties and early thirties, a woman's menstrual cycle tends to be fairly regular, unless altered by lifestyle (e.g., extreme dieting, strenuous athletic activity) or the presence of endocrine or other medical disorders. Fertility usually peaks by age twenty-five, and the body is at its physiological optimal point for childbearing during the early and mid-twenties. That does not mean that women cannot become pregnant at a later age; it simply means that in the decade of her twenties a woman's circulatory, respiratory, and digestive systems are at their peak to meet the physiological demands of pregnancy with the least stress on the mother's system.

Hormone production during the twenties and early thirties is more predictable than during either puberty or perimenopause and typically follows the pattern I outlined: estrogen levels high in the first half, and progesterone dominating the second half of each cycle.

By the mid-thirties, the menstrual flow may begin changing, at first imperceptibly, and by the late thirties, more noticeably as flow may become lighter and shorter, and cycle length may become a day or two longer. By the later thirties, women often begin to notice more pronounced premenstrual mood, energy and appetite changes, which are described as the "Premenstrual Syndrome" (PMS for short). For some women, there is no PMS at all; others experience a minor degree of discomfort; still others have more bothersome symptoms lasting a week or more. For a small percentage of women, PMS may be severely disruptive of work, family, and social relationships. I describe these changes and some of their causes, in Chapter 7.

"Perimenopausal": The Forties

Between the ages of approximately 35 and 50 women enter the phase called the "climacteric" or premenopausal years when the ovaries' production of estrogen and progesterone begin declining as the woman's follicles are diminishing. Depending on your lifestyle habits and your genetic make-up, the climacteric may start in the early thirties or may not begin until the mid-forties. During this time, the hormonal levels begin to decline, cycles become more erratic, there are more cycles where you don't ovulate, and there is more fluctuation in the actual amounts of estrogen and progesterone produced. In cycles when you do ovulate, you will have higher levels of progesterone, and those cycles are usually ones when you have much more PMS: feeling bloated, headachy, irritable, tearful, and just generally awful. In cycles when you do not ovulate, there isn't much progesterone, so you sail through and don't notice any PMS-type changes.

As estrogen declines, many body functions are affected: sleep, memory, mood, energy level, immune system, body fat distribution, circulatory system, digestive tract, bone metabolism, sexual function, bladder function, and many others that I will be addressing throughout this book. These changes are gradual and take place over several years; they do not all occur at a single point in time and suddenly you wake up and say "that's it, it's menopause." The final menstrual period happens at a definite (albeit unpredictable!) point. Leading up to it for a decade or more are hormonal changes that cause a wide variety of physical and psychological experiences. For example, intermittent palpitations and premenstrual migraines may begin to occur for the first time or may suddenly get worse if you have had problems with either in earlier years.

Another frequent early indicator of declining estrogen, characteristically occurring in the early to mid-forties is changes in sleep patterns. Has anyone noticed waking up multiple times during the night? I found that for a while I was waking up, looking at the clock, then going back to sleep; an hour later I'd wake up, look at the clock, and go back to sleep. Disrupted sleep is one of the earliest effects on the brain of decreasing levels of estrogen. Mood swings, episodic tearfulness for no reason, irritability, angry outbursts, and brief spells of feeling depressed prior to your period may also occur as a result of estrogen-triggered changes in the mood-regulating chemical messengers in the brain.

Other effects of decreased estrogen are the changes in cholesterol production and ratio of HDL to LDL cholesterol that lead to heart disease, and an increased loss of bone that can result in osteoporosis. I've had a lot of women in their late thirties and forties who were told categorically, without any further evaluation, that they were too young to be having any menopausal symptoms. This is the time that we need to be checking these various health measures so that we can take preventive steps for the future. If you're someone in a premature ovarian decline at age 39 or 40, you need to know that so you can take the necessary steps that will help reduce your risk of heart disease and bone loss in the next five to ten years.

Menopausal Transition: The Fifties

Menopause is defined as the "last menstrual period." Ovarian function has been declining for several years, and now the decline is sufficient to mark a transition from the cycling pattern of hormone production in the reproductive years to the noncycling hormone pattern of the post-reproductive years.

Menopause is a rather unique situation because it's the only thing I know of in the medical world that is defined *twelve months after it has happened!* This means its a little hard to take proactive steps to address health risks if you don't define it until twelve months after the last menstrual period. Most of the time women won't know when their last menstrual period will be until sometime after it has happened.

At menopause, the ovary does not cycle any longer, and the overall hormonal production has decreased considerably. After menopause women lose about 66 *percent* or more of their estrogen production and anywhere from 50–60 *percent* of their androgen or testosterone production. All of us have testosterone; men have a lot more than women do. Yet, the female ovary does produce testosterone, and as the estrogen declines more dramatically after menopause, we begin seeing the "unmasking" of the testosterone that is present. That's when you notice some changes in facial hair, you may notice some changes in body fat, the "pear" shape female (gynecoid) fat pattern around the hips and buttocks suddenly begins moving up toward the middle of the body to become the "apple" shape (android) more typical of men. Then you wonder, "Gee, what happened to my waistline?" I've shown this change in Diagram 3.5. These are some of the testosterone effects that begin the body changes that are characteristic of the male pattern. During these years, the enzyme *lipoprotein lipase* starts to decrease in the lower body fat tissue and increase in the upper body fat, which further adds to the pattern of increasing body fat around the waist, chest, shoulders, hips, and thighs. We see a rise in blood pressure that is similar to that in men. We see changes in the cholesterol pattern similar to men as the testosterone effects become more prevalent and estrogen declines.

As women lose the biologically active estradiol, we begin to see one of the gender *differences* become a gender *similarity*: the incidence of cardiovascular disease (CVD) increases dramatically for women. Regardless of age at menopause (whether it's a *natural* menopause at age 45 or a *surgical* menopause at age 40) the rate of CVD increases. It is based upon *menopausal status*, not just *chronological age*. It is important to know a woman's endocrine status in order to more completely assess her risk of CVD. You cannot go by age alone, since women experience declining estradiol levels at a variety of numerical ages.

Diagram 3.5
WOMEN'S MID-LIFE BODY SHAPE CHANGES

FEMALE (GYNECOID)
"PEAR" SHAPE

MALE (ANDROID)
"APPLE" SHAPE

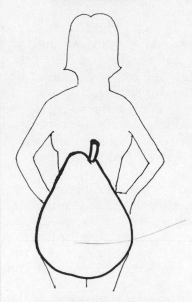
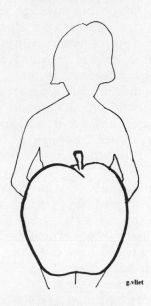

g.vliet

Characteristic of women prior to menopause, when estradiol (E2) greater than estrone (E1).

Characteristic of women after menopause (if not on hormone Rx); E1 > E2 now. Associated with higher risk of heart disease, hypertension diabetes, insulin resistance

Postmenopause—The Sixties, Seventies and Beyond

Let me share with you a different perspective on menopause and the years that follow. I think we've heard many conflicting points about menopause and it has been treated with a sense of taboo as well as fear and apprehension. Part of that has to do with the fact that at the turn of the century the average age of death for women in this country was forty-eight; the average age of menopause was fifty-one. That means as recently as 1900, most women did not live very long after menopause and ovarian decline. Five hundred years ago, women, on average, died by age thirty-five.

When we read books about the wise women of Native American cultures, Asian cultures, the Celtic traditions and others, the wise, elder women were typically those over *thirty*, past the age of childbearing in those times. Yet you and I are reading that material in the context of an *unparalleled increase in longevity* in the human population. It has only been in the last two to three generations that we have had large numbers of men and women living long enough to begin to see some of the effects declining ovary hormones in women, and the declining testicular hormones in men.

When I talk about menopause and women's health needs, I am discussing it from the perspective that we now have an unparalleled amount of time—perhaps thirty to fifty years—to live beyond menopause. For many of us that means that if we look at our adult life, we have the potential to live *at least half* of it after the ovaries have stopped producing the normal quantity of biologically active estradiol.

My clear statement to you is straightforward: **menopause is not a disease,** it is a natural transition in our lives. We now have the opportunity to go through this transition and *live an extended period beyond.* That was not the case for our great grandmothers and their ancestors; most of them died before or shortly after menopause. Menopause as a biological change is not seen in primates such as monkeys, chimpanzees, and gorillas because the females of these species die at the end of their reproductive years. I think the most critical point for women to understand is that we want to learn what we need to know about maintaining our long-term health and reducing our long-term individual disease risks so we can live these additional thirty or forty years with the best possible quality of life and good health. Don't just focus on *treating* or *bearing with symptoms* NOW; look at your big picture and make decisions based on what is needed for you over the long haul.

The Thyroid:
The Great Imitator Often Missed in Women

Thyroid disease has sometimes been called "the great imitator" because a myriad of symptoms that can be confused with many different illnesses are produced by both *hyper*thyroid syndromes (an excess of thyroid hormones, such as Graves' Disease) and *hypo*thyroid disorders (too little thyroid hormone production, or interference with normal hormone action, such as Hashimoto's thyroiditis). Thyroid disorders of all types are far more common in women, as much as *eight to twenty times the frequency found in men*. The incidence of thyroid disorders increase with age in both sexes, but there is a more dramatic increase in women in the decade of the forties and on into the seventies. There are a variety of laboratory tests that can identify these problems. What often happens for women is that only the thyroid hormones themselves are checked without looking also at the brain hormone, TSH (thyroid stimulating hormone) that is a much more sensitive indicator of excessive, or declining, thyroid function.

One facet of thyroid disease not generally recognized is its tendency to cause disturbances in mood and in menstrual cycles. Menstrual irregularity, worsening PMS, atypical depression, new onset depression later in life, post-partum depression, anxiety syndromes, excessive fatigue—all of these are "red flags" for me to also probe carefully for an underlying thyroid problem, especially in female patients. Yet, all too commonly, women with these symptoms are given a psychiatric label, referred to a therapist for "stress management" and are not evaluated medically any further than a cursory exam and basic blood chemistries. Studies of patients admitted to psychiatric hospitals have repeatedly shown a high incidence of previously unrecognized thyroid disorders that were thought to be the causative factor in the mood disorder. Women at mid-life in particular need careful evaluation of thyroid function as part of their medical check-ups.

A comment I hear frequently is "you couldn't have thyroid problems because your TSH (thyroid stimulating hormone) is normal." When the cluster of symptoms I described above are present in women, I think it is important to go one step further in evaluating the thyroid. I have a series of more than a hundred patients, all but *two* are *women*, who had a *normal* TSH and turned out to have significantly *elevated thyroid antibodies* that meant they needed thyroid medication in order to feel normal. This type of oversight is particularly common with a type of thyroid disease called

Thyroiditis, which is about *25 times* more common in females than males. There are several different types of thyroiditis, but in general this is an inflammation of the thyroid gland that can result in production of antibodies to the gland tissue (microsomal antibodies) or antibodies to the thyroid hormone itself (thyroglobulin antibodies).

These antibodies act like "blocking agents" to keep the hormones from working properly, and the patient begins to experience the clinical symptoms of declining thyroid gland function described above. For some period of time, that can vary greatly from person to person, there is a gradual or abrupt elevation in the thyroid antibodies *before* there is a compensating rise in TSH produced by the brain in response to the failing gland. This means a woman may experience the symptoms of disease *months to years before TSH goes up.*

The prevailing "dogma" among endocrinologists and thyroid specialists is that you don't test for thyroid antibodies if the TSH is normal, even if the patient has classic symptoms of hypothyroidism. That's where we often run into trouble and fail to diagnose thyroiditis. All too often, and particularly with females more than with males, the clinical problems are present and the antibodies are elevated even when TSH is normal. Adding low dose thyroid medication can be dramatic for these women.

I do *not* advocate using thyroid hormone if *all* of the laboratory studies are completely normal, *including* thyroid antibodies. There are *adverse* effects of taking thyroid when you don't actually need it: heart rhythm disturbances, and bone loss are the two most important. The problem I have found is that too often women are told their thyroid is normal *without having the complete thyroid tests done.* Of course, what most people, and many physicians, don't realize is that

1. a "normal range" on a laboratory report is just that: a *range*. A given person may require higher or lower levels to feel well and to function optimally. I think we must look at the lab results *along with the clinical picture described by the patient* and
2. one or more lab measures may still fall in the normal range and yet other, more subtle measures, may be abnormal.

I think we have to listen to the woman and her descriptions with an open mind and with trust in what she says and knows about her body. Several cases from my practice illustrate this point very clearly.

Arla was 32 when I first saw her. Her last child (of two) had been born five years earlier. Over the past three years, she had been experiencing marked loss of energy, decreased concentration at work, premenstrual mood swings, and severe chocolate cravings. She described feeling "so tired I can hardly make it through the day, that just isn't like me; my memory isn't as sharp as usual, I get dark circles under my eyes all the time, I can't lose weight no matter how much I exercise, and I just feel so loggy all the time. I thought there might be a thyroid problem, but my family doctor said my thyroid hormones were normal. What's wrong with me?"

Her routine lab studies were normal, and there was nothing particularly unusual on her physical exam except for the moderate degree of obesity. Her standard thyroid profile was normal for the T3, T4 hormones and her TSH was 2.21 (normal range is 0.3 to 5.0 and the standard teaching is that no thyroid treatment should be given until the TSH reaches about 7 or 8). The striking *abnormality* was the thyroid antibody result: her antithyroglobulin antibody was 370 when the normal range is 0.00 to 0.30 units/ml. She had a level of 1,660 on a later check of her antithyroglobulin antibody, even though her *TSH was still normal* at that time also.

The antibody to the thyroglobulin was acting like a "blocking agent" keeping the thyroid hormone from being able to attach to the receptor sites and work properly, even though the thyroid gland was making enough of the hormone. She was certainly relieved to know what had been causing her diverse symptoms, and I once again appreciated the value of listening to what the patient describes. I started her Synthroid, initially at a small dose of only 0.025 mg. She felt better fairly soon, but had to have several more dose adjustments before she reached the optimal level. A year later, she described feeling "back to my old self!"

Another woman, a twenty-year-old college student, illustrates the potential for marked effects on brain phenomena when the thyroid function is diminished. Her father asked if I would do a consult for her because they had not been able to find help for her severe "PMS" and she had not been doing well in school although previously had been an excellent student. When I saw her, she described having a lot of difficulty keeping her concentration focused to be able to study, her memory was much worse than normal, and she had a deterioration in her grades even though she was studying *more* than usual. She talked about feeling embarrassed by the severe anger outbursts before her period, "I'd be so irritable I thought I would explode and then I would cry over little things and couldn't stop." Her family described her as usually very energetic and vivacious, but over the past year, she said she could barely make it through the day and often cut class to take naps in the afternoon because she was so tired. She had gained about twenty pounds over the past year and had not previously had a weight problem.

There was no evidence of a major depression. Her primary doctor had told her that all her tests, including the thyroid hormones were normal, except **TSH, which was not done.** The physician suggested she see a counselor to help her cope with the stress of being away from home at college. When I interviewed her with her parents, I did not find any indication that she had problems adjusting to the school setting. I did, however, find out an interesting point in the family history: my patient's mother had thyroid disease and had been on thyroid medication for many years, as had her maternal grandmother.

Shellie had a complete evaluation, that came back normal *except* for the thyroid antibodies and TSH. Her antithyroglobulin antibody was 6,000 IU/L (the normal range this time was 0 to 100 IU/L), her antimicrosomal antibody was 475 (same normal range of 0–100). Her TSH was 7, a level that often would have probably been "watched" for six months and rechecked if we had not also had the critical information about the marked abnormalities of the antibodies. Clearly she was significantly hypothyroid, even though the T3 and T4 were normal. A thyroid scan showed a diffusely enlarged gland typical of thyroiditis. She was started on thyroid medication and gradually increased to the right amount for her. The brain symptoms have resolved, and her PMS is no longer the major problem it had been. She is gradually losing weight with exercise and a healthy meal plan in addition to her medication.

Both of these women show how important it is to pay attention to changes like this in brain function when the person has previously not had such difficulties. The brain is often the first organ to show the effects of subtle changes in either thyroid or ovarian hormone function because the brain is so exquisitely dependent upon normal balance for optimal function. When I talk with physicians about these issues, I emphasize that the overall "pattern" is what helps determine the tests to do. We are treating *patients*, not lab values. Since space is limited in my book, you may want to read *What's Wrong With My Hormones?* by Gillian Ford for an excellent and much more in-depth discussion of thyroid problems.

COMMON SYMPTOMS OF HYPOTHYROIDISM

- severe fatigue, loss of energy, feeling "sluggish"
- weight gain, difficulty losing weight
- depressed mood, usually not as severe as major depression, but may be mistaken for primary depression
- menstrual irregularities, difficulty becoming pregnant
- "PMS" symptoms, with premenstrual mood changes common
- dry, scaly, itchy skin and scalp
- dry, brittle hair and nails
- losing hair (alopecia)
- chronic constipation
- puffiness of face, lower legs, and feet
- slowed heart rate, diminished reflexes
- difficulty tolerating cold environments, climate ("can't get warm")
- sleeping much more than normal
- tingling in wrists/hands, mimicking "carpal tunnel syndrome"
- clotting problems
- multiple joint aches (arthralgias)
- achy muscles (myalgias), leg cramps
- diminished or lost sexual desire (libido)
- decreased memory, concentration (also brain effect of low thyroid— may be misdiagnosed as dementia in an older person)
- ABNORMAL LAB TESTS: high TSH, low thyroid hormones, high total cholesterol, lower than normal HDL, possibly elevated liver enzymes

CHAPTER 4

Hormones and the Brain: Identifying Unrecognized Connections

The Brain: Master Conductor of Our Body's Orchestra

What is the brain? To look at it, not much! To live with? Ah, that's another story entirely! Although it is out of sight and we often take it for granted, the brain is truly the organ that most defines each of us as an individual, unique person and personality. With it, we perceive the world, we laugh, we cry, we scream, we talk, we joke, we learn, we relate to others. It governs our eating, sleeping, breathing, heart beat, immune function, water balance, hormone output, and our sex drive, sexual fantasies and sexual function. The heart may beat with a mechanical pump, and we still survive. If the brain dies, which it will in the absence of oxygen for more than just a few minutes, we lose all dimensions of who we are as an individual; indeed, perhaps our very soul is lost.

The brain is a powerhouse organ, more creative and adaptable than the world's fastest computer, yet soft enough to crush with the pressure of your fingers without the protection of its bony case (the skull) and tough fibrous sac (dura mater) inside the skull. It is often compared to a computer, but that analogy hardly does it justice. If a computer is faced with a new command or task or is given incorrect directions, it simply shuts down; overloaded, it quits. Our brain, however, responds rapidly with new solutions; almost without even realizing it, we adapt and change to meet the new tasks or directions. The brain is able to remember and to forget; your computer can only remember. The computer operates only in an either-or, on-off, "binary" mode. Our brain appreciates infinite "shades of gray" along a continuum of choices and options. In many ways, it is far too complex for me to find a good metaphor or analogy for its functions.

When talking about fears of disease in my seminars, I have commented on the way in which many magazine articles lump women together by calling breast cancer our greatest fear. It isn't for me. My greatest health concern would be developing a disease that destroys my brain, since it is the organ that makes ME who I am. I could work and be ME without my breast. I can no longer work, and I no longer *exist as ME* without my brain. It has only been in the last decade or so that we have truly come to appreciate just how completely the brain defines our total being.

As I mentioned in Chapter 3, *the brain is the master conductor of the "orchestra" made up of all the "instruments" of our body.* Without the conducting, coordinating functions of our brain, there would be no "music" from our existence; all our body parts would be chaotically playing individual notes and pieces of tunes, like the discordant notes we hear as an orchestra is warming up, with all the musicians playing individual parts of songs and scales. Not the sort of music you attend a symphony to hear. But when the conductor appears on stage and with skill and flowing awareness of all the parts brings the orchestra to life as an entity, the symphonic music begins. As we listen to the orchestra, we often forget how crucial the conductor's role is or how many different individual instruments are being guided into playing together to create the drama and beauty of the music. The essence of the brain (and of woman) lies not in the parts, but in the *connections between the parts* that create the totality of the whole.

To give you an adequate appreciation of the many functions of the brain and its complex structure would require an enormous textbook. I would like to give you an overview of the major areas of the brain and some of the broad areas of function that are orchestrated by these key areas. This information is based on current understandings of the brain; keep in mind, however, that neuroscience research is an exploding area of new knowledge, increasing almost daily, so there will be more that we know about this marvelous organ in years to come. The brain diagram below will help you understand where these areas are and will serve as a reference point for the discussion of the connections that follows.

Diagram 4.1—THE HUMAN BRAIN

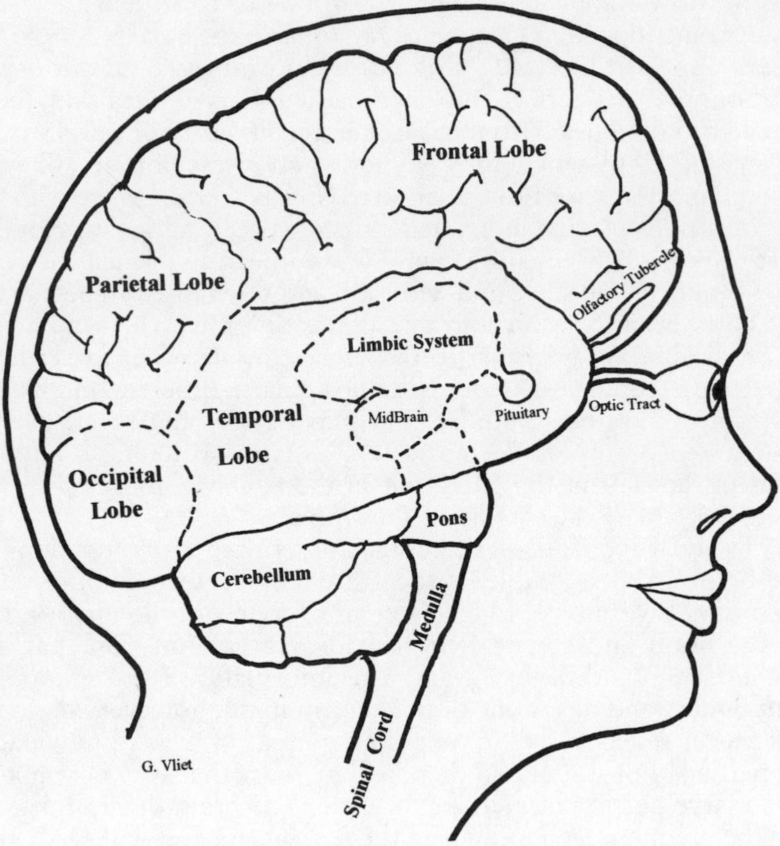

Frontal Lobe

Olfactory Tubercle

Parietal Lobe

Limbic System

Optic Tract

Temporal Lobe

MidBrain

Pituitary

Occipital Lobe

Pons

Cerebellum

Medulla

Spinal Cord

G. Vliet

The brain rests inside the bony protective cover of the skull, with a number of openings in the base of the skull for nerves to enter and exit, as well as for the spinal cord, which carries the large bundles of nerve tracts from the head down the back to the lower body. The *cortex* mediates thinking functions and is divided into two halves, the left and right *cerebral hemispheres*, which have different specialization of functions. The *left* hemisphere specializes in *verbal, analytical, and sequential (or linear)* information processing; the *right* hemisphere specializes in *visual-spatial, nonverbal, intuitive (or nonlinear), and Gestalt* information processing. Both hemispheres are further divided into areas called *lobes* named for the overlying skull bones: *frontal, temporal, parietal, and occipital*. The cortex is the part of the brain that makes us uniquely human, since it governs speech, reading, and writing of language. There is overlap among many of the brain areas to a significant degree, both structurally and functionally, which gives us an enormous capacity for adaptability.

At the interior center of the brain, lying below the cortex, is the area of structures collectively called the *limbic* system, which is the primary integrative center mediating emotion, memory, pain, sleep, appetite, sex, and other drives. The *brainstem* group of structures (lying below the cortex) regulates the "vegetative" functions, such as breathing, blood pressure, and heart rate, that keep us alive. The *cerebellum* lies somewhat above the brainstem but below the cortex and is the primary movement-regulating center. Bundles of nerve fibers leaving the cortex, limbic system, brainstem, and cerebellum come together to form the *spinal cord*, which extends to the base of the vertebral column in the lower back area. Chart 4.1 summarizes these major functions; you may find it helpful to refer to it as I discuss the chemistry of mood and hormonal effects.

Chart 4.1 BRAIN AREAS AND THEIR KEY FUNCTIONS

Brain Area	Functions
FRONTAL Lobe	• integrates thinking, feeling, creative imagining, decision making; • oversees "social appropriateness" of behavior, insight-judgment abilities • has role in expression of personality • helps control body movements
TEMPORAL Lobes	• processes auditory information, controls language (usually left hemisphere) and memory, helps in modulating emotion
PARIETAL Lobes	• receives information about body sensations ("somatosensory area"), • modulates spatial orientation ability
OCCIPITAL Lobe	• receives and processes visual information
BRAINSTEM: Midbrain, Pons, and Medullaas:	• regulates "survival functions"; such as: respiration, heart rate, blood pressure • receives information via multiple connections (brain and spinal cord)
LIMBIC SYSTEM: Amygdala, Hippocampus, Mammillary Bodies, Fornix, Basal Ganglia (BG), Thalamus, Hypothalamus, Pituitary, and Cingulate Gyrus	• memory processing • mood-emotion regulation • attention, alertness, focus • human "drives": appetite, thirst, sex, aggression, sleep-wake cycles • governs "starting and stopping" behavior • hormone regulation (esp. hypothalamus, and pituitary) • has role in modulating *chronic* pain, acute pain paths bypass limbic area • integrates sensory information and role in movement (basal ganglia)
CEREBELLUM	• integrates and coordinates movement (with cortex), balance, coordination
SPINAL CORD	• carries nerve tracts and chemical messengers back and forth between brain and body; • origin of nerve tracts to body areas

New Understandings of the Brain's Chemical Messengers

How do all these areas of the brain communicate with each other? We talk about "nerves," which are fibers. But how do messages get from one nerve cell to another? I have found it helpful to think about the brain as an enormous three-dimensional network of many different "communication centers" that turn on and off rapidly and send out bursts of electrical impulses, which then communicate further by releasing chemical messenger molecules called *neurotransmitters*. The visual image that pops into my mind is the large flashing network of fibers in the TV commercial for a worldwide communications company. There are billions of nerve fibers, all with hundreds of potential connections to other nerve fibers. To try to comprehend all this complexity is overwhelming to most of us.

The basic process of communication between nerve cells, or neurons, and other body cells is both electrical and chemical. The electrical impulse travels along the neuron to the end of the cell called the *synapse*, or junction point, where it fires off the release of the chemical messenger molecules that have been made in the cell and stored in little sacs called *storage vesicles*. The chemicals are released to travel across the space between cells, called the *synaptic cleft*. The messenger molecules fit into a receptor site, which "unlocks" the next nerve cell to allow the message to be processed and acted upon. This is often illustrated as a neuron connecting with only one other neuron, but in reality, each neuron has perhaps hundreds of connections with other cells. What I have described is a *greatly simplified* version of a very complex, multi-dimensional continuous process occurring every second of every day we are alive. It is awesome to consider the incredible intricacies of the body.

There has been an exponential growth in our understanding of the actual modes of communication between the brain and body since Dr. Candace Pert and Dr. Solomon Snyder first discovered the opiate receptor in the brain in 1973. This is the site where drugs such as morphine, heroin, and their derivatives plug into brain cells to produce their pain-relieving action. It seemed logical to these researchers that the brain would not be equipped with a special "lock" (receptor site) if it did not also produce a "key." In 1975, they found the natural "key" for this "lock" in the discovery of the endorphin and enkephalin neuropeptides, which are the pain-killing molecules produced in the brain and body. Since that time, researchers have identified many more "molecular messengers" that provide the "courier information service" between the brain and various body sites. These biochemical information substances produced in the body have been grouped into various categories including, *neurotransmitters, neuropeptides, hormones, growth factors, and lymphokines.* They all have powerful effects on multiple aspects of body function, *including mood and emotion.* You can think of these informational molecules as "biochemical words" or messages that are used by the brain to "talk" directly to body cells and organs and by the body to "talk back" to the brain. These molecules link the brain and immune system, the endocrine and immune systems, the brain and the endocrine system, the brain and the gut, the brain and the heart, and so on throughout all the possible connections between brain centers and body organs.

Some of the most important chemical messengers I will be describing with regard to hormone influences on mood and physical symptoms are:

- Serotonin (5-HT)
- Norepinephrine (NE)
- Dopamine (DA)
- Acetylcholine (ACh)
- gamma aminobutyric acid (GABA).

These molecules function to convey and modulate information going back and forth between the brain and the body. They provide an important link between emotional and physical health. This link is not surprising in view of the critical role of emotions in regulating behavior that ultimately affects our very survival. These information-carrying substances are made in the brain and body from "building blocks" called *amino acids* found in the food we eat. The body's metabolic processes to make the neurotransmitters require the presence of various vitamins and minerals as catalysts and cofactors for the synthesizing enzymes to work properly. Perhaps you are beginning to see why a healthy, balanced diet is so crucial to your good health and optimal function.

We are just beginning to discover the incredible diversity of roles and functions the neurotransmitters have. Serotonin research, for example, has given us extraordinary new insights about the biological basis of many behavior problems we previously thought were caused by psychological conflicts—everything from compulsive shoplifting to gambling, from compulsive sexual behaviors to handwashing and hair-pulling (*trichotillomania*) behaviors. Overeating is mediated by serotonin imbalances, and so are pain and sleep patterns. Anxiety syndromes have been found to be set off by changes in serotonin function, as well as by excessive production of norepinephrine. Mania results from excessive levels of norepinephrine and dopamine, while depression occurs when these and serotonin are either produced in inadequate amounts or the receptor sites are not functioning properly.

We now consider major depression to be a *biological* disorder occurring as a direct result of marked changes in these chemical messengers and an alteration in the receptor numbers and sensitivity. Attention deficit disorders are also affected by the balance between serotonin and norepinephrine. Abnormalities in dopamine production and function is thought to be the primary disturbance causing Schizophrenia and Parkinson's Disease. Loss of acetylcholine is the primary deficiency leading to Alzheimer's dementia. Irritable Bowel Syndrome and Fibromyalgia are two of many so-called "vague" medical problems aggravated, if not caused by, serotonin and norepinephrine imbalances. As you can see, these deceptively simple molecules have a profound impact on many aspects of our health.

SUMMARY OF THE ROLES OF
TWO KEY NEUROTRANSMITTERS

♦ *Increased* Serotonin (ST, or 5HT)
- diminishes **anxiety**
- improves **pain**
- improves **sleep**
- improves **depression**
- decreases **obsessions**

♦ *Increased* Norepinephrine (NE)
- improves **depression**
- worsens **anxiety**
- intensifies **pain**
- causes **restless, fragmented sleep**

Another fascinating connection that has been overlooked and underappreciated in women's health is the existence of specific estradiol, progesterone, and testosterone receptor sites in key areas throughout the brain and body. These hormone receptor sites are found *throughout* the body's organs and tissues, far beyond reproductive organ sites you would expect to respond to circulating ovarian hormones. Changes in hormone levels, in turn, affect the *amount* of neurotransmitters produced as well as the *sensitivity* of neurotransmitter receptors to the chemical messengers. In the brain, the estrogen receptors in particular are heavily concentrated in the cortex and in the limbic system areas. As I described, the limbic system is the major center for regulating **mood, memory, sleep, sex drive, appetite, and pain**. There are multiple connections between the limbic system and all the other parts of the brain and spinal cord, which carries messages to all parts of the body. The rise and fall of estrogen alters serotonin, which affects pathways in the limbic system, which then produces changes in mood, sleep, memory, pain, appetite, and many other mind-body functions. No wonder changing hormone levels at puberty, in pregnancy, after delivery, and at menopause can produce such a wide variety of physical and emotional changes.

We have only begun to scratch the surface of appreciating how widespread are these connections. You may have been told that mood changes aren't due to your hormones, but I will help you to see clearly that what you experience is **very real and has profound hormonal connections**. Contrary to popular opinion, the brain and the body really are connected! It is not all in your head in the "imaginary" sense; it is "in your head" in the real physical changes that take place regularly between the hormone messengers and the brain's own mood-altering messenger molecules.

It's NOT All in Your Imagination!
The Biology of Mood Changes

Since it has been observed in world-wide studies that both depressive syndromes and anxiety disorders are two to three times more common in women than in men, I think it is important to begin to link the women's hormone make-up with our expanded knowledge about mood-regulating mechanisms in humans. The *cause* of mood changes that occur around and during the menopausal transition has been hotly debated in scientific journals and the lay media for a long time. There is a lot of intense emotion on both sides of the debate: Is it hormonal change? Is it the combination of life stresses? Consider this example from a nationally syndicated column by Jane Brody, published in late September 1994. The headline in my newspaper was "Menopause doesn't have to be depressing." The article began this way:

> In her newly published memoir, Barbara Bush reveals that in the mid-1970s she was overcome by depression so severe that she feared she might purposely end her life by crashing her car. The former first lady attributed her emotional distress to the hormonal changes of menopause compounded by the stress of her husband's job as director of the Central Intelligence Agency. By linking her depression to menopause, Bush perpetuates a centuries-old belief that the hormonal swings that accompany this life stage can touch off what had long been called involutional melancholia (involutional is a term referring to the body's changes at menopause).

Ms. Brody then goes on to say that "studies show there is no particular link between depression and menopause; if anything, it is far more common among younger women than in those from 45-55 when most women enter menopause."

But in reality, *we do not have adequate studies that have addressed this issue. None* of the studies Ms. Brody referred to measured hormone levels, a fairly critical factor, if you are trying to see whether there's a link between hormones and depressive symptoms! Most studies did not even determine whether a woman was still menstruating or whether she had undergone a hysterectomy. Many have based menopausal status on age alone, which you will find as you read further is not at all accurate in identifying which women are actually menopausal by *endocrinological measures.*

Under Barbara Bush's picture is this quote (in large type and bold letters), which I think reflects even worse stereotypes of women and certainly is not based on well-done studies:

> Barbara Bush had led a traditional family life with her major role being raising children. As her children left home, the loss of this role may have made her more vulnerable to depression at that time. When women are not in the work force, depression may be more common at menopause, reflecting the woman's stage of life, not necessarily her hormones.
>
> —Dr. Myrna M. Weissman, as quoted in the nationally syndicated column by Jane Brody, September 27, 1994

How does this quote make you feel? Is Dr. Weissman perpetuating the old stereotype that women "can't cope" with life-stage changes and become depressed? Personally, and from a professional point of view as well, I find this attitude an appalling stigma to perpetuate in 1994. I also think it is rather arrogant to suggest that women who are "in the work force" somehow cope better with menopause because they work. Any woman who is a full-time homemaker will tell you she has a full-time job, even if she isn't paid for her labor. Moreover, Dr. Weissman's view hasn't been confirmed by sound research.

Dr. Philip Sarrel of Yale has found the opposite: Women in the work force describe *more severe* symptoms of menopausal distress than women who do not work outside the home, perhaps related to the higher levels of stress, experienced by women who are juggling multiple roles of home and career. Such stresses can further *decrease* ovarian hormone levels. Dr. Sarrel reported his research findings at the inaugural meeting of the North American Menopause Society in the fall of 1989. He said, "Most important in impairing a woman's capacity to function [at her optimal ability] in the workplace are *symptoms due to hormone deficiency*: sleep disturbance, hot flashes, anxiety attacks, depression, and altered [i.e., decreased] short-term memory. In approximately 67 percent of women who work outside of the home, and approximately 50 percent of homemakers, menopausal symptoms [such as above] have a moderate to severe effect on the ability to do work."

I do not take offense at these comments, rather I think it provides a helpful explanation of factors women suspect but which many researchers in a variety of fields have ignored. As one woman so eloquently said it, "I survived the depression era, I raised six kids, my parents died when I was in my twenties. When I was 32, my husband was killed. I have had lots of stress in my life. Why did everyone say it's "stress" causing my sleep problems and irritability when I went through menopause? Relative to what I had already lived through, menopause was *not* a stressful time, but I certainly had a lot of bothersome symptoms." Many women I see tell me that they feel *validated* in their own perceptions when I find low hormone levels contributing to their unpleasant symptoms.

Perhaps the hormonal changes, along with life stresses, were factors which aggravated Mrs. Bush's symptoms around the time of her menopause. In addition to overlooking the reality of hormone effects on brain function, I do not think any of us should *assume* that Barbara Bush became depressed because her role as a mother had changed. This statement is made as if it were an established fact, but Dr. Weissman's quote was not based on a confirmed causal connection. So, once again, a stereotype is perpetuated and possible physical factors are discounted. I think there are at least two possible *endocrine* causes for Mrs. Bush's depression: her thyroid condition, which has been known for 100 years or more to cause depression; and the changing ovarian hormone levels around the time of menopause that affect brain chemicals regulating mood. Instead of such an "either-or" mentality evident in the Brody article, why not approach these issues with a "both-and" mindset and look at all the *interrelating* factors that make women unique and contribute to the observed higher frequency of depressive symptoms and disorders in women?

If we look at the patterns of major depression, we have known for *many* years that there are several *common predisposing factors* (this is true world-wide):

- prior depressive episodes
- family history of depression
- **female gender**
- **postpartum state**
- severe, prolonged, or unanticipated stress

Two of the five factors that have been known for ages as being factors predisposing to the medical (biological) illness of depression are directly related to being female: female gender, and the postpartum state. Since these patterns of female dominance have been noted in primitive and industrialized cultures, there must be some biological reasons for this. Why do we continue to stigmatize and blame women as being "weak" and "not coping well" because they have a higher frequency of depression?

I find it hard to fathom why researchers and physicians haven't made, or paid attention to, these hormonal connections long before now. It almost appears to me that perhaps they don't want to see it. Perhaps that's a product of the concern expressed by many feminists that if we acknowledge the hormonal influences, we may lose some of the gains women have made to move into new occupational fields. I understand such fears. We have all suffered long enough from the stereotype of the bitchy, cranky, moody woman. But on the other hand, if we *don't* acknowledge possible hormonal factors, we cannot develop the most effective therapies to help women who *do* have these problems. Such women will continue to suffer from lack of recognition or from overuse of other medication or surgery which may have more side effects or higher costs. I believe these are crucial issues that must be addressed.

A good example of how profound hormone effects can be is seen in the post-partum phase. A woman's hormonal levels drop over a hundredfold in the twenty-four to thirty-six hours after delivery. That's a major adjustment for both the brain chemistry and the chemical messengers that regulate sleep and mood. Then add to that the fact that there is now have an infant who's keeping you up much of the night, so you're not sleeping very well. But a woman who becomes significantly depressed following her baby's birth is still more likely to be told she has *psychological* conflicts about being a mother, and the biological factors overlooked. Clearly, there are social and cultural factors involved, and these have been studied exhaustively.

I think we have not paid enough attention to the obvious hormonal connections that have to do with the biology of being *female*. In Europe, and in my own practice, there are good reports of the positive response to estradiol therapy for a short while after delivery in women who have a post-partum depression due to hormonal decreases. Some of these women do not need antidepressant medication, and some benefit from the combination of estradiol and a serotonin-augmenting antidepressant. We need to consider *individualization* of the best options for a given woman.

I have long been struck by the repetitive, commonly occurring pattern of mood changes and physical symptoms and their relationship to the normal changes in estrogen and progesterone hormone levels throughout the menstrual cycle. Most women who have menstrual periods (or ovarian cycles if they have had a hysterectomy) have *some* physical or emotional cues that alert them to their periods about to begin, as well as to the beginning of the mid-life transition, the *climacteric*. In my medical practice, I have found a significant percentage of patients who have luteal-phase symptoms severe enough to interfere with optimal function at home, at work, and in relationships. These women would like some constructive, well-thought out options to help them feel better on these days. I don't think that is too much to ask of a health system that can now achieve successful organ transplants and other wonders.

Even for women who have had a hysterectomy, most of the ones I talk with (who still have their ovaries) can describe quite well the body-brain markers of the residual ovary cycle. They tell me they have breast tenderness and bloating, food cravings, constipation and other markers, just like they did the week before

menses began. Or they will describe a few days of restless fragmented sleep, emotional changes, crying easily, loss of energy,
feeling mentally "foggy" like they did the first few days of bleeding (when estradiol is at its lowest point of the cycle). All I have
to do is ask them to describe what they feel and experience! I think
one problem is that many physicians don't think to ask these
questions if a woman has had a hysterectomy.

It has been my hypothesis from years of observing patients
and *listening to the way women describe their experiences* that
there is a unrecognized and unaddressed connection between
declining estrogen levels in mid-life (or perimenopausal) women
and the pattern of female dominance in depression and anxiety
disorders. Consider these observations (based on women who still
have regular menstrual cycles):

- PMS symptoms commonly become worse in the late thirties and
  early forties
- the late thirties to early forties represent the peak age range of
  new onset depression and anxiety syndromes in women, but not
  in men
- the late thirties to mid-forties is the time frame for onset of
  erratic and *declining* ovarian hormone production, creating the
  potential for effects on brain neurotransmitters to destabilize
  mood regulating mechanisms.
- By the time menses have stopped (menopause), hormone levels
  are stabilzed at a new *lower* level, and no longer cycle, making
  "mood swings" less likely.
- Researchers, however, have focused only on the time of *menopause*
  in trying to correlate hormone changes and depression.

I think a key factor in the connection between hormones and
mood effects is **the *degree* of fluctuation, or rate of change, in hormone levels.** In all the studies I have reviewed, this crucial factor
has *not been addressed*. I have studied this connection by measuring hormone levels at times in the menstrual cycle when women
describe their most distressing mood symptoms, and at times in
the cycle when estradiol is at its lowest point and its highest point.
Then I "connect the dots" to see the pattern that emerges as I
show the symptom clusters side by side with the actual hormone
results. It has been striking to find that approximately 80-85%
percent of these women in their mid thirties and early forties who
described "worsening PMS" had *below normal* estrogen levels at
these points during their menstrual cycle.

The prematurely low estradiol levels were *even more likely* to be present in women who had experienced a surgical procedure that affected blood flow to the ovaries, such as *tubal ligation* or *hysterectomy* (even when the ovaries were left in place). According to the currently accepted age-based definitions, these women were *too young* in most cases to be considered peri-menopausal. When I measured the hormone levels, however, I confirmed that they indeed had reached the *endocrinological* stage of perimenopause. I offered these women treatment with low-dose estrogen supplementation to restore their estrogen levels to more normal levels instead of using antidepressants as I might have done earlier in my career. I have been astonished at the results. Women who fit this profile described a consistent pattern of improved mood, diminished irritability, improved sleep, improved libido, improved energy level, and diminished mood swings prior to their periods, after starting on a low dose of native human estradiol. Only a few of these women required the addition of antidepressants once hormone levels were returned to the usual levels for a menstruating woman.

A variety of studies in recent years have demonstrated that neuroreceptors respond to circulating hormones of all kinds, including the sex hormones estrogen, progesterone, and testos-terone. Researchers have shown that hormones can increase or decrease the release of neurotransmitters. Hormones have both presynaptic and postsynaptic nerve cell actions, as well as indirect influences that modify the function of neurons. Both the central and the peripheral nervous systems contain cells with receptor sites sensitive to 17-beta estradiol, and the brain clearly responds to the withdrawal and absence of ovarian hormones. There are a wide variety of physical phenomena and psychological effects of estrogen decrease or withdrawal, and I discuss these connections in the next sections, as well as in Chapter 7. But first, I think it is important to clarify some descriptions of terms you will see in various articles, which may be one of the reasons there is so much confusion about hormone effects on mood.

Clarification: Depressive and Anxiety Symptoms versus Psychiatric Disorders

As you read the upcoming sections, it is important to keep in mind the difference between (1) experiencing *symptoms* on an episodic or cyclic basis with your menstrual periods and (2) having sustained physical and emotional changes that would be severe enough to be considered a *disorder* or an illness. Many women have mild to moderate symptoms or experience mood, sleep, and energy level changes around the time of hormonal changes or in conjunction with situations that are stressful. When I talk about this cyclic type of pattern, I am not referring to the *illness* of major depression, which indicates a more severe, debilitating degree of depression. The same is true with anxiety. The term anxiety may be used in many different ways, so it is important to know how it is being used in a given context. Some people mean in as a "mood"—"I'm in an anxious mood now," or "I'm feeling anxious." Others use it to mean a characteristic or trait of a person— "He's always been anxious and uptight." It may mean a brief symptom: "I had an attack of anxiety over that." It may be used to mean a sustained pattern of physical and emotional changes that we call "Generalized Anxiety Disorder."

In these chapters on hormone connections, I am generally referring to fairly short-lived, episodic anxiety *symptoms* that occur in relation to *changes* in physiological variables such as levels of glucose, thyroid hormone, estrogen, and progesterone. As a global observation, I have not found the hormone shifts of the menstrual cycle to be a *primary cause* of the psychiatric syndrome Generalized Anxiety Disorder, since this illness typically is present on an almost daily basis. On the other hand, I do commonly see women who have panic attacks only around the menstrual cycle phase of dropping estrogen and progesterone levels. I think this type of menstrually-related pattern of panic attacks is different from the psychiatric syndrome we call Panic Disorder. The cluster of symptoms (I sometimes use the nonmedical, descriptive word *phenomena* instead of symptoms) are often the same because the same brain-body pathways are involved.

In my view, the *pattern* of a particular symptom cluster provides the most important clues to contributing causes. I certainly am *not* saying that all women who experience premenstrual depressed moods or feelings of anxiety are suffering from a psychiatric disorder. Quite the contrary. I think *far* too many women are given a psychiatric diagnosis and psychotropic medication, *without the realization that the "symptoms" are occurring around the menstrual period and may be triggered by hormonal changes.*

Estrogen Effects on Serotonin and Other Mood Regulators

There have not yet been good systematic, prospective studies of the effect of rate of change in estrogen levels on the frequency and severity of mood symptoms in perimenopausal women. We have known for a long time, however, that estrogen does affect many brain-mediated phenomena. Experimental data indicate that the sex hormones (estradiol, testosterone, progesterone) are the *most potent* body-generated chemical signals affecting nerve cell activities in the brain. All three major sex hormones alter the electrical and chemical features of cells in the central nervous system (CNS), especially in the hypothalamus and limbic system (check your chart for what these areas regulate and you'll have a better idea of the potential effects). *Changes* in levels of estrogen and progesterone have been shown to influence multiple brain chemical messengers: dopamine, norepinephrine, acetylcholine, and serotonin, all of which are *powerful* modulators of mood.

Dr. Malcolm Whitehead and his associates did an excellent study that showed marked improvement in memory, anxiety, and irritability in menopausal women taking estrogen compared with menopausal women not taking estrogen. This information isn't exactly hot off the presses; it was published in the *British* medical literature *in 1977.* So we've had this kind of information in the medical literature for a long time; it has just been ignored. Women tell me every day that they have been told *categorically* by their doctors: "Hormones don't affect mood. Your memory changes aren't due to hormones. It's just stress. See a therapist and learn to relax."

Since the 1950s at least, a number of clinical reports have indicated that estrogen supplementation helps alleviate mood swings and depression as well as the physical symptoms such as hot flashes, headaches, insomnia, and memory disturbance associated with the mid-life phase. Most have been dismissed because they were not double-blind, placebo-controlled studies. Instead of ignoring these important findings, researchers *should have been using those early studies as guides for well-designed double-blind studies.*

With the development of the first modern psychotropic drugs in 1954, however, the brain effects of all kinds of hormonal influences have been forgotten and overlooked as the focus shifted to using antidepressants, antianxiety agents, neuroleptics, and sedatives. With exciting new information from neuroscience research in the past decade, and with the use of more refined diagnostic criteria rating scales to systematically assess mood characteristics, there is increasing measurable evidence that mood symptoms and physical reactions described by perimenopausal women *are* related to their hormone changes and may respond to supplemental estrogen even before menses stop.

Dr. Sarrel of Yale said in 1989 that "estrogen addition over a six-month period appeared to relieve sleep disturbance most significantly, and resulted in a marked improvement in *all* categories of perimenopausal symptoms in 40 percent of women." He went on to say that it was "of concern that women don't realize how much their quality of life may be improved with proper estrogen therapy and that *only 15 percent* of *all* menopausal women received hormone therapy at all. Many women simply do not seek medical help, even though hormonal therapy may be a benefit to them." (Italics mine).

Bruce McEwen, Ph.D., at Rockefeller University, has done extensive basic science research on the brain-hormone connections and has found that estradiol and progesterone affect the brain directly, acting at specific hormone receptors unique for each hormone. These receptors are concentrated in areas of the brain that are highly hormone-sensitive, and dense with receptor sites: the hypothalamus, limbic system, cortex, pre-frontal regions and others. There are receptor sites for progesterone in these areas also, but they must *first be "primed" by estrogen in order to work properly.*

Dr. McEwen has shown that hormone effects on the brain can be *gradual and long lasting,* i.e., on the order of hours, days, or even weeks in some cases; or may be *rapid onset and shorter duration of effect.* The rapid hormone effects typically occur at the cell membrane receptor, while the longer lasting effects occur at the cell nucleus receptor. All of these observations have many profound implications for an *interactive* model of thinking about the role of women's perimenopausal hormone shifts in producing psychological phenomena. The brain mechanisms and pathways already exist. We need to put the pieces of the puzzle *together* to see the complete picture, not have some pieces left in the "box" of gynecology, and some in the "box" belonging to psychiatry!

Acting at their specific receptor sites, hormones influence the production, release, and breakdown of the mood-regulating neurotransmitters. Antidepressants and antianxiety medications are also frequently given to influence neurotransmitters and lift or stabilize moods. The ability of these medications to work optimally appear to be affected by circulating hormones, especially estradiol and progesterone. Kendall and co-workers found that the pres-

ence of estrogen increased the binding of the antidepressant drug
imipramine (Tofranil) to serotonin-2 receptors involved in mood.
In animals, this imipramine receptor-binding effect was *abolished
if the ovaries were not present* and was *reestablished by giving
estrogen*. Many case reports describe changes antidepressant
response based on a woman's phase in her menstrual cycle.

Early in my career, as I listened to women describe side effects
with antidepressants, I found that I frequently needed to make
dosage adjustments depending on menstrual cycle phase. Women
often needed *higher* doses in the *progesterone-dominated* luteal
phase and *lower* doses in the *estrogen-dominated* follicular
phase. I never saw anything about this in the medical literature
until 1993, but my patients taught me what they needed. This fits
with what we know about estrogen having its own *antidepressant*
effects on the brain centers, so less additional medication is
needed when estrogen levels are high. Progesterone, on the other
hand, has more of a "dampening-down," sedative, or for some
women, a depressant effect on mood-regulating neurotransmitters. Thus, when progesterone levels are high in the second half
of the cycle, it is reasonable that more antidepressant medication
may be necessary.

Ovarian hormones also have been found to have effects on
several other mood-altering neuropeptides: endorphins ("morphine within" pain-reducing chemicals), oxytocin, vasopressin,
and prolactin, which are involved in modulating memory, motor
coordination, and a variety of behaviors. Recent studies have
demonstrated a decrease in some serotonin measures (either
plasma-free tryptophan or platelet serotonin) in the menopausal
and perimenopausal years that correlates with the age of peak suicide rate for women (a comparable peak has not been seen in
men). Recent studies have found that brain levels of 5-hydroxyin-
doleacetic acid (5-HIAA), a serotonin breakdown product, are
low in patients who attempted or completed suicide. If 5-HIAA is
low, it indicates that brain serotonin levels are also low.

Decreases in serotonin production and increases in serotonin
breakdown are seen in (1) the human aging process, (2) as an effect
of *declining estrogen in women*, and (3) as an effect of prolonged
stress, chronic alcohol overuse, and cigarette smoking. Numerous
world-wide studies over the past two decades have shown that
reduced serotonin levels are a primary cause of depressed mood,
increased irritability, increased generalized anxiety, increased pain
sensitivity, eating disorders, obsessive-compulsive disorders and
disruption of normal sleep cycles.

If you then add, for women, the impact of declining estrogen *also decreasing serotonin*, the symptoms of the perimenopause and menopause make even more sense *physiologically*. Many factors affect serotonin balance, but the loss of estrogen may be a key gender difference that contributes to a greater susceptibility to depression and suicide in women. Along this line, Dr. Susan Ballinger in Australia found a greater incidence of psychological symptoms in women aged 45 to 49, when estrogen is decreasing *most rapidly*, compared with both younger and older women. You *aren't* being a hypochondriac. Your body *is* changing. Much later, after all the "ups and downs" of hormone change, women reach a new balance point with overall lower hormone levels, less estradiol, and more estrone. But while the changes are occurring, some women tell me they feel like they are on a roller coaster emotional ride. Most of us don't like to feel so out of control and unable to explain what is happening to us.

Such mood changes, which are clearly cyclic and related to the menstrual cycle, often respond better to **native human 17 beta estradiol** than to antidepressant or antianxiety medication because the addition of estradiol actually normalizes the body chemicals that are out of balance. A number of clinical studies that monitored psychological measures along with physical changes in perimenopausal and early menopausal women have found that giving estrogen *does* result in marked improvement in women's sense of well-being, energy, clarity of thinking, short-term memory and quality of sleep. At the same time, women report marked decreases in hot flashes, vaginal dryness, and other typical physical symptoms.

I have certainly seen these kinds of dramatic improvements in the women I treat for these problems. In addition to the open clinical studies such as the work I have been doing, recently published randomized double-blind placebo-controlled studies have also shown that estrogen therapy effectively improves general well-being, reduces the frequency of hot flashes, and objectively improves the quality of sleep as defined by increases in length of rapid-eye-movement (REM) sleep and total sleep time.

Changes in endorphins have also been shown to play a role in premenstrual and postpartum mood disorders, particularly the anxious-agitated depressive subtypes. Estrogen has an effect on levels of endorphins: high levels of endorphins occur in the late stage of pregnancy in rats and in human females when estrogen levels are at their peak. At delivery, when the sharp drop in both estrogen and progesterone happens, there is a rapid decline in endorphin levels. The withdrawal of endorphins produces effects similar to withdrawal from morphine: irritability, tearfulness, anxiety, stomach upset, diarrhea, and sweating. I think it is reasonable to think that declining levels of estrogen associated with either postpartum, perimenopause, or menopause can cause reductions in endorphin levels and thereby play a *contributing*, if not a *causative*, role in the onset of the anxiety, depressive and pain symptoms described by women in these phases.

To summarize: Estrogen has multiple effects on the brain, that collectively act in ways similar to antidepressants and nerve growth factors. Overall, estrogen's neuropharmacological profile fits well with current theories of antidepressant actions and the action of potent neuromodulator molecules.

It has always made sense to me that changes in any aspects of body chemistry, *especially changes in such potent chemical messengers as hormones* and neurotransmitters, might *first* be evidenced by changes in brain-mediated phenomena such as irritability, depression, anxiety, and sleep. These are symptoms women notice *earlier* in the climacteric, I think because the brain is so exquisitely

---

ESTROGEN EFFECTS ON THE BRAIN

- enhances CNS availability of norepinephrine and dopamine
- increases production and/or prolongs action of serotonin
- regulates sleep centers
- improves pain tolerance
- inhibits the monoamine oxidase (MAO) enzymes that break down serotonin, dopamine, and NE (prolongs mood-lifting action of these chemical messengers)
- increases production of the enzyme needed to make acetylcholine, a crucial memory-enhancing neurotransmitter
- prolongs neuronal responses to excitatory amino acids in the cerebral cortex, cerebellum, hippocampus, hypothalamus, midbrain, and pons
- acts directly on glutamate receptor binding and inactivation
- enhances attention mechanisms and increases sensory perception for fine touch, olfactory, and visual stimuli
- increases dendrite connections between nerve cells in memory centers
- has effects that alters seizure threshold, dependent upon type of seizure

sensitive to small changes in its biochemical balance and so sensitive to alterations in the *interactions* of the various neurotransmitter systems. I believe we have to completely get away from what I consider to be an outmoded "split" between psychological and biological. **Neither model alone has all the answers.** Both are clearly part of the same human body system and have to be seen as operating *together* in an *integrated* manner. There is much more to come in our understanding of this key female hormone, but it is clear that estrogen plays a major role in maintaining our sense of well-being and zest.

The Brain's Alarm Center: Hormone Triggers of "Anxiety," "Racing Heart," and "Flutters"

You hit age 39, have been in good health, maybe you exercise three or four times a week, and wham! All of a sudden you start having horrendous palpitations, and pounding sensations as if your heart were going to literally jump out of your chest. Maybe you start feeling anxious; your stomach is a little upset; your skin is clammy. "What's going on? This can't be me? I'm healthy, and I never had these problems before. What is happening? I must be having a panic attack. Maybe I'm having a heart attack. No, that can't be; I'm too young. What is this? I'd better see the doctor." So you see your family doctor, who checks you over and says you're fine, but you need to relax more and reduce your stress. With a deep sigh of relief, you leave and go on about your daily routine. Then, a few weeks later, it happens again. *What is this?*

If you have been checked out and do not have heart disease or thyroid problems or another medical condition that can trigger such episodes, it may be hormone changes that begin in the late thirties and early forties. Have you noticed *where* in the menstrual cycle these palpitations or panicky episodes occur? You might find it helpful to keep track of this pattern. If your physical symptoms (heart flutters, heart racing or pounding, feeling queasy or nauseous, sweating, feeling anxious for no apparent reason) come right *after ovulation*, a day or so *before your period starts*, or the first *two or three days of bleeding*, these are times in the cycle when estrogen is falling or low. You may be experiencing one of the *brain* effects of *dropping estrogen levels*. I can hear you saying to yourself as you read this, "How does *estrogen* affect the *brain* to cause *heart* symptoms?" Well, by some of those chemical messenger molecules I was just talking about. A drop in blood

levels of estrogen affects the brain in several ways. Take a look
at the following sequence of events:

Deceased estradiol (ovary)→ Deceased estradiol (at the brain)
→ decreased brain endorphins→ burst of brain adrenalin
(increased Norepinephrine)→ brain-body responses to the
stimulation from norepinephrine: *increased heart rate, palpitations, rise in blood pressure,* being awakened suddenly from
sleep, dilation of body blood vessels triggering the "hot flash,"
sweating, "butterflies" in the stomach, diarrhea, headaches.

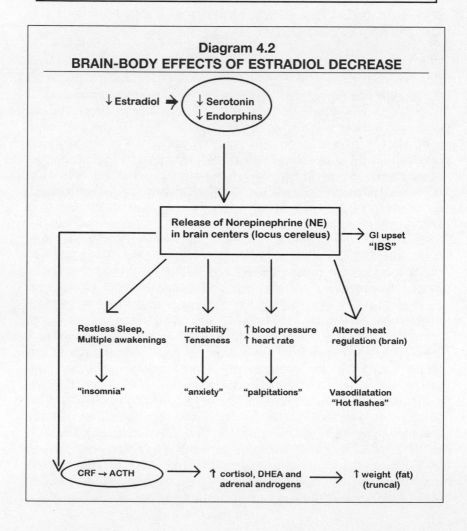

Diagram 4.2
BRAIN-BODY EFFECTS OF ESTRADIOL DECREASE

So there you are, a whole *cascade* of events spreading over the body from a direct hormone-triggered release of brain chemicals. Remember that endorphins are the body's natural pain killers and mood regulators, so you see how *psychological* symptoms can be related to the *physical* hormonal drop. This is such a common occurrence, many women don't even notice it until the hormone drops become greater during perimenopause. As estrogen production declines, a fall in estrogen before menses triggers a much more pronounced physical response. Suddenly, we are aware of something new happening. Most doctors have *not* been taught these hormone-brain-body connections, so they don't realize these are *clues* to hormone shifts for women. Women tell me they *know* "it's a physical, chemical kind of thing," but they have been told that it's "all in your head" and so their *intuitive* (and I would say more often *correct*) *knowing* has been dismissed.

In fact it wasn't until very recently that doctors accepted scientific proof that women's hot flashes were a real physical phenomenon. They had been assumed to be psychological. Menopause researcher, Dr. Rebar, said at the 1992 meeting of the North American Menopause Society (NAMS, 9/19/92): "It wasn't until the **late 1970s** that physicians realized that the hot flashes were REAL physiological phenomena, *not just a figment of the woman's imagination*!" (italics mine). The surging hormones prior to menopause trigger pulses of LH and drops in estradiol which fires off norepinephrine (NE) in the limbic system, and this burst of NE disrupts the normal function of the heat-regulating center in the hypothalamus. The thermoregulatory center then sends its chemical messengers to the arteries, dilating them to allow excess heat to dissipate. The dilation is accompanied by sweating, body temperature begins to drop, and you feel a chilly sensation sweeping over you. If it happens at night, this whole sequence wakes you up, often soaked in sweat.

When estrogen is dropping, it triggers a decrease in serotonin. Since serotonin helps maintain sleep and decrease anxiety, a drop in serotonin *adds* to the episodes of awakenings at night, and aggravates the adrenalin-induced feelings of irritability, tension, palpitations, and chest discomfort. It is important to have palpitations and chest discomfort evaluated and the possibility of heart disease ruled out. It is *also* important that in women's health checkups we look at changing hormone levels as contributing factors and not immediately jump to the conclusion that it's just psychological stress. This just makes so much sense to me, I don't understand why it's not routinely done in the women's medical care.

Situational and psychological STRESS obviously makes all this worse by further suppressing ovarian function along with its many other effects on the body. I will discuss the stress-induced connections in greater detail in Chapter 7. A lot of the mood swings women experience are not due *only* to external stresses; mood swings also result from the *interaction* of external stresses and our internal body changes (which are also stressors requiring the body to change and adapt). So, when you experience heart flutters and palpitations, keep in mind that it's not all in your imagination or just due to anxiety, it can also be your hormones changing. This sequence of physical sensations is very real, and once again shows the connections between hormone changes, the brain, and the body.

Progesterone and the Brain

With all the headlines talking about progesterone as a "wonder hormone" to prevent osteoporosis and solve all of women's problems, I think it's time to clarify what we know about this hormone. Some of the promoters of the natural "wild yam" progesterone cream have got it backwards as to which hormone does what in the female body—but then most of these promoters are men who don't live with our body experiences every month! A recent sales flyer a patient sent me from Florida had this headline: "Estrogen's Lethal Effects." Of course, this newsletter was selling...you guessed it, natural progesterone as a wonder hormone cure-all. I wrote a humorous note back to my patient thanking her, and made the observation wondering when the guys would ever get it right. We women live with estrogen all our lives, and most of the really serious health problems that affect our quality of life and our longevity don't start to really show up until the primary active estrogen (17-beta-estradiol) is *decreasing*. So if estrogen were truly "lethal," as this newsletter proclaimed, most women would be dead long before menopause, since estrogen levels are their *highest* from puberty until menopause. I found the newsletter so ridiculously inaccurate as to be humorous, but the tragedy is that too many women believe it. Obviously, this important hormone plays a critical role in sustaining pregnancy, but being pregnant is not a woman's *only* function. And as every *woman* knows, what's crucial for our sense of well-being is the *balance* of our primary hormones.

Progesterone, as you recall from earlier chapters, is the primary hormone designed to prepare the female body to support a pregnancy. "Pro-gestational" hormone tells you a lot about its functions, which I reviewed in Chapter 3. Progesterone has some rather interesting effects on the brain. It acts as an anti-estrogen (similar to Tamoxifen) and an antitestosterone by several mechanisms. Significant new research into these brain effects have given us a better understanding of these neuroendocrine functions. Progesterone "down-regulates" or "dampens down" the estradiol and testosterone receptors in the brain, so that it offsets some of the usual mood-*lifting* effects of both estradiol and testosterone.

Progesterone also increases the flow of calcium ions into nerve cells, *decreasing* the release of important chemical messengers (neurotransmitters) that boost mood. At high levels, it actually acts very much like the benzodiazepine antianxiety medications (e.g., Xanax, Valium, and others) by binding to the GABA receptor sites and facilitating the release of the inhibitory neurotransmitter GABA. This is the same receptor site where Xanax and Valium bind in the brain by the same mechanism and produce their antianxiety effects.

Boosting the action of GABA is, I think, one of the primary reasons that high doses of progesterone help decrease anxiety in some women with severe PMS. Such high doses are actually providing a *pharmacologic* effect on the brain rather than a *physiologic* one. I think there is a place for use of progesterone in certain patients with PMS, but I think it has to be individualized, based on the type and pattern of the woman's symptoms. Many women become **more depressed** on large doses of progesterone. This is to be expected due to progesterone's effects on the brain. In fact, several metabolic breakdown products of the natural human progesterone molecule are *very potent* depressants of brain (CNS) function.

One of the metabolites of progesterone (3-alpha-OH-DHP) has been found to be about *eight times* more potent (as an antianxiety and sedative agent) than the most potent barbiturate known today, methohexital. Studies looking at the anticonvulsant actions of 3-alpha-OH-DHP have found it to be more potent than clonazepam (Klonopin), a high-potency benzodiazepine used for epilepsy and panic disorder. There is clearly a lot of additional information we need about the varied brain effects of progesterone before we can in good conscience suggest that women buy over-the-counter progesterone creams to use on a daily basis.

If you are wondering about sex drive, it turns out that progesterone also *competes with* testosterone for uptake from the blood into the brain and decreases the conversion of testosterone into its most active form. This reduction in the amount of active testosterone at the brain has the result of further decreasing sexual interest (libido), particularly if estrogen levels are also low. In addition, both estradiol and testosterone have mood-elevating effects, so when progesterone diminishes the binding of estradiol and testosterone at brain receptors, it's not surprising that you may notice your mood is grumpy, irritable, tearful, and depressed.

This is what is typically observed in women with PMS: the moods become more consistently negative when progesterone rises in the second half of the menstrual cycle, especially if estradiol production is diminished. Some women find the "calming" effects of progesterone pleasant. Other women really are uncomfortable and "out-of-sorts" with the depression-producing effects of progesterone. This has certainly been widely observed in menopausal women on HRT, who report feeling very well on the estrogen-only phase of hormones, but then become depressed, lethargic, bloated, and miserable during the days when progesterone or progestin is added. We once again come back to the importance of a healthy balance of the ovarian hormones Mother Nature provided us. There's no quick fix, no magic bullet, and rarely is anything going to give us 100 percent positive effects, without the possibility for some offsetting negatives. If you have begun using a wild yam or progesterone cream and experience *a decrease* in energy, sex drive, or mood, you may feel better by stopping the progesterone product.

Testosterone and the Brain

In Chapter 6, you will read how testosterone is crucially important for normal sex drive in women, since it activates the brain "sexual circuits" in both women and men. For now, I just want to emphasize that it is another hormone produced by the ovary that helps to improve a woman's sense of well-being, energy level, and stimulates normal bone growth and muscle development. Thanks to more recent neuroendocrine research, we know that a certain level of estradiol (estrogen) must be present in our brain areas in order for testosterone to function properly. It is now thought that the *brain testosterone receptor is <u>created</u> by the presence of estradiol*. Without enough estrogen to "prime the pump" so to speak, testosterone produced by the ovary cannot attach properly in brain centers to stimulate sexual arousal for women. So your level of estradiol also plays a role in how well your body's testosterone can work! When I have explained this biology to women and their partners, it has helped improve many hurts in relationships when the partner thought she was no longer attracted to him.

As another illustration of the connection between estradiol and testerone, we have seen in women who have had breast cancer and cannot take estrogen, that providing supplemental testosterone may only *partially* improve their sexual desire and ability to have an orgasm. The important role of "estrogen-priming" for optimal testosterone response may explain these clinical observations. Other studies have demonstrated a mood-lifting or anti-depressant effect of testosterone, which many women in my center also describe after testosterone therapy is added to their program. It is rewarding to me to hear my patients describe how they feel after taking natural testosterone, when they have typically experienced low testosterone levels for quite a long time: "GOSH, I FEEL LIKE MY OLD SELF AGAIN. I have my energy back. I'M INTERESTED IN SEX AGAIN. I have my get-up-and-go feelings." Using natural testosterone at doses designed for women, it is uncommon that I see unwanted side effects. I will describe in Chapter 6 the different types of testosterone available and how I use blood levels and women's descriptions to find the right amount for a given person.

Future Directions

For centuries, medical observation has written about the connection between reproductive hormones and changes in mood and behavior, but these observations have been largely dismissed due to problems in methods, lack of "adequate" biological evidence, and lack of the necessary interdisciplinary studies. Recent developments in the study of the endocrine system and brain function have certainly shed light on the ways that changes in hormones through the menstrual cycle may contribute to perimenopausal mood *disorders* and *symptoms*. Mood disorders and milder mood-change symptoms are a significant source of distress to many women in the perimenopausal years; yet, they often fall between the cracks in our fragmented health care system.

The model I have developed for *HER Place: Health Enhancement and Renewal for Women*™ Centers in Tucson and Ft. Worth at All Saints Hospital are one example of the integrated approach we crucially need for women's health care services, as well as educational and research paradigms. Just as new research on unipolar and bipolar mood disorders has replaced the former cause-effect model with an *interactive* one which addresses abnormalities in the *balance* of mood-regulating mechanisms that may lead to mania (elevated moods) or depression, we need to view hormonal effects on mood from an *interactive* perspective. We need to focus on the internal biological factors, such as hormones, that interact with external events to increase the likelihood of *exaggerated* or *abnormal responses* to *normal* hormonal changes. Areas of future research need to also include evaluation of the

- possibility that different types of estrogens, progestins and testosterone, as well as different doses, likely have very different effects on the brain
- mood effects of estrogen and progesterone in women who have never had previous depression
- effect of different hormone preparations in women who have a history of hormone-related depressions
- different types of estrogens' effects in various subtypes of depressed patients (unipolar, bipolar, those with normal estrogen levels, those with proven low estrogen levels, etc.)
- differential effects of brief and ongoing estrogen use along with how it is taken;
- evaluation of estrogen's possible role as an augmentation approach to traditional antidepressant medications
- evaluation of the role that stress plays in possibly suppressing ovarian function
- the effects of hormone interactions with other medications.

There is a great deal of exciting work to be done to understand our awesome female body and these intricate interconnections. The need is great, and the list of unanswered questions is long. At *HER Place*, we are among the leaders in these endeavors. Speak out in your community and encourage the development of integrated clinical research and health enhancement services among Gynecology, Endocrinology, Psychiatry/Psychology, and Preventive Medicine. All of us working together can make a difference in understanding women's health needs. It is crucial, in my view, that we *combine* our understandings in ways to provide effective and safe symptom relief for women *so that we may have healthy, enjoyable, and productive lives for the next half of adult life!*

CHAPTER 5

The Big Question: Has Anybody Seen My Estrogen?

... And Will Someone Help Me Look For It? What About Blood Tests for Hormones?

Women having been asking me these questions for years! It makes so much sense to measure a baseline level of almost anything before starting a medication designed to *change that particular parameter*. Clearly, one of the important advantages of modern medicine is our ability to measure objective parameters in the laboratory, with X-rays, MRI, bone density tests and other techniques. We then combine this information with the clinical description from the patient about what she is experiencing to determine a diagnosis and a meaningful course of action or treatment plan.

For example, if you have clinical symptoms which suggest low thyroid function, we measure the level of thyroid hormones in your blood, both those produced by the gland (T3, T4), the brain (TSH), and possibly thyroid antibodies. If you need thyroid medication, we then prescribe a low dose and gradually increase it. Then we check a follow-up blood level of TSH to see if the dose is right for you and if not, make further adjustments in the amount you take. This process is routinely done with diabetics on insulin by monitoring the blood levels of fasting glucose and postprandial (after meals) glucose. It is also used in patients on heart medicine, such as digitalis, by monitoring blood levels of the medication at a certain number of hours after a dose. By monitoring blood levels of hormones or medications, doctors are able to use the right amount for your body and minimize the possibility of unwanted side effects. Makes sense, right?

So why isn't this same standard of medical practice used in helping postmenopausal women find the right dose of estrogen therapy? Why have we had in the U.S. what I call the "cookbook" approach, with the same Premarin-Provera "recipe" for all postmenopausal women, even giving the *same doses* to better than 90 percent of patients? I simply cannot fathom this practice. We do not use the same dose of blood pressure medication for everyone with high blood pressure, or the same dose of insulin for all diabetics, or the same dose of anticonvulsant medication for everyone with seizure disorders. So why take such a cookbook approach to women's hormone therapy after menopause? Could it be that older women just aren't seen as that important, or their "complaints" aren't taken seriously?

I estimate that over the last 15 years of my medical practice, *9 out of every 10* women I've seen who were already taking hormone therapy were on 0.625 mg of Premarin for 25 days a month, and 10 mg of Provera (rarely I would find someone who had been given 5 mg) for days 16-25 every month. Some women said they felt wonderful, others described having "nothing but problems" since starting on these hormones. I was bothered by the fact that almost every woman I saw was on the same dose and type of hormones.

Since not everyone was *feeling well* on the recipe, I began to ask more questions. Why the same dose? *"That's the amount that's needed."* Why always the same type of estrogen? *"That's what we've always used."* Are there any others? *"Don't know of any."* What if women are having side effects? *"She can stop, or just take less."* What about rechecking FSH after a woman is on her therapy and see if she has the right amount? *"That's not needed, the FSH never comes back down to normal after menopause."* How do we know; are there any studies on this? *"No, there aren't any studies, we just know that's the way it is."* Can't we check blood levels to see if the amount is right? *"No, blood levels are useless, hormone levels vary."* **That's my point!** They *do* vary, and we need to know *how* they vary in relationship to what a woman is experiencing.

I wanted to scream, it was all such nonsense. How could we *know* if there aren't any studies? Why doesn't FSH come back down when a woman is on the right amount of estrogen? That's how *other* hormone feedback systems in the body work. This "reasoning" (or lack of it!) simply did not make either physiological or medical sense to me. With my patients who were taking hormones and yet were still not feeling well, I started letting them know that checking FSH, estradiol, and testosterone blood levels was an option for them even though we did not have a lot of good information about correlation of blood levels and physical symptoms. Many women elected to have this done—it made intuitive sense to them (and to me). Well, amazing results began to unfold.

I found that there was a very *good correlation between* desirable blood hormonal levels in women who were doing well on their regimen and suboptimal hormonal blood levels in women who were still describing symptoms.

As I continued to research this issue, I found that Dr. Philip Sarrel at Yale had been finding the same thing, as had some European researchers. Dr. Sarrel studied the women who came to the Yale Menopause Center and tabulated the percentage of women who described problems with sexual function as one of the reasons they were seeking a consultation. The numbers speak for themselves as to the magnitude of the impact on women's lives:

SEXUAL DYSFUNCTION AFTER MENOPAUSE: YALE MID-LIFE STUDY

Problems Patients Reported:	*Patients Experiencing It*
Decreased sexual desire	77%
Reporting of sexual problems	68%
Bothered by sexual problems	64%
Intercourse (less than/=)1/month	50%

Ref: Sarrel: *Obstet Gynecol* 1990; 75 (suppl. 265–308)

Dr. Sarrel further showed that there seems to be a **threshold level of about 50 pg/ml** for estradiol with regard to women having sexual problems at menopause: women with estradiol levels *greater than 50* had **minimal** reports of adverse changes in their sexual function; however, women whose estradiol levels were *below 50* had a *dramatic increase* in sexual problems of all types, including decreased lubrication, burning and pain with intercourse, difficulty having an orgasm and diminished quality of orgasm. This was one of the few studies I could find in the literature that clearly demonstrated a relationship between estradiol blood levels and the clinical problems women were describing. Finally, someone had *listened to the patients*! Dr. Sarrel has done groundbreaking, well-documented research in this area and has been effective in helping other physicians understand the importance of these connections. I felt validated in my own observations when I discovered the results of his studies.

The more I listened to my patients and tried to help them feel better, the more I found that blood level information helped guide me in my recommendations for each individual woman. It also helped *her* feel that a more rational, logical approach was being used to determine her individual needs.

I decided that taking the systematic approach of making treatment decisions based on *both* clinical symptoms and objective laboratory results made good sense, and provided better medical care for my women patients. This approach means that the doses are then designed for the individual woman, and she and I have objective measures of what is the right amount for her. I think this approach is also more cost-effective in the long run, since everyone is looking at health care costs these days. Women quickly discover that many vague symptoms, for which they may have had to see multiple physicians, often went away when the type and amount of estradiol was right for their individual needs.

If you want to request these blood tests from your physician, what should you be looking for as a desirable target range for estradiol? In my clinical experience, women typically experience their usual energy level, mood, sleep, and memory when serum (blood) **levels of estradiol are** *above* **90-100 pg/ml**. Levels above this range, up to about 200 or so, are the *normal estradiol levels* reached in the first half of the menstrual cycle before women reach menopause. Levels below this are generally too low to maintain a normal feeling of well-being. Recent research has found that estradiol levels below about 60 pg/ml result in *increased bone loss after menopause*. There now appears to be a threshold level of about 50–60 pg/ml for estradiol, and below this level women lose more bone and have more loss of sexual function.

I have been criticized by other physicians for recommending that women have both FSH and estradiol levels checked. They have often said to me that it is "too expensive," "unreliable," or "doesn't tell us anything." **I disagree.** Clearly, having this information has made an enormous difference to the women who had been told their symptoms were "all in their head" and who now have a hormone regimen right for them. Many of my patients have also been able to stop the expensive medications for lowering blood pressure and cholesterol, as well as eliminate psychotropic medications when their estradiol levels were again in the optimal ranges.

Furthermore, it is difficult to put a price tag on improving someone's quality of life. I think in the long run it is less expensive to check hormone blood levels than to do all the myriad tests and evaluations that end up being done when hormone problems are *not* recognized, or for women to undergo a long series of psychotherapy sessions thinking that the mood changes are just stress or empty nest or a bad relationship. In my opinion, this blood test is extremely efficient, cost-effective, and psychologically helpful in identifying a physical cause of disturbing symptoms women frequently experience at mid-life and around menopause. *I feel strongly that such tests of hormone levels should be available to women, especially those who have had their ovaries removed.*

I am in the process of collecting outcome data on larger numbers of patients to be able to demonstrate to insurance companies that such tests are in fact useful and cost-effective. This research, underway at HER Place at All Saints Health System in Ft. Worth, Texas in addition to my Tucson center, will help clarify these important issues, and I hope change the way health services are offered to mid-life women. Instead of operating on **unproved assumptions**, we really need to look at the whole woman and evaluate her endocrine system carefully to rule out hormonal factors contributing to her symptoms as well. *If your doctor isn't listening to your requests, find one who does.*

Types of Estrogen

There is so much confusion about *estrogens*, I would like to describe some of the differences between various types. Bear with me for the "chemistry lesson." I hope you will find this information very eye-opening. There are *three* estrogens found in human females, and the relative amounts of each one present is determined by several factors: genetic make-up, age, amount of body fat, pregnancy, diet, and the presence of any medical condition or lifestyle habits condition that alter ovary function. Many women at my seminars think "estrogen" equals "Premarin." A recent cover of a major newsmagazine perpetuated that confusion by showing a Premarin tablet under the headline about ESTROGEN. This is not the case. Premarin is only *one* brand of estrogen among many brands available. I will describe the estrogens commercially available in the U.S. First, some definitions:

HUMAN ESTROGENS:

- **17-beta estradiol (E2):** The predominant natural human estrogen produced by the human ovary *prior to menopause*; it is the primary *biologically active* estrogen at cell surface receptor sites, and also inside the cell at the nucleus receptor site as I described in Chapter 3. It is the major *functioning* estrogen for our bodies from puberty until menopause, and it is the one responsible for over 400 functions in the female body. After menopause, it is the **17-beta estradiol** from the ovary that **declines**, resulting in the post-menopausal changes in skin, bone, hair, heart/blood vessels, brain, and other organs.

Ideally, if a woman decides to take estrogen therapy after menopause, she would take a form of 17-beta estradiol to provide exactly the same chemical molecule her ovary had previously made. *Three brands of 17-beta estradiol are commercially available in the U.S. for estrogen therapy (ET, or ERT)*: **Estrace** tablets and vaginal cream (approved by the FDA in 1976), **Estraderm** skin patch, and **Climara** (released in 1995), also a skin patch. It surprises me that Estrace has been on the market so long and most women have never heard of it.

- **estrone (E1)**: The predominate estrogen found in *post-menopausal* women. Before menopause, estrone is made by body fat *and* in the ovary. Estrone is also produced from conversion of estradiol, and vice versa. It serves primarily as a reservoir for the body to make the biologically active 17-beta estradiol. Estrone continues to be produced in the body fat (adipose) tissue after menopause. The more body fat a woman has (before or after menopause) the more estrone is present.

  This is the form of estrogen which many researchers now think may be related to the higher risk of endometrial and breast cancer in older women who are obese. One brand of estrone is commercially available in the U.S. for postmenopausal therapy: **Ogen** (piperazine estrone sulfate), which is *chemically similar to, but not exactly the same as*, human estrone. If you are taking a form of estrone for a postmenopausal estrogen, you may still have some residual symptoms due to the lower amount of estradiol present.

- **estriol (E3)**: The weakest of the human estrogens, it is the one produced during pregnancy, Estriol is not available in an FDA approved brand for ERT in this country, but it may be made up to your individual needs by pharmacists. Estriol is biologically the weakest estrogen and has not been shown to provide the degree of protective effects on bone, heart, brain, and nerves as does the normal premenopausal 17-beta estradiol. Estriol may relieve some of the milder symptoms of menopause, but it does not have the significant effects on improving memory, mood and sleep that I find with the primary active estrogen, 17-beta estradiol. Keep in mind that estriol is **not** normally present in measurable amounts in non-pregnant women. We do not know what its effects would be if it is taken continuously during and after menopause.

ANIMAL ESTROGENS (NOT FOUND IN HUMANS):

- **equine estrogens:** Extracted from the urine of pregnant mares to produce a mixture known as *conjugated equine estrogens* (CEE). The most commonly used brand of CEE is **Premarin** (<u>Pre</u>gnant <u>Mar</u>e's Ur<u>ine</u>). Actually, the equine estrogens are *not* just one estrogen as many women think; CEE refers to the entire group of about 10 or more different chemical molecules that have different "attachment strengths" for the estradiol receptor sites. Many doctors consider that Premarin is the "gold standard" for estrogen therapy because it is the one which has been on the market longer, and most of the research studies have used only this one type of estrogen to determine estrogen benefits, side effects, and risks.

  Since the equine estrogens have several components which attach more strongly to the estradiol receptor than does human estradiol, and some of the equine estrogens stay in the body far longer than does estradiol, it only makes sense to me that we should study the potential for different effects of horse-derived estrogens on human females. To date, there have not been *any* significant prospective, double-blind controlled studies in this country *comparing* the equine estrogens with the native human estrogen 17-beta estradiol to see whether there are *differences* in side effects, blood pressure changes, breast cancer incidence, uterine cancer rates, brain effects, and/or joint-muscle pain syndromes. I will talk more about these issues later in this chapter.

"SYNTHETIC" ESTROGENS (NOT NATIVE TO HUMANS):

These estrogens have slightly different chemical structures than does the human estradiol, and therefore have somewhat different effects on the body.

- **ethinyl estradiol:** The most common form of estrogen found in the birth control pill. Ethinyl estradiol is not used much in the U.S. for postmenopausal ERT because it is so much more potent than the 17-beta estradiol and provides more estrogen effect than is needed after a woman reaches menopause. Available by itself as one brand, **Estinyl**, which is *only* estrogen and is **not** a birth control pill.

- **estradiol valerate:** About 100 times more potent than 17-beta estradiol, it is rarely used in the U.S., but it is common in Europe for postmenopausal ERT. This is the type of estradiol which was used in a Swedish study and was thought to *possibly* be a factor in the slightly higher breast cancer cases reported by that research. (I elaborate on the flaws in that study in chapter 14). You need to keep in mind that the *estradiol* referred to in European research can be *either* the native human form (17-beta-estradiol) *or* the synthetic and more potent estradiol valerate.

PLANT ESTROGENS:

- **Phytoestrogens:** Estrogenic compounds found in a variety of plants, including soybeans, dong quai, ginseng, and others. Biologically weaker than the native human estrogens, these are sometimes used as precursor molecules for producing 17-beta estradiol. Plant sources vary in amount of estrogenic effects and potency. This may help explain the apparent discrepancy in reports that in China and Japan, where diets are high in phytoestrogens and herbal sources of estrogen are widely used, women do not typically describe hot flashes but *do continue to have bone loss* after menopause. Japanese menopause researchers have shown clearly that there is an epidemic of osteoporosis in their country; their research indicates that phytoestrogens alone do not provide enough estrogen effect to protect against osteoporosis and decline in cognitive function, even though the plant sources may be helpful for mild symptoms. Ginseng is often recommended by herbalists as a "natural" source of estrogen. Ginseng, however, can cause high blood pressure, insomnia, anxiety, and agitation if taken in large amounts.
- **Xenoestrogens:** A group of synthetic organo-solvents, pesticides and other compounds that mimic some of the actions of estrogen in humans, but are not native to the human body and also produce toxic effects. These chemicals, such as DDT, PCB and a variety of others are not normally found in nature, and as a group are responsible for a great deal of environmental damage to animals, plants, and water sources. Their potent effect on living organisms is one of the factors responsible for reproductive abnormalities in wildlife, and is also postulated as a cause of lower average sperm counts found in human males in recent years. I talk more about these compounds and what we know about their potential car-

cinogenic effects in Chapter 14. The important thing to keep in mind is that although these chemicals may have some *estrogenic* effects, they are *not* the same estrogen produced by our bodies.

What Do We Mean by Natural or Synthetic?

I hear a lot of women talking about wanting to only take *natural* hormones, which is the reason often given for wanting to use the "wild yam" skin cream advertised as a source of progesterone, or dong quai (an herb with estrogenic compounds), or estriol (weakest of the three primary human estrogens) instead of "drugs," which are "synthetic." Use of the words natural and synthetic can be very confusing, to patients and doctors alike. Actually, something *synthetic* can also be *natural*, while something *natural* may be *foreign (not native to)* the human body. The key here is not whether a compound is "natural" to plants or horses or whatever, but **is the compound natural to the human body and identical to compounds made by the human body** so that it will fit properly as a "key" in the body's receptor sites. Don't be misled by clever wording in advertising!

The term *"synthesis"* comes from the Greek meaning "a putting together, composition." In other words, it means "to make something." *Synthetic* simply means "produced by synthesis." In common usage today, "synthetic" has *come to mean "artificial,"* but that is not always correct. For example: We previously used insulins derived from cows (bovine) and pigs (porcine, or pork insulin) to treat diabetics who needed insulin, because we did not have a way to obtain human insulin. These animal insulins were "natural" in that they came from biological sources, but they were not "native" molecules for the human body, and many times, human diabetics developed allergic reactions or a "resistance" to the animal insulins.

In recent years, scientists have determined the makeup of the human insulin molecule and have been able to make (synthesize) the exact same molecule of human insulin in the laboratory, so that we can now give human diabetics the *native* human insulin (one brand is Humulin). So, here is one example of a "synthetic" medication being used because it is the natural one for humans and, therefore, is better tolerated, more effective, and has fewer side effects. Insulin derived from cows and pigs is used less often today as a result of the availability of the natural human form. **We need to do more of this with female hormones.**

The same is true with estrogen. In the past, we did not have a way to give estrogen orally, because it would be broken down and lost in the digestive process before getting into the bloodstream. About fifty years ago, scientists developed a way to extract estrogens from the urine of pregnant mares, purify the extract containing "conjugated equine estrogens" (CEE), and then coat the estrogens in a matrix of binders (called enteric coating) that allowed the tablet to survive digestion in the stomach, reach the small intestine, be absorbed into the bloodstream, and then produce an estrogenic effect on the body organs. This product, Premarin, has been the primary type of estrogen used in the United States since that time, accounting for about 85 to 90 percent of the prescriptions written for estrogen in the U.S. An oral dose of Premarin produces blood levels of the two primary estrogens also found in humans: estradiol and estrone; but it also produces *high blood levels of equine estrogens native to horses, also called "equilin estrogens."* A typical oral dose of 0.625 mg Premarin produces about 2/3 of the total circulating estrogens as equilin compounds; only about 1/3 of the total estrogen present is the estrone and estradiol found in humans. I have shown some comparisons on blood levels in the graphs on the next page.

In **1976**, the FDA approved a new product (brand name: Estrace) that had been developed as a form of native human estrogen, 17-beta-estradiol (derived from soybeans), in a *micronized* form, which will survive digestion and be well absorbed into the bloodstream. Micronization means making the molecule particles small enough that they can be rapidly absorbed into the bloodstream before being broken down by digestive acids and the liver. Many recent studies have shown that the smaller the particle size, the better the absorption and the more reliable the blood levels obtained. Micronization is used to make many therapeutic medications and has been particularly helpful in developing native human forms of estradiol (estrogen), progesterone, and testosterone because these hormones typically were inactivated or destroyed by digestion when taken orally.

The sources for most of these natural human hormones are actually plants such as soybeans and yams, with the purified, concentrated extract producing chemical molecules *identical to those is made in the human body.* **This resulting 17-beta estradiol, progesterone, or testosterone is then compounded into standardized tablets to regulate the amount of hormone given. Standardization of the dose in each tablet also allows for tailoring the amount given more closely to each individual woman's needs.** I feel this

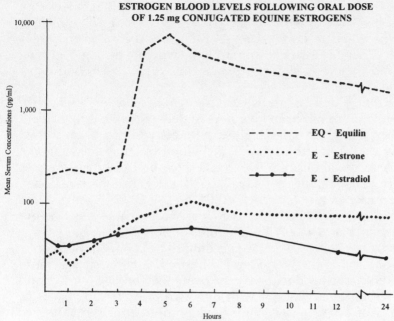

ESTROGEN BLOOD LEVELS FOLLOWING ORAL DOSE OF 1.25 mg CONJUGATED EQUINE ESTROGENS

EQ - Equilin
E - Estrone
E - Estradiol

Equilin (EQ) estrogens are derived from horses and are not native to human females
Blood levels of EQ after an oral dose are higher than levels of human E and E2
Effects of EQ on human females are not well known

Adapted from Yen, Martin, Burnier, et al, as cited in Whittaker

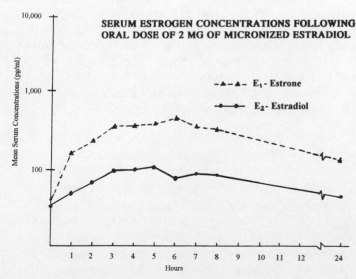

SERUM ESTROGEN CONCENTRATIONS FOLLOWING ORAL DOSE OF 2 MG OF MICRONIZED ESTRADIOL

E_1 - Estrone
E_2 - Estradiol

Adapted from Yen, Martin, Burnier, et al, as cited in Whittaker

approach is better than trying to get enough active hormone from plant/herbal sources alone, since you really are not able to *determine how much you are taking and whether the amount is right for you*. There is also the question of whether you are getting additional chemicals *native to plants* that your *human* body may not need.

The two brands of transdermal estrogen patches, Estraderm and Climara, are recent innovations to deliver the human 17-beta estradiol. The patch system allows the estradiol to be absorbed through the skin, directly into the bloodstream, bypassing the "first pass" metabolism in the liver (which breaks down some of the hormone, making it unavailable for its normal functions). Estraderm looks like a circular (0.05 mg) or oval (0.1 mg) clear Band-Aid and is left on the skin for two to three days before changing to a new one. Climara (0.05 mg) is similar, but is supposed to last a full week before needing to be changed. Both are a means of keeping the blood levels of estradiol fairly steady, more like the hormone production by the ovary. Patches are a very good option for estrogen therapy, with only two primary drawbacks to this form of estradiol: (1) the skin irritation from the adhesive, which bothers many women, and (2) since it bypasses the liver, the patch does not trigger as much of an increase in the HDL (good) cholesterol as do the oral forms of estrogen. *Oral* estrogens produce a *pharmacologic* effect on the liver that stimulates production of more HDL cholesterol. The transdermal forms of estrogen (the patch in this country, skin gels and patches in Europe) produce only the *physiological* effect of estrogen to maintain the normal level of HDL cholesterol. This may be all that is needed for women who have a normal cholesterol profile. For women who have *high* total cholesterol and *low* HDL, however, an *oral* form of estradiol provides more *decrease* in total cholesterol and a more significant *increase* in HDL for cardiovascular protective effects.

New Research on Estrogen and a Woman's Body

I have talked about the concept of the body's chemical messengers (hormones, neurotransmitters, etc.) acting like a "key" in a special receptor site "lock" on the cell membrane. The molecules made by the human body are the specific "key" which fit our cell receptor sites. Similar chemical molecules, either from other animals or made in the laboratory, may also work the "lock" at least partially the same as the human molecules do. But some of these other chemical molecules may get "stuck" in the lock, and actually block the action of our own human molecular "keys." That's why it is important to understand the different types of hormone preparations, and know that the different forms available may have very different effects in your body.

For the steroid hormones, there is an additional receptor site located in the cell nucleus. These receptor sites have been identified for all three primary ovarian hormones. In particular, estrogen receptor sites are found throughout the brain and all organs of the body-skin, blood vessels, bone, heart, intestinal tract, urinary bladder-not just the organs of reproduction! The blood levels of human estrogens include predominately estradiol and, in lower amounts, estrone. Most of an oral dose of estrogen is converted in the blood to estrone or estrone sulfate. But there are important differences between the estrogen circulating in the blood and the estrogen that acts at the cell receptor site. 17-beta estradiol is needed at the receptor site to actually work properly.

Estradiol is the estrogen in humans that declines so rapidly after menopause, causing the *symptoms* of declining estrogen. Estrone is still present in post-menopausal women since it is made in the adrenal glands and in the fat tissue. If estrone were the primary hormone activating the receptor site, then we would NOT expect to see postmenopausal women having the symptoms of estrogen decline. Make sense?

So far, researchers have identified two types of estradiol receptors in the body: one is found inside the *nucleus* of cells, and another type is found on the *membrane* surface of cells. The body's estrogen receptors need the proper "keys" of 17-beta estradiol molecules to fit in the "locks" but the nucleus and membrane receptors each act by a different mechanism to influence the biochemical processes of cells.

The estradiol receptor in the nucleus works in a more complex manner than the membrane receptors. The estradiol molecule fits into the nuclear receptor and then binds with the cell's DNA to regulate gene expression. These genes are involved in the synthesis of particular proteins that make up neuropeptides, crucial enzymes, and other chemical messengers. This process is called the *genomic* hormonal action. An example important in memory regulation is the action of estradiol to trigger the formation of *choline acetyltransferase*, the enzyme that makes the memory-enhancing chemical messenger, *acetylcholine*. This effect cannot be investigated in living humans with our current techniques, but it has been shown in studies of rat brains. Estradiol also acts at the

---

SUMMARY: Estradiol Receptors in the Nervous System

- CNS: Concentrated in limbic system
- PNS: Found in spinal cord, peripheral nerves
- Specific for 17-beta-estradiol (E2)
- Nerve function is affected by *changing E2 levels*
- 17-beta-estradiol is the *active* form at E2 receptor
- equilin estrogens: higher affinity at receptors *than human E2*
- equilin estrogens *may displace* 17-beta-estradiol at receptors

---

nucleus receptor to stimulate messenger RNA inside cells so that neurons in the brain can make *proenkephalin*, an opiate "messenger" peptide important in pain-reducing pathways. These are just two of many examples of estrogen action at the *genomic receptor*. Many of the sites of estradiol's action in the brain, as well as other body organs, work by this process.

Another mechanism of action for estradiol and other hormones is called the *non-genomic process*. Here, the estradiol binds with a specific "lock" or receptor site *on the cell membrane* rather than inside the cell. We have not yet discovered the many ways in which these membrane receptors work, but we do know that this mechanism produces *much more rapid effects* than does the process of gene regulation directed by the nucleus estradiol receptors. Examples in this category seem to be the estradiol stimulation of various neurotransmitters, such as serotonin, dopamine, and GABA. Recent studies in mice indicate that pain pathways in males and females are functionally distinct, and that estradiol is an important regulator of these pathways. Such a significant finding means that we now need to take into account the sex differences in nerve mechanisms regulating pain when we are treating women patients, as well as when doing basic scientific research on pain mechanisms.

Different Estrogens, Different Effects

Although many physicians think all the estrogens for ERT are essentially the same, and the manufacturers of the leading products would like you to *think* they are all the same, **they are not.** Over a decade ago, two leading menopause researchers in England, Dr. Malcolm Whitehead and Dr. Campbell, did studies of the potencies of the different types of estrogens and the effects of the various estrogens on different target organs in the body. What they found was quite disturbing and has profound implications for women taking various products. They raised some critically important questions back then (1978–1982), but practically speaking, *none of their questions and concerns* have been addressed with further studies in this country. In fact, as I travel and speak to physician groups, very few of them even know these studies were done and what the outcomes were. Dr. Campbell and Dr. Whitehead's work has languished in the literature, and their questions are left unanswered.

How does this issue relate to women at risk for heart disease? The work done by Campbell and Whitehead shows that the conjugated equine estrogens are about *three times more potent* in stimulating the liver production of *renin substrate*, which is used to make angiotensin in the body, a factor that causes *increased blood pressure*. Increases in the circulating levels of renin substrate have been proposed as the possible mechanism by which conjugated equine estrogens may elevate blood pressure in some women. Two other estrogens used in this country, micronized estradiol (brand name: Estrace) and piperazine estrone sulfate (brand: Ogen), did **not** show this elevation of renin substrate. This finding also fits with work published by Geola in 1980 who observed that 1.25 mg of conjugated equine estrogens (brand name: Premarin) daily, caused *supraphysiologic* (greater than normal) effects on the liver synthesis of renin substrate, physiological (normal) actions on the vagina lining tissue (epithelium), and *subphysiological* (less than normal) effects on the brain hormones FSH and LH.

This correlates with what I have been seeing clinically: the dose of equine estrogens that is adequate for vaginal lubrication may produce a rise in blood pressure, and inadequate effect on brain phenomena like memory. It has to do with *different target organs* (in this case, liver, vagina, and brain) having very *different sensitivities* to the various molecular types of estrogens. The findings from studies such as those by Campbell and Whitehead are an additional argument for *individualizing* the estrogen options for women, rather than using one kind of estrogen and one dose *for every woman*.

Based on work such as that done by Campbell and Whitehead, it appears that women with existing hypertension would be better served to use one of the native human forms of estrogen, rather than the equine estrogens, in order to avoid the potentially harmful production of high levels of renin substrate. I recently presented this information at a Grand Rounds program for Internal Medicine and Family Medicine physicians at a major medical center. The physician who was head of the hypertension clinic was shocked to hear about these differences in various estrogen potencies on angiotensin. He had not heard about the studies from England and now wants to design a research project in his clinic that will compare blood pressure effects of several types of estrogens. This is the important kind of cross-fertilization of ideas and questions that helps us find better approaches for women.

I have seen many women for evaluation who clearly have had allergic-type reactions to the horse-derived CEE. I also have a significant number of patients who had had problems with vague joint pain syndromes that resolved when I took them off the CEE and prescribed a native human form of 17-beta estradiol. These women had already been evaluated by rheumatologists for possible rheumatoid arthritis, osteoarthritis, lupus, and other diseases which cause joint pain, and had been told "there was nothing wrong." To me, that statement means simply that there were *no laboratory abnormalities* that provided a diagnostic label for the joint pain. The joint pain was definitely real for these patients, and it improved with the change in type of estrogen.

Whether the pain was due to an adverse allergenic or auto-immune reaction to the horse-derived estrogens, or whether it represented the kind of joint pain that is seen with estrogen deficiency (meaning the dose wasn't right for these women), I cannot say at this point in time. I am suspicious that the joint pain syndrome I have seen so commonly in women on CEE is related to an immunological reaction to the equilin estrogens, similar in theory to the immunological reactions seen in diabetics on the animal-derived insulins. Until more physicians and basic science researchers take seriously the descriptions women give about their body experiences on different estrogens, we will not be able to answer these questions.

The data from Campbell and Whitehead, as well as other researchers, has indicated that the equilin (horse) components of conjugated estrogens (equilin and 17-alpha-dihydroequilin) in themselves possess estrogenic activity in the human female, but this has not been studied further to determine whether this activity is beneficial or adverse. I find it incomprehensible that the Campbell-Whitehead research has not prompted more investigation in this country on the potential adverse effects of the equilin estrogens. Even the recently published PEPI studies (Postmenopausal Estrogen and Progestin Intervention trial) *used only Premarin as the estrogen*, even though this important study compared *natural micronized progesterone* with a *synthetic progestin*

(Provera) for the first time in the U.S. *Why aren't such studies also including a native human form of 17-beta estradiol?*

I will give you even more food for thought: recent media attention focused on reports of an increased risk of breast cancer in women in the Nurses Health Study who had been on estrogen longer than 5 years. What was **never** addressed by any of the physicians or health writers commenting on this disturbing information is that the overwhelming majority of women in the series were taking the conjugated equine estrogens, **not 17-beta estradiol**.

With what we know about (1) how long the equine estrogens stay in the human body (anywhere from 8–14 weeks after the last dose), and (2) the stronger "attachment strength" (affinity) of the equine estrogens for the body estradiol receptors (especially the breasts, where estrogens may concentrate in the fat tissue), it seems incredible to me that *no one is talking about* a possible link between accumulations of equine estrogens in breast tissue and the observed higher risk of breast cancer with long-term use. I think this is such an important question that it deserves careful attention and research, but prescribing habits and research protocols are so dominated by the use of one type of estrogen that no one seems to even consider that there may be crucial differences which women need to know.

Even in 1995, with other options available for a number of years, conjugated equine estrogens (usually Premarin) *account for about 85 percent of all estrogen prescriptions in the U.S.* Recently an animal rights group has been boycotting Premarin due to objections about the way the mares are treated in the process of obtaining the equilin estrogen. While I may understand the concerns expressed by this organization, *I find it ironic that we don't have a similar concern for the well-being of <u>human</u> females*, since we really have not studied the potential long term effects of taking equine estrogens, which are not found in the female body. *This is an area which desperately needs to be addressed in good research.*

CHAPTER 6

The Overlooked *Women's* Hormone: Where's My Testosterone?

Myths About "The Male Hormone" for Women

Testosterone? That's the MALE hormone isn't it? *Testosterone?* That's the one that makes you grow a mustache, isn't it? **Testosterone?** That's the one that causes your voice to get deep, isn't it? TESTOSTERONE? That's the one that causes liver damage, isn't it? How often have you read or heard these warnings about testosterone?

These are all old myths, based on synthetic hormones in doses designed for men, not women! Women need testosterone too—it is the hormone that activates the sexual circuits in the brain for men **and** women!

So now that I have your attention, here's *the latest important information for women.* I find that most women have heard all the negatives, but know very little about the beneficial roles testosterone plays in a woman's body. Listen to the voice of this young woman:

> I just don't have any desire for sex. I feel terrible about this. I would *like* to be interested in it, I love my husband and I am very attracted to him. I enjoy sex when we have it, but I just don't feel interested. It frustrates me and it frustrates my husband. It's like somebody turned off a switch.
>
> —MG, 33 years old

Her blood level of testosterone turned out to be *less than 10 ng/dl.* Her low blood level corresponds with the way she described feeling. For women to have an optimal sex drive and interest in sex, testosterone blood levels need to be about 30 to 60 ng/dl. For comparison, men's testosterone levels run about 450–900 ng/dl, and most men don't experience a loss of libido until testosterone drops down to around 500 or less. Because women are more sensitive to small amounts of testosterone, a slight drop of only 10–15 units can make an enormous difference in whether a woman will feel her usual sexual spark.

When she talked with her primary physician about these problems, she said he told her: "Well, I guess you'll need some marital therapy. It must be a problem in your relationship." When she asked about having her hormones tested, she was told "there's no way to do that, and it doesn't mean anything anyway." When she had her consultation with me, an integral part of my evaluation was to actually measure the blood levels of testosterone. Not only is this very helpful in determining *whether* a testosterone supplement may be indicated, it also helps guide me in planning the appropriate amount for each patient. This all made a great deal of sense to MG and helped her see that there is a systematic way to evaluate her needs. She was quite willing to *consider the necessity of* marital therapy, but not until the *hormonal* aspects of her problem were assessed. In her body wisdom, it appeared more likely to her that the problem was a physical change, since she honestly felt her relationship was a good one, and her previous enjoyment of sex had been high.

Women's Sexuality: An Overlooked Concern in Health Care

It sometimes appears that the men who have dominated the hormone decisions, medical research, and the rest of women's health have been a little *afraid* for us women to have access to testosterone and a vital, normal, healthy, active sex drive as we grow older (after all, *their* testosterone, and erectile function, is often declining as they grow older). And, for generations, the standard medical teaching was that it was *abnormal* for women to have a sex drive. Women ("good girls" and "ladies") were supposed to be *passive recipients* of the sex act and were considered "loose" if they appeared to actually *desire* sex!

Many of these myths and age-old stereotypes lie just beneath the surface in women's encounters with health professionals today. I know that seems like a strange idea, given the relatively open sexuality of our culture today. But these hidden messages about women's sexuality, and how women are "supposed" to act are deeply embedded in our culture (notice the mixed messages about women's sexuality in many ads—women are supposed to be "innocent" and sexy at the same time) and especially in the traditional medical teachings. Take a look at these examples, some from a long time ago and some more recent:

Dr. W.W. Bliss (1870), in keeping with the thinking of the times, made a rigid distinction between a woman's *reproductive* ability and a woman's *sexuality*. Female sexuality was seen as unwomanly and *detrimental* to the supreme role and function of *reproduction*. Dr. Bliss in his writings warned against "any spasmodic convulsion" (i.e., orgasm) by a woman during sexual intercourse to avoid interfering with conception.

Dr. Mary Wood-Allen, a woman physician of the same era, wrote that women should embrace their husbands "without a particle of desire." Doctors were taught that women were not meant to enjoy the sex act, and a "ladylike" woman should certainly never *initiate* the sexual act. Even though the physicians of the time denied that there were female sexual feelings and desires, there still appeared to be an undercurrent of male fear of women's potentially *insatiable lust*, which, if ever aroused, might then become uncontrollable.

Things haven't gotten much better in more recent medical textbooks. Consider these quotes from a textbook of gynecology used when I was in medical school in 1977 (and think about all the physicians practicing medicine today who were trained when such textbooks were in use):

> There seems to be little doubt that libido, which is well-developed among normal males, appears to be less highly developed among females. Certainly the majority of cases of dyspareunia [painful intercourse] or frigidity, or both, undoubtedly fall into the psychogenic category. The treatment for frigidity must usually stress the educational and psychotherapeutic aspects rather than the patient's pelvic or endocrine [hormonal] status. The female should be advised to allow her male partner's sex drive to set their pace and she should attempt to gear hers satisfactorily to his . . . . The importance of the [sex] act to her husband in both physical and emotional aspects should be stressed [i.e., by the physician].

The emphasis on the man's sexual needs being met, and a woman's sexual problems as primarily psychogenic, viewed from our perspective today seems quite strikingly unbalanced. As a third-year medical student, I was, like the rest of my classmates, appropriately deferential to the teachings of the "authorities," the "experts in the field," even though these teachings did not fit with my own experience or what I was hearing from my patients.

Listen to the voice of this *recently married* 67-year-old woman who had a consultation about her problems with vaginal dryness and decreased sexual desire:

> My gynecologist just seemed to dismiss my concerns. He just told me that's what happens when you get older. I don't want to lose the sexual part of my life. I have a new husband, I love him, and we want to enjoy our sex. I just don't seem to have the interest I used to, and it hurts because I'm so dry.

She reported that she had been offered a vaginal estrogen cream and counseling had also been recommended. When she asked about having her hormones checked, her physician's reply was "That's not necessary. It won't tell us anything." When I evaluated her, her estradiol level was *less than 30* pg/ml (a desirable level would be at least 80 pg/ml), and her testosterone level was reported as "non-detectable" (recall that it should be about 30 to 50 ng/dl). Finding out that her hormone levels were so low certainly helped validate for this woman and her husband that her problems were hormonal and not due to the relationship.

Now, I ask you, is it reasonable to ignore these concerns and to dismiss a patient's request for a perfectly appropriate blood test? Particularly when, in this case, the patient has concerns so easily alleviated with readily available hormone treatments. This woman should have at least been given the information that we do have helpful tests, and potential therapeutic options, to enhance her sex life for this new phase of her life. After being started on a low dose of supplemental testosterone and estradiol, she came in a month later and described *"I feel like a new woman. I have my old spark back, and now I want—and enjoy—sex again."* She also told me that her quality of orgasms had improved, it was easier to have an orgasm, and she now had no difficulty with arousal and lubrication. Her estradiol level at the three month follow-up visit was 98 pg/ml, and her testosterone level was now 25 ng/dl, which were good levels for her.

Women's Bodies DO Make Testosterone

Testosterone is one of a group of hormones called "ANDROGENS" which are made from cholesterol by the female ovary and adrenal glands. Androgens are also made from precursor "building blocks" in body fat tissue, muscle and other sites. The word androgen is derived from the Greek andros meaning "male-like" and refers to any steroid molecule with 19 carbon atoms that is able to bind to the androgen hormone receptor sites in the brain and body. The amount of circulating active androgens in women is obviously much lower than in men, but these compounds are important for many normal functions of the female body.

ANDROGENS

- *dihydrotestosterone* (DHT)
- *testosterone*
- d*ehydroepiandrosterone* (DHEA)
- *dehydroepiandrosterone-sulfate* (DHEA-S)
- *androstenedione*

Over the course of a woman's life, the ovary makes on average about one-third of a woman's circulating androgens, in addition to producing the female hormones estrogen and progesterone. If the ovaries are surgically removed in a *premenopausal* woman, concentrations of testosterone fall markedly within 24 to 48 hours after surgery. There are potentially significant effects from the loss of testosterone: *loss of sex drive, fatigue, declining muscle mass, decreased bone density, and changes in feelings of well-being to name a few.*

I am convinced that many of the problems women attribute to having a hysterectomy are actually due to *not having adequate testosterone and estradiol replacement* after the surgery. How do doctors really know what a woman needs after surgery if no one ever checks hormone levels or relates these changes I have described to the loss of crucial hormones?

When the ovary decreases its hormone production after menopause, women lose about 50 percent of their androgen source. I wonder how many men would like to go around for the last thirty or forty years of life with only *half* their normal testosterone! One reason there is less of the active form of testosterone after menopause is that an important precursor molecule, *androstenedione*, decreases more than 50 percent when the ovary ceases its hormone production. Many doctors do not realize that when women have a decline in *estrogen* production, it also results in a decrease in *testosterone* production as well, due to the loss of precursors usually made by the ovary.

There are noticeable effects of the changing hormone balance during the climacteric or mid-life years: lower estrogen *relative* to the amount of testosterone present allows for the testosterone effects to be "unmasked," producing changes in facial hair, voice, sex drive, energy level, and distribution of body fat. With more androgen influence and less estrogen, women experience their bodies shifting from the "pear" or gynecoid (female) fat pattern to the "apple" or male fat pattern of body fat around the waist and "trunk" or upper abdomen/chest. I have a diagram of these body shape changes in Chapter 3. It may not be just that you "don't have the willpower to lose weight;" it may be that your hormone ratios are now working against you.

Contrary to the popular myths about hormones perpetuated in magazine articles, it *isn't* the *estrogen* that is typically the culprit in weight gain at mid-life. It's the changing *ratios* of the ovarian estrogen and testosterone, combined with less physical activity, lower metabolic rate and usually more food intake than is needed as we age. Without the proper balance of estrogen, androgens from the adrenal gland and fat tissue begin to produce unwanted body changes for women: *increasing blood pressure*, *increasing total cholesterol*, and *decreasing HDL* ("good") cholesterol, along with *increasing LDL* ("bad") cholesterol. All of these changes contribute to the increasing risks of heart disease, hypertension, and diabetes in women in their forties and beyond. You will read more about this in Chapter 13. The characteristic *premenopausal* balance of estrogens and androgens is needed in order to reduce these undesirable body changes in later years.

Throughout a woman's life, testosterone has important functions in maintaining muscle tissues in women (that wonderful "fat-burning" machinery of the body!) and helping to *build bone*. Maintaining bone density is one of the crucial roles of testosterone for women, particularly as women grow older and lose the effects of estrogen in maintaining bone density. Furthermore, testosterone plays a key role in keeping a woman's energy level optimal. Decline or loss of this critical hormone is one of the frequently unrecognized factors in the mid-life problem of "chronic fatigue." Many women have multiple medical evaluations, tests, and therapies to diagnose and treat "chronic fatigue" (or CFS, CFIDS) and *never have a blood level test for testosterone!*

Mrs. C., a delightful woman in her early sixties who loved to ski every winter, had noticed a significant decrease in her stamina and energy on the slopes over the past two or three seasons. During her consultation to discuss her questions about hormone therapy, she mentioned that she had experienced a noticeable decline in her strength and endurance for skiing. She had never had anyone check her hormone levels, although she had asked about having this done. Along with a suboptimal estradiol level on her Premarin dose of 0.625 mg, she also had a testosterone level of less than 10 according to the lab report. She has been on 2.5 mg of natural micronized testosterone for the past two years.

Within the first six months, she described a marked increase in her energy level, and what she described as "my old spark coming back." The next year at her follow-up visit she gleefully told me that when she returned to the ski slopes the season after starting testosterone, her ski instructor commented on the noticeable improvements in her strength and stamina. He asked her what her new training regimen had been over the summer! She smiled and said "I never told him what *really* made the difference!" There had not been any adverse side effects on this dose and her cholesterol profile had maintained a healthy balance. She also commented "I just *felt better*. It's hard to describe, but I just have such a good change in my overall feeling of well-being and energy again. I didn't realize I had lost some of that until I got it back!"

Our psychological sense of well-being is also enhanced by testosterone. In some women, what appeared to be a depression turned out to be a deficiency of testosterone. Yes, this hormone does lift moods when the amounts are present at normal levels for women. As testosterone levels rise higher than needed for optimal balance, (whether from overproduction in the body or from supplemental hormones) women report increased facial hair usually above the lip, increased dreaming and/or nightmares, difficulty falling asleep, and perhaps more sex drive than usual. At high levels, and in doses used in steroid abuse for muscle-building, *both* men and women develop toxic behavioral effects such as: extreme irritability, volatile/explosive moods, aggressiveness and assaultiveness. So again, *balance* is the key.

Synthetic versus Natural Micronized Testosterone

Most of the women I see have already heard comments like those I made at the beginning of this chapter: testosterone causes a mustache, a beard, deep voice, liver damage, "oversexed women." A key factor most women don't know, because it isn't addressed in books and magazine articles, and doctors have not been taught this: *all of the above problems are related to the DOSE and TYPE used, not just testosterone itself*. In the U.S.A. until very recently, we have only had **synthetic** methyltestosterone or androgens available, which are far more potent than the natural hormones made by the ovary and adrenal gland. And until recently, doctors did not realize that women needed *much* less supplemental hormone than doses used for men. In the United States, we have not even had commercial tablets *available* in doses low enough for women. As an example, 10 to 15 mg has been a typical dose of methyltestosterone prescribed for women.

On average, I am using doses of 1.25 mg to about 3 mg a day of the natural micronized testosterone. Quite a difference! At these lower doses, which are obviously much more appropriate for women, my patients tell me they feel more energy, have a return of their normal sex drive, and do not have the unwanted side effects described above. In addition, I monitor cholesterol blood levels and have not had any patients who have had a negative effect on their cholesterol levels using these lower doses of testosterone.

Remember from my discussion in Chapter 5, *"synthetic"* simply means "produced by putting together," not *"artificial,"* as it has come to be used. Remember the example of human insulin from the previous chapter? Another illustration is human growth hormone, which scientists have been able to synthesize in the laboratory, so that we can now give the human form to children deficient in this hormone. These are examples of *synthetic* (i.e., made in the laboratory) medications being used because they are the *natural* ones found in human bodies. Molecules which are the same as those made by the body, even if synthesized in a laboratory, are better tolerated, more effective, and have fewer side effects.

The same is true with testosterone. In the past, we did not have a way to give natural testosterone orally because it would be broken down and lost in the digestive process before getting into the bloodstream. So, scientists developed similar but slightly different molecules: one type is methyltestosterone, and it is the addition of the methyl group which appears to have the increased potential for liver toxicity. Methyltestosterone survives the digestion, is absorbed into the bloodstream, and produces a testosterone-like effect on the body organs. This has worked well for the majority of *male* patients who needed testosterone but not as well for women, because the commercial doses available, designed for men, were simply too high for women.

Today, there are pharmacists who have begun making a form of natural testosterone in a *micronized* form producing particles small enough to survive digestion and be absorbed into the blood-stream. Micronization is also used to make native human preparations of progesterone and estradiol, since all of these hormones are inactivated or destroyed by digestion when taken orally.

The source for these natural forms of human hormones is actually from plants: soybeans and yams. The chemical precursors are extracted, purified, synthesized into molecules *identical to those made in the human body*, and then compounded into standardized tablets so that you know the amount of hormone you are getting. This approach, I feel, allows better "fine-tuning" of hormone therapy than trying to get enough active hormone from plant/herbal sources, since you really are not able to determine how much you are taking, and whether the amount is right for you.

Testosterone can also be made by pharmacists in a wide variety of other forms: skin cream, skin gel, sublingual tablets (to dissolve under the tongue), and vaginal suppositories. I have listed in Appendix 2 several experienced, reputable pharmacists who will work with you and your physician to determine the proper amount of natural testosterone for you, provide educational resources and telephone question/answer services to assist patients and physicians in determining the most appropriate options.

Finding What's Right for You: Options Available

To help you make the important decisions about what is best for you and your health needs, I have summarized in the following table *benefits of adding testosterone* to a hormone therapy regimen, and also compared the effects of too little and too much testosterone. Most women need only *very small amounts* of testosterone to achieve these benefits. I generally start my patients on 1.25 mg of oral micronized tablets, and then gradually increase the dose based on the woman's description of how she is feeling, until we reach a dose of 3 to 4 mg a day. At that time, I recommend checking the testosterone blood level before going higher on the dosage. Sometimes oral doses may still not be absorbed well enough to give desirable blood levels and I will suggest changing to a sublingual capsule or a skin cream to improve absorption.

SUMMARY OF TESTOSTERONE EFFECTS

Too Little	*Just Right*	*Too Much*
• low energy	• normal energy	• hyper feelings
• loss of sex drive	• normal libido	• increased libido
• slowed down	• alert, interested	• "scattered" thoughts
• mildly depressed mood	• positive mood	• irritable, anxious
• fewer dreams	• normal dreams	• intense dreaming
───	───	• aggressive dreams
		• violent dreams
• thin, fine hair	• hair thicker	• facial hair
• dry, thin skin	• normal skin	• acne

Options for Testosterone Supplementation

In addition to the natural micronized testosterone that can be compounded for you by pharmacists who provide this individualized service, there are a number of commercial methyltestosterone products, available in the U.S. These are summarized in the tables below.

A *word of* **caution** *about the* **injectable** *testosterone preparations*: it is more difficult to achieve the right dose for women with these, and as a result, they are more frequently associated with the unwanted side effects I have described. These preparations also wear off unpredictably, and make it harder to keep you feeling on an even keel without having the risk of getting too much testosterone. I have *never* used these preparations for women, and I do not recommend them for most men either. *In my opinion, there are much better and safer options now available.*

COMMERCIAL TESTOSTERONE PREPARATIONS

TESTOSTERONE ALONE: **Doses Available**

Oreton, Metandren (methyltestosterone):   5mg, 10mg, 25 mg
                                            (oral tablets)

Halotestin, Ora-Testryl (fluoxymesterone):   5 mg, 10 mg
                                              (oral tablets)

Testopel (Testosterone pellets)   75 mg (inserted under skin)

Delatest, Testone LA, Depo-Testadiol
(testosterone enanthate)   100 mg/ml (injectable)

Depo-Test (testosterone cypionate)   50 mg/ml (injectable)

TESTOSTERONE-ESTROGEN COMBINATIONS:

Estratest: esterified estrogens . . . . 1.25 mg (oral tablets)
           and methyltestosterone . . . . 2.5 mg

Estratest HS: esterified estrogens . . . . . . 0.625 mg (oral tablets)
              and methyltestosterone 1.25mg

Premarin: conjugated equine estrogens (CEE)—oral tablets: two strengths
          with methyltestosterone (T) . . . 0.625mg (CEE) with 5 mg T
          . . . . 1.25 mg (CEE) with 10 mg T

Depo-Testadiol: estradiol cypionate . . . . . 2 mg (injectable)
                with testosterone cypionate . . . . . 50 mg

In my opinion, Premarin with testosterone has **way too much testosterone** for most women and I think that's how testosterone has gotten such a bad reputation for causing problems. As you see from the table, one tablet strength has 5 mg methyltestosterone, and the other has 10 mg methyltestosterone. I have *never* used 10 mg *of methyl*testosterone, and *very rarely* even 5 mg, when I have prescribed androgen therapy for women. I rarely use the *fixed-dose* combination estrogen-testosterone preparations because, in my opinion, these fixed-dose products do not allow for *individualized* adjustments of hormone therapies. I have found that with the fixed-dose combinations there is not enough estrogen, and often not the *right type* of estrogen, and there is *too much* testosterone so that the balance just isn't right for most women.

A way I have found effective to use these combination products if a woman wants to have the convenience of getting a commercial tablet from her local pharmacy, or who just likes the idea of taking occasional testosterone, I will first stabilize the woman on a native human estrogen like 17-beta-estradiol (tablets or patches), and then suggest use of the combination estrogen-testosterone tablet (for example Estratest) 2 to 3 times a week. This approach seems to work well for some women. Other women can use these combination products daily and find that they provide the desired benefits without unwanted side effects. *The key is finding what is best for you, and I would expect your "recipe" will likely be slightly different from what works for your friends.*

If you decide to take hormones, remember that each woman's body is different. Trust *your* body wisdom, and what *you know* about how you feel. You may also check the summary chart on indications of too much versus too little testosterone, ask your doctor to check a blood level and to work with you to adjust your dose to one that feels good for you. You and your physician need to be *partners* in the process of *maximizing* your benefits from hormone therapy and *minimizing* any undesirable side effects. There are good options available now to help you achieve your goals for enhanced well-being.

The Role of Blood Level Testing

Objective laboratory testing allows hormone doses to be specifically tailored to meet the your needs as an individual. What should you be looking for as a desirable target range for testosterone? In my clinical experience, women typically experience their optimal normal energy level and libido when serum (blood) levels of *total* testosterone are between 30 and 60 ng/dl. Levels below 20 ng/dl are generally too low to maintain your usual libido, and energy. The majority of menopausal women I have evaluated, particularly those who have had surgical removal of the ovaries in their thirties and forties, have had testosterone levels of less than 10! This is certainly an understandable factor in fatigue and decreased sexual desire. A more accurate, but also more expensive, way to evaluate testosterone is to check the blood level of *free* testosterone as well as the *total*. Free testosterone is the biologically active, unbound, portion circulating in the blood and it gives a more reliable indication of the active hormone present. I do not order this for everyone; I use this test when I have a patient who isn't responding the way I would expect with the usual amount of added testosterone.

In my opinion, hormone tests are helpful, efficient, cost-effective, and provide psychological benefit by identifying a physical cause of the disturbing symptoms women may experience at midlife and around menopause. *I feel strongly that such tests should be available to women, especially those who have had their ovaries removed.* There are too many "hidden" medical, psychological, and relationship costs if you don't know your physiological measures. You may find that it is too expensive **not** to have this information as you plan how to best achieve your health goals.

Sexual Vitality As You Age

A healthy, vital, invigorated sexual response and enjoyment is an important dimension of your optimal well-being throughout your adult years, whether it results from being with a partner or pleasuring yourself if you are alone. There are many books totally devoted to this subject, so I will only be able to hit the highlights in my discussion of sexual vitality here.

What about your lifestyle habits? Cigarette smoking (and use of chewing tobacco) is a big culprit robbing you of sexual vitality. Nicotine in all forms of tobacco products constricts blood vessels and decreases blood flow to the pelvic organs in men and women, which causes impaired sexual arousal and performance. Vasoconstriction from nicotine particularly affects men adversely by decreasing blood flow to the penis, which markedly diminishes fullness and firmness of erections, especially as men get older and there has been more vascular damage from use of nicotine. Talking with men about this effect of tobacco has been one of my effective motivators to get men to stop smoking! Most of my male patients had *never* had a physician tell them that cigarette smoking adversely affects quality of erections as men grow older.

Another thief of sexual vigor is alcohol: in excess, it robs you of your sexual desire and your ability to respond normally. Alcohol is a *depressant drug* and dampens down the brain centers for arousal and orgasm. A small amount of alcohol may *initially* release your inhibitions and make you feel relaxed and "in the mood for sex." After that, alcohol begins to make it harder to reach full arousal and orgasm. Men who have had too much alcohol often have difficulty achieving an erection that is full and rigid enough to allow satisfying intercourse.

A frequently overlooked thief of sexual interest and responsiveness is too much stress in a hectic lifestyle. You may be simply too exhausted to relax and become aroused. Remember, the "flight or fight" adrenalin response evolved to help us *escape danger*, not relax and become aroused for sex! If your adrenalin system is working overtime to keep up with the demands in your life, your sexual drive will be nil. Take time out to "get away," slow down, relax, and enjoy the physical pleasures of relaxed foreplay and sexual exploration. Notice I said **take** time, not **find** time. You have to establish your priorities and *take* the time for what is important to you—it doesn't just happen, given the busy lives we all lead today. And another thing: *get up and move your body*! Exercise has a lot of well-publicized health benefits, including revving up your sexual energy, and clearing away the loggy feeling from stress overload.

It is also important to have a thorough medical checkup if you have noticed a significant change in your sexual desire; painful intercourse; vaginal dryness, burning or itching; diminished ability to have an orgasm (or for men, diminished ability to achieve an erection). This checkup should include a physical examination, laboratory tests of general blood chemistries, sexually transmitted diseases, and hormone blood tests (especially thyroid, estradiol, and testosterone). If your hormone levels are too low, talk with your physician about an appropriate hormone regimen to help you regain your sexual vitality. More information on hormone therapy regimens is found in Chapters 5 (on estrogen) and 15 (about hormone therapy). Healthy lifestyle changes I described above are your primary foundation, so be sure to address these. Hormones do help many women immensely, as my patients tell me after they experience the balance right for them: "It's like someone turned the light switch back on! I *just feel better*."

Relationships often change at mid-life, and many women find themselves back in the dating arena after many years in a stable relationship. I feel it is important to address the issue of sexually transmitted diseases (STDs), all of which are far more common today than when many of us baby-boomers were becoming sexually active. Bacterial vaginitis, trichomonas, chlamydia, herpes, human papilloma virus ("venereal warts"), gonorrhea, syphilis, and now AIDS. The list is daunting. While AIDS is the most feared STD, the others are many times more common and may result in a variety of symptoms which rob you of sexual pleasure and vitality. And yet, women are still frequently too shy about asking male sexual partners to wear a condom for fear of hurting their feelings.

Women, wake up and protect yourself! I will bluntly tell you that if a man is worth having sex with, then he should be concerned enough about *your* health to wear a condom. This is particularly true in new relationships, or even in long-standing relationships if there is any indication that your partner has had sexual encounters outside of your relationship. With *proper* use of a latex condom, you markedly decrease your risk of getting STDs, unless you have unprotected oral sex with a partner who has an active infection. For best protection against STDs, use of a high quality *latex* condom should be combined with use of a spermicidal foam or jelly. In recent studies, the most widely used spermicide, *nonoxynol-9*, has been shown to kill all of the bacteria and viruses listed above. If you are concerned about whether your partner will have a condom available, you can always carry your own supply and be in control of having one when you need it.

The incidence of AIDS *in women* in this country has been largely underestimated until recently due to the fact that women in the early stages of the disease suffer different manifestations, such as chronic vaginal infections. This wasn't even initially included as one of the criteria symptoms of AIDS. Another factor is that virtually all the research on AIDS has been done on homosexual *men*, the population in which it first developed. Women with AIDS also frequently die of different causes and infectious illnesses than do men. Men with AIDS have been **twice** as likely to get AZT as women, a drug which clearly prolongs survival. Not surprisingly, the survival rate of women with AIDS is significantly lower than that of men, according to a study conducted by the Maryland Department of Health in Baltimore. If the current trends continue, AIDS will be the fifth leading cause of death next year for women between the ages of 15 and 44. Not using a condom may be potentially life-threatening. Be aware, and be prepared.

Resources for Rekindling the Sexual Fires!

Often, patients tell me that their doctors have never asked about their sexual activity or changes in sexual function. Many physicians are still embarrassed to initiate this discussion with patients, particularly women in mid-life and beyond. Then I hear physicians say that they assume their patients will tell them if they are having sexual problems, but most women tell me *they* are too embarrassed to bring this issue up when they see their doctor. So it ends up being a stand off, and the discussion doesn't happen. I urge you to be proactive and bring up your sexual questions and concerns when you see your physician. Take responsibility for your health and ask. Before you visit your doctor, you may find it helpful to explore your feelings about your sexuality in the self-check questionnaire in Chapter 18: "How's My Sexuality?" Jot down whatever comes to mind about each of these questions. This will give you a list of topics when you go in for your medical visit and may help you focus your questions in the time you have with your doctor. If your physician doesn't seem interested or knowledgeable in these areas, then seek other resources for help. Don't just suffer silently!

One of the most common problems I encounter in my medical practice is primarily a lack of knowledge about the human sexual response in men and women; concerns over what is "normal" and culturally derived unrealistic performance expectations. Consequently, I have included a list of resources in appendix II which will give you additional ideas for enhanced sexual vitality and rekindling the sexual fires! My patients, men and women of all ages, tell me that the ones listed have been helpful, well written, and beautifully descriptive of the wide variety of sensual pleasures. Dr. Miriam Stoppard's book, *The Magic of Sex*, is the best I have seen as a comprehensive, beautifully illustrated and sensitively written guide for sexual enjoyment for men and women.

Another resource you may find helpful is the *Sensate Focus Experience*. This series of sexual pleasuring exercises is designed to help you and your partner explore each other's bodies and communicate your feelings to each other so as to help each of you learn what is most pleasing, arousing and desirable for the other. You may also do this alone if you do not have or want a partner. This series of exercises is described in more detail in many of the books I have included on the resource list. Briefly, the Sensate Focus Experience establishes a structure to help both of you relax and not feel pressured to perform sexually. You and your partner commit to a specified amount of time, for example 30 minutes or an hour. Select a time and place when you won't be interrupted, and are able to "tune out" stressful stimuli. You may want to help create the desired mood with music, candles, pleasant fragrances, sensuous fabrics. One person begins as the *receiver* of the sensate pleasuring, and the other person is the *giver*. In the next time together, you alternate roles. During the entire time of the session, the *giver* caresses, touches and explores the *receiver's* body. The *receiver* gives positive feedback about what feels pleasurable, what is less desirable and what is uncomfortable. What does one *do* during these pleasuring times? Be creative! You may also have to redo the "mental tapes" from childhood prohibiting touching various body areas. Nothing is "off limits" for you as an adult unless it causes discomfort or pain for the partner. You may find ideas in some of the resource books in Appendix 2.

I encourage couples to proceed, *at your own pace*, through the following levels of Sensate Focus Experience:

- Level I: non erotic, non-genital pleasuring
- Level II: erotic, non-genital pleasuring
- Level III: erotic and genital pleasuring
- Level IV: pleasuring which proceeds to intercourse.

Prior to reaching Level IV, couples agree to abide by the guidelines of no intercourse, no matter how sexually aroused you become. Keeping this agreement helps build trust and reduce performance anxiety. If you commit to this process, and communicate with each other positively and sensitively, you will likely find the "fires" rekindled in your sexual encounters.

Depression, PMS, or Perimenopause? Hidden Hormonal Links

Listen to the voices of these women who have called our center for a medical consultation. Each of these women had seen other physicians, (both male and female physicians, I might add). Each woman described on our initial health form that she had felt dismissed, like her problems were trivial, and had felt that the physicians "just weren't listening to me, he/she just seemed to want to get me out the door, I felt like I was on an assembly line, I felt like I was just being patted on the head like a little girl and my problems weren't important." I know there are good, competent caring physicians out there—both men and women—but I am greatly concerned with the overwhelming frequency with which I hear comments like those above. The trend seems to be getting worse, not better, as more and more patients are thrust into HMO settings where many physicians are on quotas as to how many patients they have to see in an hour. Do any of these descriptions sound familiar?

> "I hit thirty-nine and all of a sudden I'm a witch before my period. I never used to have PMS, and this is terrible. My mood! What's happening to me?"

> "I used to sleep so soundly a train coming through the bedroom wouldn't wake me up. Now, I wake up five or six times a night, wide awake, my heart racing, and I get up in the morning feeling like I never went to bed. I'm just forty-two, and I asked my doctor if I was starting into menopause, but she said I'm too young."

"Could I have PMS? I go through these awful moods—bitchy, cranky, irritable, yelling at my kids—the week before my periods, and then it seems to go as quickly as it came on after my period starts. And my hip joints, knees and shoulders seem stiff and achy so much. Am I beginning to get arthritis?"

—Forty-one-year-old mother of two

"I never had headaches, and last year I started getting fierce, stabbing, pounding headaches the day before my period. I feel like my head is coming apart, and I've missed work more, I just can't function when a headache hits. I've seen three doctors. They tell me there's nothing wrong to worry about, but nothing has helped stop these headaches. What can I do to get some relief?"

—Forty-seven-year-old woman

"My bladder is acting up, I have more problems with infections, and I want to see if you have any ideas to help me. I've been having these strange times each month before my period when I feel like somebody pulled a curtain over my brain, I feel foggy, my memory is shot, I can't sleep and wake up a dozen times a night soaking wet, I don't have any energy and I feel really blue and bad about myself. Is this stress or am I getting depressed? My doctor told me it's just PMS and not to worry about it, but I never had this before. Is there anything that will help?"

—Thirty-eight-year-old woman

"My sex drive is gone. Zip. Zero. Just nothing there. I love my husband, we have a great relationship, I enjoyed our sex life. I have less stress in my life than I have had for years, so things should be good. I don't understand it. My periods are getting lighter and some months I don't have one. My hair is falling out in clumps and I always had such great hair. I'm not sleeping very well anymore, and my energy seems shot. I feel like I've been run over by a truck a lot of the time. I try to keep going, but inside I'm worried about what is going on. My doctor said I couldn't be starting menopause because I am too young, and she said my thyroid was normal."

—Thirty-seven-year-old woman

PMS. Perimenopause. Panic. Premenopause. Stress. Uncertainty.

What does all this mean? One thing is clear. There are a *lot* of unanswered questions out there. There are a lot of women who are confused by the terms, unsure of when to be aware of changes that might mean menopause is beginning. There are also a lot of women who are experiencing premenstrual problems, who are seeking help and having difficulty finding it. I hope you will find some answers as you read this chapter. I also hope that if you are having problems like this, you will learn options for feeling better!

Is It PMS or Perimenopause?

Premenstrual syndrome (PMS) was first described in *modern* medical writings in 1931 by Dr. Robert T. Frank, an American gynecologist, (unfortunately his work appeared in the *Archives of Neurology and Psychiatry*, a journal not widely read by gynecologists). Incredibly, it was also described in the writings of Hippocrates in ancient Greece. It is 1995, and medical science *still* says we aren't sure what causes it or what helps it, or even *if* the mood changes are caused (or contributed to) by hormonal changes! Of course, as I have listened to women's descriptions over the years, I have to say it seems pretty obvious that there *has* to be *some kind* of hormonal connection in something that happens cyclically before menses on a consistent basis and resolves after the period is over. Just because we physicians and scientists may not have *found* the connection doesn't mean it isn't there. I do find it curious, however, that medical science has considered the hormonal-mood connection "controversial." Most studies I have reviewed do not even measure hormone levels—the reason given is usually something inane like hormone levels aren't reliable (they *can't* be if you don't check them!), or hormone levels vary. Of course. That's the point. They *do* vary, throughout the menstrual cycle! I think the question is: HOW do they vary, and in what relationship to the pattern of mood changes and physical symptoms?

Well, now you've heard me on my soapbox again. *"All these women can't be wrong!"* I said to myself. I knew that what I was seeing, and hearing my patients describe, was clearly different from the biological disorder of major depression. So I began to try and figure it out based on what I was hearing, and what I knew *could* be measured. I systematically checked hormone levels at specific times in the menstrual cycle, and used daily mood rating scales, depression inventories, and other measures. The patterns of hormonal change I have identified as being connected to the premenstrual mood and physical changes are:

1. declining estradiol levels in the luteal phase (relative to levels seen in women without PMS),
2. changing ratios of estradiol and progesterone in the luteal phase,
3. lower than expected levels of testosterone, and,
4. in women in their mid-thirties to mid-forties, lower than expected estradiol levels in the first one to three days of menses, but with FSH levels still in the premenopausal ranges.

Women in this last category are still menstruating (unless they have had an hysterectomy) and most are still ovulating, but their estrogen is declining and appears to have a marked and consistent connection with the symptom clusters such as those described at the beginning of this chapter.

Now, do we call it PMS, premenopause, or perimenopause? One of the reasons this becomes confusing is that these terms are used in many different ways in the media and in scientific articles. Generally, but not always, **premenopause** refers to a woman *still menstruating* regularly; **perimenopause** refers to a woman who has begun to have *erratic, inconsistent periods* with changing flow-patterns (may be heavy one month, lighter and shorter the next), and she is also beginning to skip periods; **PMS** refers to the *symptom cluster* of physical and emotional changes occurring *between* *ovulation and menses*, which then clears for a symptom-free interval each month. **Menopause** technically means *cessation of menses*, although as I pointed out earlier, it is difficult to know when the last period is until a woman has gone an extended time without any menstrual periods, usually at least a year. **Postmenopause** refers to the years after the complete cessation of menses. Now that I have defined the terms, it may not really tell you all that much, because they are often used interchangeably. Rarely is there a discussion of age ranges, and even if there is, the *chronological* age doesn't necessarily correlate well with the *endocrinological* age (although you will often see it written about as if the chronological age was the *primary* indicator of what to expect with menopause changes).

The climacteric, pre- or perimenopausal years are a normal phase of a woman's reproductive life cycle. Many women make this transition to menopause without difficulty; however, approximately sixty to eighty of women DO experience mild to moderate symptoms, such as insomnia, worsening premenstrual tension, irritability, mood swings (lability), and tearfulness.

Approximately 60 to 80 percent of women DO experience mild to moderate PMS symptoms during their thirties and forties. How serious are such symptoms? They are usually not serious enough to cause significant disruption in home, work and social relationships and activities. Another 15 to 20 percent of women, however, experience *marked* luteal phase (PMS) symptoms, which are severe enough to disrupt optimal function at home and work, and are a significant source of distress for the individual woman. Several recent studies have shown that these brain-mediated symptoms are actually more numerous during the premenopause (ages forty to forty-nine years) than after menopause.

When articles say "there's no evidence that women become more depressed at menopause," they are missing the important *time frame* in which to look for these mood changes, as well as to look for major depression. Based on the *existing* studies that have asked this question, and included women in their late thirties and early forties, such distressing symptoms are extremely common and do appear to correlate both with *declining* hormone levels and with *widely fluctuating* hormone levels. Many women know or suspect this connection, but have had their observations devalued and discounted.

Early effects of estradiol decline usually manifest as restless sleep, premenstrual migraines, chronic fatigue, declining libido, the premenstrual mood changes I listed above, and irregular menstrual cycles with changing flow (lighter *or* heavier). While women in mid-life may also be experiencing many *life* changes—balancing home, career, children, aging parents, community roles—I find that their changing *physiological hormone balance* often increases their susceptibility to situational stressors and contributes to an increasing degree of bothersome symptoms, as well as to increasing health risks for future problems like bone loss. This can become a "vicious cycle" in that physiological and psychological stressors further suppresses ovarian function, which then exacerbates bone loss, particularly if the woman is a smoker or lacks adequate dietary calcium and weight-bearing exercise.

These are not just the "worried well" women, as they have been labeled when health professionals (and sometimes other women) perceived these kinds of symptoms as "minor." I have not encountered many women who take time off from work or away from their families and busy lives to come for a medical appointment just because they are "worried but well." I think this is another paternalistic attitude about women, whether it's a male or a female physician who voices such a view. In my experience, the women who come in are having health changes that are a significant source of distress, or they wouldn't be making the effort and spending the money (and time, which may be even more valuable to many women these days) to come and see a physician. I think we in medicine sometimes forget that point and think women have nothing better to do than come see the doctor. I do think there is something important going on; I just don't think our present healthcare settings have *really listened* to what our mid-life women have been trying to tell us. This next woman's story will give you some insights as to why I think these issues should be taken seriously.

Sue was a thirty-six-year-old married woman, with no prior history of depression, who came in for an evaluation of "worsening PMS" over the past several years. She was very concerned that her mood changes and angry outbursts were getting out of hand, both at home and at work. She was worried that because she had gotten angry at her boss several times, and had "popped off" at a co-worker, she might be in danger of losing her job. She was also beginning to realize that during her PMS time, she was craving alcohol in a way that she had never experienced before, and was consuming more alcohol during that week than she felt was healthy. She had not had any pattern of daily alcohol abuse and had not experienced any alcohol withdrawal episodes, but she was worried about her increasing tendency to drink too much in the week before her period. She also described herself as "a raving maniac for chocolate" during the premenstrual week, and had even gone to the store at 2:00 A.M. to buy chocolate candy. She knew that wasn't particularly safe, given where she lived, but she said "it was such an overwhelming urge, I thought I would fly out of my skin if I couldn't get some chocolate right then!"

In getting a complete and more detailed picture of her symptoms, both at the initial visit and then with the daily symptom logs she kept for the next two cycles, it was clear that she had a well-documented, progressively intensifying pattern of premenstrual (luteal phase) mood changes (lability), tearfulness, anxiety, irritability, anger outbursts, depressed mood, decreased energy, restless sleep, nightmares, cravings for sweets and alcohol, breast tenderness, bloating (with a 3- to 5-pound weight gain), and constipation. She described feeling "almost suicidally depressed" just prior to her menses, although she had never made any suicide attempt and had not been treated for a primary depressive disorder. She said "the weird thing is, once my period starts, the feeling of wanting to die seems to vanish almost as fast as it came on, and it's gone completely until next time before my period, and then it all starts again." She also described difficulty functioning at work the week before menses, due to her mood changes, diminished energy, and a decreased ability to concentrate, along with changes in her short-term memory and word recall.

She did not have a sustained pattern of depressive symptoms present throughout her menstrual cycle, and described feeling "my mood lifting, and I felt normal again" soon after menses began. In her words, "I hate this merry-go-round of being this way . . . two weeks of the month I'm fine, and ten days of the month I'm a lunatic. Isn't there anything I can do to get this under control and feel better?"

Her past medical history was unremarkable for major medical illnesses. She had a pregnancy at age fifteen, but later was unable to conceive. She was found to have marked endometriosis and underwent laser surgery treatment at age twenty-eight, which appeared to solve the menstrual pain and cramps she had previously experienced. Menses continued to be regular. She took no medications except Tylenol occasionally for premenstrual headache or back pain. She started to smoke cigarettes at about age eighteen and was soon smoking two packs of cigarettes a day. She did not have a history of illegal drug use.

Both parents were alcoholic, and her three sisters had all suffered from PMS. Two sisters had undergone hysterectomies, and it was no longer clear whether they had a cyclic pattern to their symptoms. Neither her sisters nor her brother had ever required treatment for major depressive disorder. Her biological father's medical history was not known, other than that he had been an alcoholic. Her mother was diabetic, not yet on insulin, and had been alcoholic but off alcohol for two years. Her mother had no history of depression. There was a strong history of diabetes in both parents' families.

Her physical examination was normal, including pelvic and pap. She was slender and had a normal blood pressure. Her blood studies showed a normal chemistry profile, normal blood cell count and normal urinalysis. Her thyroid profile, including TSH was also normal. Day 1 estradiol was low at 20 pg/ml; her Day 20 estradiol was also quite low at 57 pg/ml (it should have been in the range of 150–250 pg/ml), but FSH and LH were still at pre-menopausal levels. Progesterone on Day 20 was 10 ng/ml, which indicated an ovulatory level of progesterone even though her estradiol was so low. Testosterone was less than 20 ng/dl, also too low.

Since she had such pronounced sweet cravings premenstrually and a strong family history of diabetes, I thought she may be having progesterone-induced changes in blood glucose regulation in the second half of her menstrual cycle. I suggested a luteal phase 5 hour Glucose Tolerance Test, which was done in my office where I could observe any major symptoms and where my staff could help track symptoms in between blood drawings. She developed drowsiness, palpitations, and fell asleep in the first hour and a half of the test; between the third and forth hours, she became cool, clammy, sweaty, nauseous, had trouble reading, burst out crying, described feeling anxious, and experienced the intense urge for alcohol "to calm me down."

About twenty minutes later, these symptoms had passed, and she described feeling extremely tired, "wrung out," and had difficulty concentrating on her magazine. When we reviewed the test results two weeks later, she showed a rapid rise in her blood glucose to 180 mg/dL at the first hour (which had contributed to her drowsiness) and at hour four her blood glucose had dropped sharply to 45 mg/dL (normal is greater than 65 mg/dL). With the adrenalin surge triggered by the dropping glucose (which had caused the symptoms she experienced between hours three and four), her blood sugar had risen to 60 mg/dL by hour five. This was still lower than her initial fasting glucose, which had been normal at 84 mg/dL. I explained that she had a reactive hypo-glycemia pattern, which is common in women who have diabetes in their families and is aggravated by the effects of progesterone on insulin secretion in the second half of the menstrual cycle. I thought this was a major factor in her premenstrual craving for alcohol and sweets.

With her long history of smoking and her current low estrogen levels, I recommended she have a bone density test done even though she was still menstruating and was only 36. My goal in recommending the test was to have a baseline evaluation, but it turned out that she was *already quite low for her age* on bone density at the hip. This meant she was at a much higher risk for early osteoporosis.

With all this information, what recommendations did I make for this woman? First, **dietary and lifestyle habit changes were crucial.** She needed to decrease caffeine to help keep her from losing more calcium and making her bone loss worse. I also urged her to stop smoking because of tobacco's many adverse health effects; but the most crucial reason for stopping smoking was the further suppression of her ovaries by smoking, which in turn caused more loss of estrogen and more bone loss. She was clearly much too young to have this much bone loss. She needed to completely eliminate alcohol during her premenstrual week, because this made her blood glucose changes even worse and contributed more to the depressed mood and angry outbursts, as well as additional loss of calcium needed for her bone health.

She had not realized how damaging the alcohol was and had thought it helped keep her from having the mood changes and anxiety symptoms. She was willing to eliminate it once she had experienced the effects of the blood glucose changes so dramatically. The nutritionist in my office went over a meal plan to control the reactive hypoglycemia, which consisted of approximately 60 percent complex carbohydrates, 20 percent fat, and 20 percent protein with three smaller meals and three healthy snacks daily during the premenstrual week in particular. She was advised to avoid salty foods that aggravated her fluid retention.

Second, I thought that **hormonal approaches** were important. This is an example of a situation where having information about the hormone levels made a difference in the treatment recommendations. Without such *definite* evidence of low estrogen, I would not have been as likely to suggest she consider adding hormones. If medication had been needed, I would probably have used one of the serotonin-augmenting medications for the second half of her menstrual cycle and encouraged her to make the dietary and lifestyle changes I had described. But given the significant *objective* evidence of early ovarian decline (bone loss, low estradiol), and the severity of the premenstrual hormonal effects on mood and sleep, we discussed the pros and cons of adding estradiol during the premenstrual and menstrual week to boost estradiol levels to more normal ranges.

I gave her several articles to read about these options and encouraged her to think about what she wanted to try. She was aware that, due to her continued cigarette smoking, she was not a candidate for a trial of oral contraceptives. When she came back for her follow-up visit to discuss her choices, she said "my quality of life for the next ten to fifteen years is more important than the remote chance of some dread disease." We also discussed the possibility that adding estradiol might have a slight possibility of triggering her previous endometriosis. She decided she wanted to try Estraderm anyway, since she had no problems with endometriosis since the laser surgery and her PMS was so disruptive for her.

Four weeks after beginning the Estraderm patch she stated she was feeling better overall, and both subjective and objective ratings of PMS symptoms had improved significantly. She continued to use the Estraderm patch premenstrually for another two years. Then she was successful in stopping smoking and wanted to change over to the low-dose birth control pills. She has continued to do well and has maintained a healthier lifestyle in addition to the hormones. She feels that hormonal stability has helped immensely to practically eliminate the disruptive mood and physical symptoms. I think the dietary changes were also significant in helping her feel better. I agree with her opinion that restoring her estrogen level to a normal range was crucial to her improvement. I believe this is a good example of the way in which our approaches need to be *individualized*, utilizing objective information combined with the patient's descriptions, to determine how best to create a woman's personalized health plan.

At this point, you may be asking yourself, "Well, did she have PMS or was she perimenopausal?" Technically, by our currently accepted definitions, Sue had PMS and was not yet perimenopausal, because her FSH and LH were still low (premenopausal levels), and she was still menstruating regularly. The window of time chronologically listed as perimenopausal is usually given as four years before menopause and four years after menopause, taken as an average age of fifty-one. Because women are all so different, I find these arbitrary age ranges useless. I also think that *what we will come to understand* in the future is that the observed pattern of "worsening PMS" in the mid- to late thirties and forties is in all probability the *beginning of ovarian decline* leading to perimenopause, and that the worsening symptoms of PMS are all part of the *continuum* of women's mid-life changes rather than *discrete* points in time.

Just What Is PMS?

Some of you may have experienced PMS, or family members with PMS—and it may have looked a little like this:

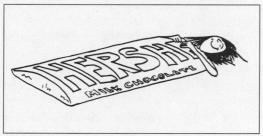

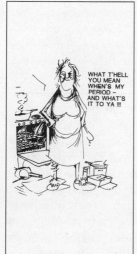 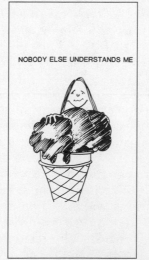 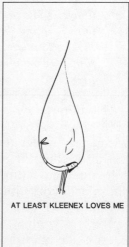

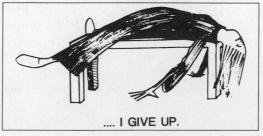

- Most women at my seminars howl with laughter and self-recognition when I put up the slides of these cartoons. I have to admit, somewhat sheepishly, that they were drawn by my husband a few years ago when I asked him to draw something funny for my talks. He asked what I wanted for PMS, and I said "Oh, just do whatever you think. You know what I get like, see what you come up with." Little did I know when I gave him such carte blanche that he was such a keen observer! So now you know some of my PMS secrets!
- I enjoy the humor, but there is a downside to it: if by joking about it, we trivialize the experiences of women who are truly bothered by symptoms of PMS each month, then it doesn't become a focus of medical study to determine the causes of and to find ways to help the significant percentage of women who suffer from PMS.

Look at these statistics:

- *Forty percent of all menstruating American women have regular premenstrual symptoms. This figure translates into 27 **million women**! The majority of these have a milder form of the disorder, with bloating, headache, irritability, and the "blues."*
- *Five to ten percent of these, or 3 **to** 7 **million women**, have symptoms severe enough to disrupt their personal and professional lives.*

Even in today, we don't have many answers to the questions I have raised above. The science of the menstrual cycle still is not adequately understood and lags behind our knowledge of body functions common to males and females. Some of the major difficulties in conducting research into PMS are the heterogeneous and amorphous descriptions of menstrually related syndromes, the multiplicity of populations evaluated, and the paucity of adequate rating instruments—among others. Studies that purport to address the question of menstrually related mood disorders have included subjects from PMS clinics; infertility clinics; women who have had gynecological surgery; patients from primary care settings, with and without complaints of PMS symptoms; college populations; "normal" women *without* symptoms; and "normal" women *with* symptoms but not seeking treatment. Some authors have excluded women with irregular menstrual cycles, even though this group is reported to have a greater incidence of symptoms. Such a "mixed bag" of study populations obviously makes it difficult to come up with meaningful and reliable data!

PMS *primarily* affects women between the ages of twenty-five to forty-eight, but it can affect adolescents as well: my youngest patient with clearly documented PMS was fourteen. I have been asked by pediatricians to consult on a number of cases of girls with PMS, and I think they may well have some parallels with the erratic hormonal balance and fluctuations seen in the perimenopause. PMS does, however, seem to be more common in older women and to worsen with age, generally becoming most marked for women in their late thirties to mid- or later forties.

The symptoms of PMS typically begin in conjunction with a hormonal change such as puberty, pregnancy, or starting or stopping oral contraceptive pills; or following surgery that affects the blood supply to the ovaries such as tubal ligation or hysterectomy without removal of the ovaries. In fact, a common pattern is for a woman to have the onset of her PMS about three or four years after a tubal ligation. This is now recognized to be related to the alterations in blood flow to the ovary resulting from having the tubes tied. Although when they ask about these connections, many women are still told that "this couldn't possibly be happening." This connection between PMS and surgical procedures has been increasingly discussed in gynecology journals. Thus, new techniques for tubal ligations have been developed to minimize any negative effects on ovarian blood flow.

Use of oral contraceptives with a *multiphasic* (many are *triphasic*) hormone content has also been found to produce a PMS-like syndrome in a significant percentage of women. A *multiphasic* pill has two or three *different* hormone doses, designed to theoretically mimic the normal cycle using synthetic hormones (some brand names are Triphasil, Tri-Levlen, Tri-Norinyl, Ortho Tri-Cyclen, Ortho-Novum 7//7/7, Ortho-Novum 10/11, Jenest). Aggravation of PMS, as well as migraine headaches, are reasons I *don't* recommend this type of birth control pill, *especially for perimenopausal women* who tend to be more negatively affected by hormonal fluctuations such as the multiphasic pills produce.

I find it fascinating to look back in the older medical literature, when the observations of patients formed the basis of clinical writings and practice. Such observations are now called "anecdotal" information and devalued in importance! I have included Dr. Frank's original description of the PMS syndrome he recognized from *observing and listening to his patients*. I think it is important for several reasons. First, dietary habits in the U.S. in 1931 included far more fresh fruits and vegetables, and less refined sugar, alcohol, and caffeine than is typical today; *yet women are describing the same experiences then and now.* So, while dietary factors play a role in *aggravating* PMS symptoms, I do not think they are the primary cause of PMS. The language Dr. Frank used in 1931 is somewhat different from words I would use today, but notice how similar his description is to what women continue to describe in 1995. Over the last sixty-four years or so since Dr. Frank's article, nothing much has changed in *women's described experiences,* so why would we even question whether PMS is real or not? Yet, you will still hear people arguing over this issue and saying PMS is a psychological problem without evidence of a hormonal cause.

DESCRIPTION OF PMS: 1931

"The group of women to whom I refer especially complain of a feeling of indescribable tension, from ten to seven days preceding menstruation, which in most instances continues until a time that the menstrual flow occurs. The patients complain of unrest, irritability, feeling like jumping out of their skin, and a desire to find relief by foolish and ill-considered actions. Their personal suffering is intense and it manifests itself in many reckless, and sometimes, reprehensible actions. Not only do they realize their own suffering, but they feel conscience-stricken toward their husbands and families, knowing well that they are unbearable in their attitudes and their reactions. Within an hour or two after the onset of the menstrual flow complete relief from both physical and mental tension occurs."

—Robert T. Frank, M.D.

It is important to note that the key defining characteristic of PMS is the *cyclicity* of symptoms, which then resolve around the onset of menses. PMS alone occurs prior to menstruation, and the bleeding phase itself is usually painless. PMS is **not** menstrual pain and cramps. The medical term for menstrual pain is **dysmenorrhea**, and it is another disorder altogether, although it may coexist with PMS in a small percentage of women. This is the widely used operational definition of PMS now:

CURRENT MEDICAL DEFINITION OF PMS

A pattern of recurring mood, behavioral, and physical symptoms which regularly occurs between ovulation and menstruation (in the luteal phase) and abates by the end of menstruation
to then be followed by a symptom-free interval each month.
Symptoms are present for at least six months, cause moderate
to severe disruption in normal functioning, and are not due to
another disorder.

PMS, which is *cyclic*, is also different than Major Depressive
Disorder, which is a *sustained* pattern of depressed, dysphoric
mood and physical symptoms. I will discuss Major Depression in
the next section. PMS as a recurring pattern of symptoms which
may *include anxiety attacks*, is also different than Panic Disorder
or Dysthymic Disorder, which are ongoing disorders without a
clear pattern of relationship to the premenstrual phase of the cycle.
Before concluding that a woman has PMS, the physician needs to
rule out other medical disorders which may mimic the symptoms
of PMS, such as thyroid problems, diabetes, and others.

Common Symptom Clusters in PMS

There have been over 150 symptoms described as part of PMS,
but can be grouped into a few common *patterns* of symptoms. I
have designated several major categories—AFFECTIVE (MOOD),
BEHAVIORAL, AUTONOMIC, FLUID/ELECTROLYTE, DERMATOLOGICAL,
COGNITIVE (BRAIN), PAIN, AND AN "OTHER" GROUP. The table below
lists some of the frequently reported symptoms in each category.
Not every patient will have all of these symptoms, but for each
patient there is usually a typical pattern, and the same symptoms
tend to recur with each cycle. Sometimes the symptoms for one
person may begin soon after ovulation and continue until menses;
in other women the symptoms begin about the peak of luteal
phase rise in estrogen and progesterone (about Day 21 or 22), a
week before the period. Pattern of onset may vary from woman to
woman but tends to stay about the same in a given person from
one cycle to another, which is why symptom logs kept daily for
several cycles are so helpful in making a correct diagnosis of PMS.

PMS SYMPTOM CLUSTERS

AFFECTIVE: depression, irritability, anxiety, angry outbursts, tearfulness, panicky feelings

BEHAVIORAL: impulsive actions, compulsions, agitation, lethargy, decreased motivation

AUTONOMIC: palpitations, nausea, constipation, dizziness, sweating, tremors

FLUID/ELECTROLYTE: fluid retention, bloating, weight gain, breast fullness, hands swelling

DERMATOLOGICAL: acne, oily hair, hives and rashes, herpes outbreaks, allergy outbreaks

COGNITIVE (BRAIN): decreased concentration, memory changes, word-retrieval problems

PAIN: migraines, tension headaches, back pain, muscle and joint aches, breast pain

OTHER: drug/alcohol abuse, food binges, hypersomnia or insomnia

---

What Are Some of the Causes of PMS?

In spite of clinical evidence of *physiological* changes as the underlying disturbance, most medical textbooks, researchers and physicians have attributed PMS symptoms to *psychological or sociological causes*—such as women's failure to accept the female role. Though psychological factors may *intensify* the patient's suffering, they do not *cause* the syndrome. Dr. Samuel Yen and other current researchers who have systematically studied PMS think that it is a *neuroendocrine imbalance.* The underlying mechanism involves neuroendocrine triggers within the hypothalamus and pituitary that then affect the function of such neurotransmitters as *serotonin (ST), norepinephrine (NE), dopamine (DA), and acetylcholine (ACh)* as I talked about in chapters 3 and 4.

The diversity of symptoms in PMS is caused by the many different brain centers and the whole series of pituitary and hypothalamic neuropeptide hormones governed by these neurotransmitters (TSH, FSH, ACTH, beta-endorphin, and alpha melanocyte stimulating [MSH] hormone and others). The neuropeptides beta-endorphin and MSH not only regulate the neurotransmitters involved in mood and behavior, but they also modulate pituitary release of other hormones, such as prolactin and vasopressin, which produce a number of physical and mood effects on the brain and body. The brain-body regulation of progesterone and estrogen in response to these changes in neuropeptides differs from woman to woman and I think accounts for the various clinical forms of PMS. As better-designed studies are done, I think we will find that **hormone ratios** and **rate of change** are key factors triggering the diverse brain-mediated symptoms of PMS.

Dr. Katharina Dalton, the British pioneer who has studied PMS patients for more than thirty years, has hypothesized that a deficiency of progesterone relative to the amount of estrogen present before menstruation triggers the syndrome. Her clinical studies have shown that some women with PMS do respond well to large doses of natural progesterone. I have not found this to be the case in my practice, and it may be that I am seeing a different age group of women in whom the declining estradiol is a more crucial factor. The clear pattern of hormone profiles in my patients is one of *low* estradiol (E2) and relatively normal levels of progesterone (P), so that there is a reduced ratio of E2 to P.

Several recent double blind, placebo-controlled studies have shown that natural progesterone is not any better than placebo in reducing PMS symptoms, and this has been my clinical experience as well. Consequently, I think there is much more to PMS, than just progesterone deficiency. In addition, the many different responses of women to a variety of hormonal approaches suggest we need a more encompassing theory of cause. I view PMS as a neuro-endocrine disorder that begins with physiological hormonal shifts affecting multiple brain centers. The brain events then trigger a variety of physical changes in multiple systems in the body, and can be aggravated by diet, substance use and life stress.

Many women describe their worst days in the cycle as being the day prior to bleeding and the first day bleeding begins. Tearfulness, crying spells, fragmented sleep, anxiety attacks, palpitations, and irritability typically are intensified for these two or three days. What causes the elevated frequency of symptoms on these two specified perimenstrual days is not known with certainty. Based on my knowledge of brain chemistry, it seems most likely that these are triggered by the *falling and low estrogen*. It is interesting that the estrogen levels reach their bottom point of the cycle close to the day before the onset of menses and are still low on Day 1 of bleeding. Low levels of estrogen are known to coincide with both *low endorphin levels* and *high* levels of monoamine oxidase enzymes (MAO), which break down catecholamines, and resulting in catecholamine depletion in the brain.

Loss of catecholamines is a significant factor in precipitating depressive mood changes. The decrease in endorphins contributes to the irritability, tearfulness, and restless sleep.

Dr. E. L. Klaiber and co-workers found that a series of pre-menopausal women with regular menstrual cycles who suffered from a major depressive illness had higher levels of plasma MAO activity (which breaks down and inactivates catecholamines and serotonin) than did *nondepressed* women. Dr. Klaiber interpreted these abnormalities as further evidence of norepinephrine/serotonin insufficiency consistent with current biological theories of depression. His study did not attempt to evaluate the therapeutic effectiveness of the estrogen therapy, but all of the patients who received estrogen therapy reported "moderate to marked" improvement in their moods. In another study of women with treatment refractory depression, Dr. Klaiber's group found that oral estrogen therapy was significantly effective in improving mood in women who had not responded to more traditional antidepressant medications. Taken together with the other evidence I have described in chapters 3 and 4, Dr. Klaiber's research lends additional support to the role of premenopausal decline in estrogen as a contributing factor in the PMS-perimenopause continuum of mood and physical symptoms.

There is an additional mechanism by which perimenopausal women may experience anxiety attacks and depressive mood changes: this is related to the drop in estrogen levels triggering hot flashes that cause multiple awakenings at night. Hot flashes causing waking episodes can be objectively measured in sleep laboratories; these waking episodes caused by surges of adrenalin trigger hot flashes that have been confirmed on EEG brain-wave recordings during sleep. Waking episodes result in sleep deprivation, a factor shown to be associated with irritable, depressive mood changes. Eighty percent to eighty-five percent of women experience hot flashes that typically occur at night for several years prior to the beginning of skipped periods in perimenopause.

The resulting sleep disturbances, coupled with unhealthy lifestyle habits, could contribute significantly to disturbances in mood (irritability and depression), loss of energy, reduced concentration and memory, fatigue and diminished sense of well-being. You may want to refer to the chart in Chapter 4 summarizing estrogen effects on the brain to see how all this works together. I have listed the four key antidepressant actions of estradiol again in the chart below. Unpleasant changes like ones I just described respond best to a *boost in estradiol*, rather than antidepressants, antianxiety medications, or sleeping pills.

ESTRADIOL: ANTIDEPRESSANT EFFECTS

- increases serotonin levels and receptors
- increases endorphin activity
- inhibits MAO enzyme activity, which prolongs activity of ST, DA, NE
- enhances binding of tricyclic antidepressants at brain receptors

---

PMS, ESTRADIOL AND SEROTONIN (ST)

- Rate of rise and fall in E2: *crucial* variable in effects on serotonin
- A more rapid rise and fall in E2, causes greater change in ST
- E2 effect on serotonin is a probable trigger for premenstrual migraine (*see Chapter 10*)

There are other postulated causes of PMS, but these may also be *results* of the neuroendocrine changes I have already described, so it is unclear whether some of these disturbances are *causes* of the syndrome, or are *results* of alterations in the reproductive hormone levels:

- altered glucose metabolism perhaps due to alterations in glucocorticoids and/or insulin activity;
- abnormal fatty acid metabolism resulting in altered tissue sensitivity to reproductive hormones
- abnormalities in the prolactin, aldosterone, renin, angiotensin, and vasopressin that govern normal fluid and electrolyte balance in the body

Other factors that may be involved in the rising incidence of PMS in recent years, and *adversely amplify* menstrual cycle hormonal changes are as follows:

1. the fact that many women are postponing pregnancy and having fewer pregnancies than women did years ago—resulting in more years of ovulatory cycles, which are clearly associated with a higher incidence of PMS;
2. the significant increase in obesity in our society—which results in increased peripheral conversion of androgens to the estrone type of estrogen in women. This alters the total estrogen to progesterone ratio but does not provide the higher level of 17-beta estradiol produced in the ovary, which now appears to be the primary active estrogen at brain receptors. **The majority of women suffering from PMS are obese** (defined as more than 20 percent over ideal body weight).
3. the fact that the typical American diet is high in fat, protein, salt, refined sugars, alcohol, and caffeinated beverages—all of which have been shown to significantly aggravate the symptoms of PMS;
4. the tendency of American women to have a deficit of magnesium in their diets, which also contributes to PMS symptoms, due to magnesium's role as an important co-factor in the synthesis of mood-elevating neurotransmitters.
5. possible inadequate intake of vitamin B_6 (pyridoxine), which is also a co-factor in the synthesis of mood-elevating neurotransmitters and is involved in the liver metabolism of estrogen and progesterone.

In summary, I think our current research findings lend more support to the integrated theory of PMS being triggered by the brain effects of ovarian hormones, with multiple brain-body systems then being affected and leading to the wide variety of symptoms. This integrated model makes more sense to me physiologically, and approaching it from an integrated point of view helps me to develop a more systematic, and physiological, approach to helping women feel better and deal constructively with the menstrual cycle hormonal shifts.

Is It the Blues, the Blahs, or Major Depression?

Nearly everyone has occasional down, moody times or bouts of sadness and discouragement that may last for a while. When do the "blues and blahs" become "major depressive disorder," a clinical depressive illness requiring professional intervention and possibly medication treatment? When a black mood settles in and remains for several weeks, sapping your energy, appetite, your interest in life and activities you usually enjoy, and altering your sleep, you may be clinically depressed.

Clinical depression is a medical illness which is now thought to have a primarily physical cause, that of a chemical imbalance in the neurotransmitter or "messenger" molecules in the brain. The illness of depression is two to three times more common in women, with the gender differences beginning in puberty and ending after menopause, when rates of depression become higher in males. This gender difference implicates a hormonal factor, which has not been addressed as an important connection in women's health.

In spite of major advances in our understandings of the neurobiology of depression, and the development of new and safer antidepressant medications, physicians and the lay public still labor under the misconception that the "chin up and get through it" approach is all that is needed. In fact, according to a recent poll by the National Alliance for the Mentally Ill, the American public still has many mistaken beliefs about mental illness in general:

- **71 percent believe it is due to emotional weakness**
- **65 percent believe it is caused by bad parenting**
- **45 percent believe it's the victim's fault, can be willed away**
- **43 percent believe it is incurable**
- **35 percent believe it is the consequence of sinful behavior**
- **only 10 percent BELIEVE IT HAS A BIOLOGICAL BASIS and involves brain chemistry (in spite of much publicity on this over the past 20 years!)**

Clinical depression is a very common disorder, which affects 20 to 30 percent of adults sometime during their lifetime. Experts estimate that at any given time, some 10 million Americans are in its throes. Unfortunately, even today with so much good information available, depression is still all too frequently misunderstood by the general public and physicians alike. Many people who suffer from depression are too embarrassed to seek help. A common expression I hear in my medical practice is "I feel like I'm weak. I should be able to handle this by myself." Such self-blaming, negative thought patterns are *often a symptom of depression but are not recognized as such* by the sufferer, who then has difficulty asking for help.

Lack of proper treatment causes not only untold suffering, lost productivity, and diminished quality of life, but is also a major risk factor in suicide. Fifteen percent of people with clinical depression commit suicide. This is a tragic loss when we consider that treatment of depression is successful for 80 to 90 percent of sufferers, with *proper diagnosis* and careful use of medication. **The lifetime risk of death from major depressive illness is greater than the lifetime risk of death from breast cancer!**

This physical, or biological, form of depression is not likely to be cured by "talk" therapies alone. Antidepressant medication to reestablish the normal chemical balance in the brain is now considered to be the most effective treatment. Proper medical diagnosis is needed to identify this form of depression and rule out other medical causes for the symptoms, such as hypothyroidism, diabetes, lupus, and perhaps a hundred or more medical problems and medications that have been found to cause a syndrome indistinguishable from primary major depressive disorders.

Overuse of alcohol, caffeine, nicotine, decongestants, phenylpropanolamine diet pills, herbal products containing ephedra, and illicit drugs (cocaine, stimulants, hallucinogens, and others) may also cause biological depressions. Severe and *prolonged life stress*, even though "understandable" may cause enough biochemical changes in the brain and body to result in depressive illness needing medication and psychotherapy. After a careful medical history, physical examination, and appropriate blood tests rule out these other causes, your physician may recommend antidepressant medication, which can alleviate sustained and severe depressions even though they may be clearly related to life stress.

How do you tell if what you are experiencing is just the normal "blues" or a clinical depression? DURATION of symptoms is one important key. If your mood remains down, blue, sad, discouraged or hopeless for *more than two weeks*, in spite of pleasant events in your life, clinical depression is likely. People with clinical depression may also describe feeling "numb," "leaden," or like "I'm just going through the motions" of life. Women have said to me "I feel like I'm trying to move my body through quicksand." Another woman said she felt like her body "weighed a thousand pounds, it was just hard to even start moving."

Presence of SOMATIC (physical) or VEGETATIVE changes occur, such as significant loss or gain of weight for no apparent reason or changes in your sleep pattern (trouble falling asleep; problems with multiple awakenings at night; or waking up very early, unable to go back to sleep). Loss of energy, feeling "keyed up" and "hyper," or feeling very "slowed down" and "sluggish" are other signs, along with changes in your ability to concentrate on tasks, loss of sex drive, fatigue, menstrual irregularities, marked decrease or increase in appetite with compulsive overeating, GI upset, constipation or diarrhea, and loss of interest or pleasure in your usual activities.

THOUGHTS OF DEATH OR SUICIDE are very serious symptoms and should never be ignored, particularly if you begin to feel that you no longer care about living and think about ways of taking your life. You *must* seek a qualified professional to help you if thoughts of suicide are present for any length of time. If a friend or family member tells you about such thoughts, even if they try to pass it off as a joke, you should take it seriously and bring it to the attention of someone who can get them to see a qualified mental health professional or physician for an evaluation. Studies are clear in showing that better than 90 percent of people who commit suicide *have told someone ahead of time that they had these thoughts*, but many were just not taken seriously and guided to professional help.

If you find that you have *five of the above symptoms persisting more than two weeks*, it is important that you see your physician for help. Many people come into a physician's office with vague physical complaints and sidestep the real reason they are seeking help. This only leads to misdiagnosis and delay of proper treatment. Be direct. Tell your doctor that you feel depressed. Depression is just as much of an illness as diabetes, high blood pressure, and heart disease are. Depression can have physical, chemical, genetic, hormonal, medication, emotional, and situational causes. Help is available, and the newer antidepressants have typically very few side effects. Depression is NOT "weak character." You should not feel ashamed about having the illness of depression.

If your physician recommends an antidepressant, the serotonin-augmenting ones have few side effects and are quite effective. The serotonin-boosters are especially helpful for women in whom depression may be caused or aggravated by estrogen changes that appear to specifically decrease serotonin. Your doctor may also recommend counseling or psychotherapy to help you deal more effectively with the stresses in your life. I think other effective, helpful approaches are professionally led support groups, healthy eating, regular exercise, relaxation training, and/or meditation.

Since the large majority of patients with depression are seen by primary care physicians (often for vague somatic complaints) *rather than by psychiatrists*, I think it is crucial that YOU know how to recognize symptoms that could indicate the presence of a biological major depression, so you can tell your doctor. I also think it is imperative that we intensify efforts to help primary care physicians recognize milder forms of depression and begin to treat these syndromes appropriately, using antidepressant medications when indicated. Patient education brochures on depression are published by the National Institute of Mental Health and are available free. Simple screening questionnaires, such as the Zung Depression Inventory, are also available free from various sources and are valuable aids to you and your physicians to identify "masked" depression. I have included one of these "Self-Tests" for depression in Chapter 18, which you may use to see where you score if you are having symptoms such as I have described.

I think it is crucial that we teach women that depression is a highly treatable biologically based disorder, and getting help early would greatly reduce suffering and debilitation, as well as help to reduce the economic burdens of excessive medical utilization and lost productivity in the workplace or at home. If you find yourself feeling overwhelmed by life and slipping into a major depression, don't feel ashamed and withdraw or hesitate to ask for help. Clinical depression is a highly treatable medical condition—one that you should NOT have to suffer through alone.

Stress: Vicious Cycle Effects on Hormones, Anxiety, and Depression

In spite of the fact that we live in a culture that often times acts as if women don't have a brain, WE DO, and the brain is a *physiological* organ, as well as the *psychological* organ of "mind" expressing our personality, psyche, and behavior. It is affected by outside stressors (stimuli) and by internal stimuli or changes in the body, so that many times what are labeled psychological symptoms and *assumed to have a psychological cause* may in fact be *caused by biochemical* changes in our body's *physiological balance*. Likewise, psychological stress causes profound changes in every cell in the body, including brain chemistry.

For both men and women, stress of whatever form, whether it's external stressors or whether it's the internal stressors of physiological changes that require the body to change and adapt, all of us have the body as our "final common pathway" through which these changes act and operate. With prolonged stress the body's balance, or homeostasis, is disrupted and we see symptoms that relate to "adrenalin" overactivity, such as headaches, high blood pressure, panic attacks, colitis, arteriosclerosis, eczema, overwhelming fatigue, and many others. We also see illnesses that are the result of long-term chronic stress having an adverse effect on the immune system, producing problems related to *hyperactivity* of the immune system such as asthma and allergies, problems related to a *hypoactive* immune system such as cancers, and problems which arise when the immune system runs amuck and attacks your own body, such as the autoimmune disorders. All of these are manifestations of the combined effects of stress-induced biochemical changes on the body pathways, occurring over time.

Another aspect of the problem of stress when it affects women is the role of chronic stress in decreasing the normal function and hormone production of the ovaries, as well as the thyroid gland. At the North American Menopause Society meeting, Susan Ballinger, Ph.D., of Sydney, Australia, reported on their study addressing connections between women's perception of the presence of life stress and levels of their ovarian estrogens. Ballinger's study assessed life events, clinical depression, and anxiety, together with measurements of urinary and plasma estrogens. This study demonstrated that a high level of urinary estrogens correlated with higher psychosocial stress scores. Her conclusion was that "psychosocial stress, emotional vulnerability, and coping skills may all contribute to estrogen deficiency in post menopause."

From my clinical observations and correlation of the estrogen levels in perimenopausal women, the *opposite* hypothesis may also be true about the connection between hormone levels and stress, but we don't yet have much information on this half of the equation: declining estrogen levels contribute to alterations in the function of norepinephrine, serotonin, dopamine, and acetylcholine, which regulate mood, behavior, and cognitive function. Declining estrogen, and the subsequent effect on brain chemical messengers, may then contribute to the observed difficulty coping with psychosocial stressors by women who have previously been able to cope successfully. Once again, the role of stress is a two-way street: life stress suppresses the ovaries, which decreases estrogen production, which affects sleep, and so on. Normal declines in estrogen affect brain chemistry, which affects ability to cope with stress. It's another one of those vicious cycles, as I have diagrammed in the next section.

How Are All of These Phenomena Related?

Since I am such a "visual" learner, I decided to draw a diagram that represents how I see these various stress and hormone factors coming together to cause some of the phenomena, or symptoms,

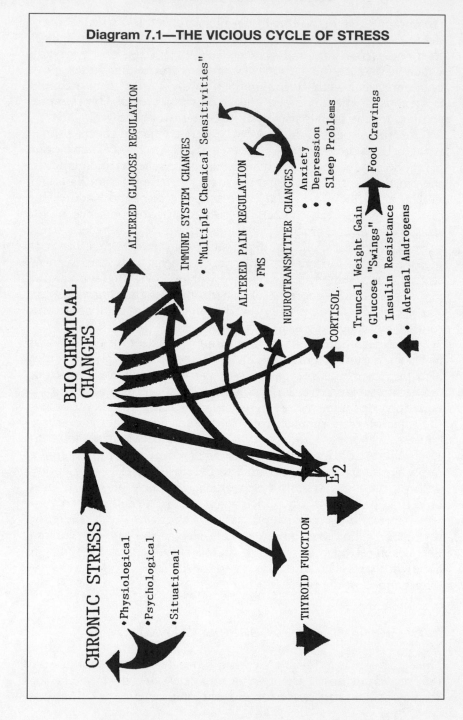

Diagram 7.1—THE VICIOUS CYCLE OF STRESS

we experience. I see it much like a "vicious cycle" with one event affecting another, until it all snowballs on us. Think about these various pieces of the puzzle as they relate to your life, and your lifestyle habits, and see if it helps you identify some healthy ways to "break the cycle."

How Can I Tell What My Problem Is? Getting Checked Out

PMS is commonly not recognized or is misdiagnosed so **thorough evaluation is very important.** There are many diagnoses given to women who in fact have PMS: some of these are dysthymic disorder, manic-depressive illness, major depressive disorder, atypical depression, chronic fatigue, chronic candidiasis, panic disorder, anxiety disorder, stress reaction, and others. The goal of a comprehensive evaluation is also to make certain that you do not have another medical problem causing similar symptoms; and to insure that any previously unrecognized secondary disorders, which may be contributing to your symptoms, are diagnosed and properly treated.

If you are having difficulty feeling that your PMS concerns are taken seriously, you may find a specialty clinic for PMS would provide more helpful resources and suggestions. Madison Pharmacy Associates is an excellent source of reliable information on PMS centers around the country, and I have included their toll-free number in Appendix 2. The chart which follows lists some of the aspects of a complete evaluation, and points to discuss with your physician.

COMPONENTS OF A COMPREHENSIVE PMS EVALUATION

I. MEDICAL HISTORY:
   Key aspects include:

1. Timing of symptoms (onset, duration, when end)

2. Symptom cluster (types of problems you encounter with your cycle)

3. Onset in relation to some hormonal change (puberty, pregnancy, starting or stopping oral contraceptives, perimenopause).

4. Time of increased severity of symptoms (usually following discontinuation of oral contraceptives, after tubal ligation, following hysterectomy without removal of ovaries, after a pregnancy, after cessation of breast-feeding, or after several months of no menses).

5. History of threatened or actual miscarriage, "toxemia" (pre-eclampsia): 86 percent of women with pre-eclampsia developed PMS in the months following birth.

6. History of post-partum depression of sufficient severity to require antidepressant treatment. In one study of 100 women treated for severe PMS, 73 percent had a history of significant post partum depression.

7. Weight fluctuations in adult life greater than 25 lb. Obesity increases the likelihood of PMS for reasons which are still unclear, but may be related to increased estrone production in body fat.

8. History of past thyroid problems and/or treatment with thyroid

9. History of painless menstruation (*painful* menses is a different problem called *dysmenorrhea* and is more often due to endometriosis)

10. Pattern of food/or alcohol cravings, and/or alcohol intolerance during premenstrual phase of cycle.

11. Inability to tolerate high-progestin birth control pills. Women with PMS often experience severe side effects and/or exacerbation of PMS with high progestin oral contraceptives, particularly the tri-phasic pills with changing hormone content.

12. Increased libido. Women with PMS frequently report increased sex drive during the premenstrual phase, compared to women with primary depression who usually report diminished sex drive.

II. FAMILY HISTORY

Note presence of similar problems, especially among women in family: such as diabetes, thyroid disease, multiple allergies, autoimmune diseases, disorders such as alcoholism, depression and/or mania, anxiety disorders, and eating disorders (anorexia, bulimia). All of these have been associated with increased risk of menstrually related mood and physical changes seen in PMS.

III. MEDICAL AND PSYCHOLOGICAL EVALUATION

1. Physical Examination, particularly any signs of hormone imbalance

2. Laboratory Tests: Blood Chemistry panel, Complete Blood Count (CBC), Thyroid Profile with TSH and possibly thyroid antibodies, Prolactin, FSH, LH, Progesterone, Estradiol. Other lab tests as medically appropriate and indicated by history and physical findings.

3. Psychological Assessment of emotional and cognitive function, with rating scales such as Beck, Hamilton or Zung Depression/Anxiety Scales; Profile of Mood States (POMS), Hopkins SCL-90, PRISM Menstrual Calendar, etc.

4. Daily Symptom Log/Journal through at least one and preferably 2–3 menstrual cycles. Should include:
    a. MENSTRUAL SYMPTOMS, WEIGHT, BODY TEMP.
    b. Dietary intake log relating food intake to time of symptoms
    c. record of alcohol, caffeine, and tobacco use
    d. record of over-the-counter and prescription medication use

You and your physician should then review this information and discuss the various options available which would be helpful to you. I find that a combination of approaches works best, using ones from the section that follows or others which your physician may recommend.

Options for Feeling Better

There are a variety of approaches that will help you recapture your sense of well-being and "zest." At the most basic level, you really can't expect *anything* to help a great deal unless you first address constructive lifestyle changes to reduce or eliminate potential "triggers" and "aggravators" that make you feel worse if you have PMS. Basic and simple, yet many times not done, are the dietary modifications that have been found to be of help in eliminating many PMS symptoms. Frequently I find that it is difficult to get patients to accept that something as "simple" as changing the way they eat can have a profound impact on the way they feel—their mood, energy level, clarity of thinking—BUT IT DOES! The following suggestions are "tried and true." They DO work, but you first have to commit to really giving it your best effort for *long enough* to see a difference. I found that when I paid close attention to these basics, I was able to eliminate just about all of my own PMS problems. I admit I wasn't perfect all the time, but these steps do make a big difference. So, before you ask your doctor for medication or rush out for a herbal "fix," make certain you try these:

I. DIETARY CHANGES TO DIMINISH PMS

1. Avoid simple sugars (you know what I am talking about: all those "sweets" that just seem to stick to your fingers!), reduce salt; cut out, alcohol, caffeine, nicotine, and chocolate—*especially just before your period.*
2. Increase intake of complex carbohydrates to 60 percent of total daily calorie intake (have a low fat, low sugar, high fiber bran muffin instead of a brownie).
3. Decrease intake of protein to about 20 percent of total daily calories, and concentrate on the low-fat protein sources—fish, chicken, low-fat cheese.
4. Proper spacing of meals. Symptoms seen to be worsened by long intervals between food intake, perhaps due to the alterations in glucose tolerance seen in the premenstrual phase. More frequent eating, with smaller portions and less of the simple sugars also reduces the tendency for women with PMS to crave and binge on sweets.

II. EXERCISE PROGRAM

I can't say it enough: MOVE THE BODY! Exercise is great medicine! When I do it, I feel like a different person; when I don't, I feel sluggish. Our bodies were designed to be active. I educate women about the physiological and psychological effects of exercise that are of benefit in PMS: *increases in beta-endorphin, stimulation of NE, reducing excess anxiety, stabilization of serum glucose, appetite suppression, increased energy, improved mood, enhanced sexual energy.*

I teach women how to safely begin an aerobic exercise activity and how to monitor pulse rate for optimum effect. You don't have to be a marathon runner to get the benefits of increased physical activity. Walking will do it, especially if you have been inactive. If you have any limitations due to medical problems, talk with your physician and get a referral for a trained physical therapist to help you get started with an appropriate program.

III. STRESS MANAGEMENT

Take a look now at the "Vicious Cycle" diagrams in Chapter 19. Stress plays a direct role in negatively influencing the chemical messengers that are out of balance and contribute to PMS in the first place. Look for ways of reducing avoidable stresses, and look for ways you can minimize the adverse effects of Unavoidable stresses. One of the techniques I teach my patients is the relaxation response, popularized by Dr. Herbert Benson but used for hundreds of years in many cultures. You can do the relaxations using a variety of techniques: visualization, progressive muscle relaxation, self-hypnosis, autogenic conditioning, meditation, and others. There are good books and tapes available to guide you.

Counseling for stress management techniques may be helpful for some women, especially during times when it feels like life is running you over! Getting an outside perspective on what you can do often helps you feel more in control, which then decreases the body's "fight or flight" stress response which intensifies PMS.

Another good stress management technique is having massage therapy during the premenstrual week. Therapeutic massage is an excellent way of improving relaxation, boosting endorphins, improving circulation, and decreasing muscle tension, headaches and back pain. Look for a registered, certified therapeutic massage therapist in your phone book under American Association of

Massage Therapists, or call the A.A.M.T. toll-free number for a member therapist in your area. Acupuncture may also be helpful for some of these stress and PMS symptoms, although this modality does not usually have the more rapid onset of beneficial effect as do the relaxation techniques and therapeutic massage. Acupuncture, to be most effective, typically requires a series of treatments.

IV. MEDICATION APPROACHES

1. VITAMINS: A variety of vitamin combinations have been reported to help alleviate PMS symptoms, but there have not been clear-cut benefits found in controlled studies. I think particularly if you are under a great deal of stress, which depletes the B group and vitamin C, adding a low dose of B complex supplement at least during the premenstrual week can be helpful for some women. Pyridoxine (vitamin B_6) has been recommended and reported to ease some of the symptoms of PMS if used in conjunction with diet and exercise. We are not sure how pyridoxine achieves these effects, except that it is a cofactor in many chemical reactions, including those involved in making dopamine and serotonin, and it inhibits prolactin metabolism. B_6 may modulate the action of dopamine and serotonin in the chain of reactions that regulate production of estrogen and progesterone. It is also involved in the metabolism of estrogen by the liver and in the metabolism of fats and carbohydrates.

The usual starting dose of B_6 is fifty mg per day. Although some herbal practitioners and naturopaths say that you cannot overdose or become toxic on the water-soluble B vitamins, it has been well-documented that excessive supplementation of the B vitamins (particularly B_6) may cause neurological problems. **Do not exceed 100 mg per day because of the risk of peripheral neuropathy (numbness, paresthesias, tingling).**

I have found it is better to supplement the **B complex vitamins as a group** in one supplement rather than taking just vitamin B_6, because the B complex needs to be present in the proper balance and ratio in order to work optimally. There are now a number of commercial vitamin formulas that have been theoretically designed for the special needs of women with PMS. Although these are usually more expensive than the general brands sold at the pharmacy, they may provide the balance of vitamins and minerals needed by some women. You may want to consider one of these options. The staff at Madison Pharmacy Associates (see Appendix 2) are a good resource to discuss vitamin formulations designed for women.

2. DIURETICS. Many doctors have used the thiazide diuretics (hydrochlorothiazide or HCTZ, Dyazide, Maxide and others) to alleviate the fluid retention some women experience in the premenstrual week. The thiazides are *not* the diuretics I recommend, because they further increase potassium loss and may actually aggravate PMS symptoms. They also tend to interfere with normal glucose balance and may increase cholesterol.

I think the only diuretic that makes *physiological* sense to use is *spironolactone* (brand name: Aldactone) if you are someone who clearly experiences documented premenstrual weight gain, bloating, and breast tenderness due to fluid retention. The usual dosage is fifty mg (25 mg twice a day) to 100 mg a day (taken in divided doses as 25 mg four times a day, because it is a shorter-acting medication). Spironolactone acts on the fluid-regulating hormone (aldosterone) which is altered by progesterone in the luteal phase of the cycle, leading to fluid shifts. I do not find that the majority of women with PMS need a diuretic if the hormonal balance and diet is improved.

3. ORAL CONTRACEPTIVES (OCs). I find that the steady-dose (monophasic) OCs can provide a marked degree of symptom relief in a large percentage of women, especially pre(peri)menopausal nonsmoking women who are experiencing diminishing estrogen production and erratic cycles.

I have found over the years that the key to using OCs in PMS is to *start* with a pill formulation with *the least possible progestin* (the culprit for most of the unwanted side effects) and a little better level of estrogen.

Many commonly recommended oral contraceptives are higher in progestin, and lower in estrogen. *This is the reverse of what a woman over thirty needs as you look at what is happening to women hormonally at this time in their lives.* The three OC pill options on the market in the United States that I have found produce the best results in reducing PMS are: Ovcon-35 (least progestin), Modicon, and Brevicon (next lowest amount of progestin).

Using the OCs during the perimenopause transition was approved by the FDA for nonsmokers just a few years ago, and the OCs have *added health benefits* of decreasing the risk of ovarian and endometrial cancers, uterine fibroids, and fibrocystic breast changes. Perimenopausal use of monophasic OCs to reduce PMS also helps maintain adequate estradiol levels to prevent bone loss. You MUST NOT SMOKE if you take the oral contraceptives, because smoking increases the risk of stroke and blood clots in women who take oral contraceptives.

Conventional teaching has been that women with PMS don't do well on the birth control pills due to the **synthetic progestin** which can aggravate PMS. I have found that this is true *if the progestin content is higher than 0.5mg norethindrone* (or equivalent progestational activity). If one of my patients decides to try the birth control pill for to reduce PMS, I *only* prescribe the low progestin formulas. There are still some women who can't take even the lowest amount of synthetic progestin, but in my experience, this has been a minority. For women who cannot take the synthetic progestins at all, natural progesterone may work, and I talk about this further along in this section.

You might find it helpful to listen to the voices of these patients of mine who have benefited from using oral contraceptives to alleviate the mid-life PMS:

A forty seven year old white female described her health as "much better, it's Christmas and I am not sick, and that's different from the past three years. I think the hormones [Ovcon-35] are helping me feel a whole lot better. It was really good to find out that there really is something there, I'm not imagining things. I am feeling really good."

A forty three year old woman who developed severe depression on Loestrin oral contraceptive had these comments several months after I changed to a higher estrogen/lower progestin pill, Ovcon-35: "I felt much better, I'm not crying, I don't feel depressed, I have my energy, I don't have those headaches. I really have noticed an incredible difference. I have been able to exercise again, and I wasn't been able to do that on the other pill (Loestrin) because I just didn't have the energy. I felt wiped out all the time."

A fifty year old woman said: "The birth control pills were heaven sent. Since I started taking them, I have not had any cramps, the bleeding is less, the depression is much better, that black cloud has lifted, and that's been wonderful. I'm as painfree as I have ever been with my periods. The minute I started taking them I could tell a difference. I have had only very mild PMS feelings, but the moods going up and down has gotten better. I am so grateful to you that I feel so good."

A thirty six year old woman, now on the monophasic oral contraceptive, said her physician was against her taking the hormones because of family history of breast cancer in her grandmother, "but I discussed it and felt like this was right for me and I decided to do this. I am much, much better. Its been three weeks on the new pills, I am sleeping through the night, the crying spells are almost completely gone even though I have a reason to cry because a family member almost died of a brain abscess and I flew to another city to take care of him. I handled it really well. I don't have the *crying-for-no-reason* spells like I used to. I'm like a different person, a great decrease in anxiety, I'm not irritable, the GI symptoms have resolved, I have enough energy I'm exercising in the morning going to the gym, my mood's even, my secretary even said I seem a lot happier, I feel more focused, and my memory is somewhat better and I am getting more organized at work. I am ecstatic about my improvement, I can't thank you enough. I'm glad to know I wasn't crazy to be with all the things I was experiencing."

There are some added benefits, and reduced medical costs for the last woman who described her experience beginning the oral contraceptives. She has been able to stop taking the sleeping pills and daily Xanax she had been using, she has had no further migraine type headaches which had required numerous trips to the ER for injections to treat the severe pain, and her moderate incontinence has resolved without her needing the urological consultation her previous physician had recommended. Pretty good results for about $20.00 a month, *and* improved quality of life, as you can see from her description.

4. PROGESTERONE. The use of natural progesterone, as opposed to the synthetic progestational agents found in oral contraceptives, has been recommended by Dr. Dalton in Britain, who has used it successfully for PMS relief in her patients. There are no controlled studies demonstrating its effectiveness. Progesterone has not yet been approved by the FDA for PMS, but then I can't think of *any* of the currently widely used medications for PMS that have been approved by the FDA specifically for use in PMS therapy! The most recently published (1995) double-blind, placebo-controlled study of natural progesterone for PMS again showed that progesterone was no better than placebo to reduce symptoms. These results are in contrast to the successes reported by Dr. Dalton; no one seems to be certain of the reasons for the differences.

Progesterone has been helpful for some women, and the rationale for its use is its effects on the brain pathways involved in producing PMS symptoms. Progesterone inhibits norepinephrine release and reuptake (an anti-anxiety action), it alters dopamine neurotransmission, and has an anticonvulsant effect at levels in the normal range for the luteal phase. At higher doses, metabolites of progesterone produce an anti-anxiety effect by also increasing the inhibitory neurotransmitter, GABA, the same way the tranquilizers Valium and Xanax work. Doses of progesterone used for PMS are in the **pharmacologic** dose range, and produce circulating levels of progesterone much higher than normal for the menstrual cycle. At these drug-equivalent doses, progesterone acts on the brain as a **sedative**, and also has anesthetic properties. **If you have a history of major depression, or a family history of depressive illnesses, be cautious about using progesterone for PMS, since it may trigger an episode of major depression.**

In my opinion, progesterone (like estrogen or testosterone) should not be used lightly or without good, knowledgeable medical supervision. Even though it is a natural hormone, taking more than you need can produce multiple unwanted side effects and does have some risks. I have treated numerous patients who had exaggerated PMS and depressive symptoms from high doses of progesterone. It takes a **slow tapering** from such high levels to avoid having marked progesterone withdrawal symptoms.

I have generally not found progesterone to be all that helpful for PMS relief in women in the perimenopausal age range, because with the declining estrogen at this time, women on large doses of progesterone are more likely to become markedly depressed. I have other concerns about long-term progesterone at this dose, since we don't have good data about the potential adverse effects on breast tissue when it is used continuously. Remember, in the normal menstrual cycle, progesterone is only present for about *half* the cycle. In addition, using progesterone for a week or ten days and then stopping with menstruation can cause mood changes that result from the combined endorphin-serotonin drops triggered by estradiol and progesterone dropping sharply at the same time. If you are using natural progesterone and have *more* symptoms of tearfulness, irritability, and anxiety during menses after stopping progesterone, you may have *progesterone-withdrawal*. Talk with your physician about ways to manage this.

In Chapter 15, I have summary charts on the comparative potencies of some of the over-the-counter progesterone creams, so you may want to check this information before you start using any of these products. Side effects can occur even from *natural* substances.

5. OTHER HORMONES. Danazol is a potent progestin with androgen properties that has been used in the treatment of PMS and endometriosis. It can be effective, but with a very high price, both in dollars and in very unpleasant side effects: depression, weight gain, acne, an increase in facial and body hair. It appears to reduce PMS and endometriosis by suppressing ovarian cycles in hormone production, which eliminates the "triggers" for PMS and the estrogen stimulation of endometrial growth. **I do not use it just for PMS because I think there are just too many severe side effects which are more disruptive of quality of life than the PMS!** I have usually been able to help women find another alternative when treating PMS. I have had patients whose gynecologists prescribed Danazol for severe endometriosis not responsive to other treatments, and for these women, the side effects may be worth the decrease in endometriosis pain, which can be extremely severe and debilitating.

Lupron (leuprolide) is an medication that mimics the gonadotropin-releasing hormones in the brain and results in shutting down the ovaries to eliminate the hormonal cycling that sets off PMS. It has been used to treat severe PMS, but it causes a full menopausal syndrome with hot flashes and even bone loss if it is used for a long period of time, since it shuts off estrogen and progesterone production. To eliminate the hot flashes, sleep problems and other negative side effects of Lupron, your physician would need to "add-back" a steady amount of estrogen. You cannot, however, take estrogen alone for an extended period of time due to the increase in abnormal bleeding and hyperplasia of the uterine lining. In addition to the careful monitoring needed, and the fact that Lupron has to be given by injection (daily, or as a long-acting shot once a month), Lupron is also quite expensive (approximately $500–$600 per month). If the PMS is so severe and incapacitating that your physician has recommended removal of the ovaries and uterus, it may be worth a two or three month trial of Lupron with "add-back" estrogen to see whether eliminating the ovarian cycling alleviates the severe PMS. I would not recommend such a major step for treating PMS unless the PMS were of extreme severity and absolutely *nothing else* had worked.

6. ANXIOLYTICS (ANTI-ANXIETY AGENTS). Buspar (buspirone) belongs to a new generation of anxiolytics that act primarily as a serotonin 1A receptor "booster" in the presynaptic neurons and a partial agonist "booster" in the post-synaptic neurons. Buspirone is not an addictive or habit forming drug, does not produce withdrawal symptoms if stopped abruptly, and there is no known abuse potential. Buspirone is not a tranquilizer; it does not cause sedation or adverse effects on memory or coordination. In a study of PMS patients at East Carolina University, Dr. Daniel David found that using buspirone (Buspar) in women with *mild* PMS resulted in an 80 percent "helpful" response, women with *moderate* PMS showed a 92 percent "helpful" response, and patients with *marked* PMS showed a 100 percent helpful response. I have not personally found such dramatic results, but I have found that Buspar does help a number of women with PMS. It provides another safe option for you to discuss with your own physician. What I find interesting about Dr. David's study is that the more severe the PMS was, the better the response to Buspirone, which is what I would expect if indeed PMS is triggered by a serotonin deficiency or imbalance.

Buspirone is *not* a medication to take "as needed" (or PRN). It takes at least seven days to effect a significant enough level in the brain to produce its beneficial effects and reduce anxiety. A method that works well with this medication is to begin taking it at the end of the menstrual period and take it daily until the next menses starts, then stop for the days of bleeding. Some physicians working with PMS patients have found buspirone to be markedly effective in reducing symptoms, with the advantage that it is non-addictive and tends to have few side effects.

The Benzodiazepines (Xanax, Ativan, Serax, Valium, Klonopin and others) act on the GABA receptor sites and have multiple effects on the brain: anticonvulsant, sedative, muscle relaxant, and anxiolytic. I find that these medications *may* have limited helpfulness for some patients, but they may also aggravate the dysphoric (or unpleasant) mood states of PMS and may also impair thinking, concentration, and memory in larger doses. I don't recommend these very often because they have an additive adverse effect with alcohol, and produce a dependence syndrome requiring careful tapering off when being stopped. They are also drugs which tend to be frequently abused. If they are used in the management of "crisis" symptoms in PMS, they should be used sparingly, and short term, with the goal being to help you make lifestyle changes that will reduce symptoms in other ways. Of the benzodiazepines listed above, Xanax (alprazolam) is the only one which has been shown in double-blind, placebo-controlled studies, to reduce PMS symptoms significantly. It can safely be taken just during the luteal phase when symptoms are present, and usually does not cause any withdrawal symptoms when you stop it at the beginning of bleeding.

7. SEROTONIN-REUPTAKE INHIBITORS (SSRI). The medications currently available are Prozac, Paxil, Zoloft and Luvox. Another drug, Serzone, was released recently, and has similar characteristics to the SSRIs, but with fewer sexual side effects. Prozac was the first one of these medications which was FDA-approved in 1988 for the treatment of depression. It has now been tested in double-blind studies of PMS patients and found to be significantly effective, even though none of the SSRIs have been FDA-approved for the treatment of PMS. The most recent (1995) double-blind, placebo-controlled study of Prozac for PMS, this time in seven centers in Canada with a total of over 400 women, again showed significant reductions in women's symptoms.

I have prescribed Prozac successfully for years to help treat PMS; in fact, I had been awaiting its release in 1988 because I had already been working with the serotonin connection in PMS for a number of years and thought that a "serotonin-booster" should be helpful for women with this problem. I have found it to be dramatically helpful to the majority of PMS patients for whom I think it may be appropriate. Other PMS specialists report equally good results, with estimates of 70 to 85 percent positive response to SSRIs. When I use an SSRI for PMS, I usually find that these medications can be given just in the luteal phase of the cycle. This is unlike the situation in major depression where the onset of therapeutic effect of these medications may take several *weeks*. With the availability now of Zoloft, Paxil, Luvox, and Serzone, this provides several options for women to try. You may respond well to one but not the others, so don't give up.

All of the SSRIs have far fewer side effects than the older anti-depressants: tricyclics (TCA) and the MAO inhibitors. Generally the side effects may be a mild queasiness, anxious feelings, loose bowel movements, and possibly headaches. All of these early side effects tend to diminish over time or with a decrease in dose. Relatively few people have to stop these medications altogether due to unpleasant side effects. The one problem that does tend to make women want to change to a different medication is that all of the SSRIs can make orgasm more difficult to reach, or blunt orgasm intensity (Serzone is reported to be less likely to cause this problem). SSRIs are also helpful for other disorders due to serotonin abnormalities: chronic pain syndromes, migraines, obsessive-compulsive disorders, bulimia, and others.

8. TRICYCLIC ANTIDEPRESSANTS (TCA). In my opinion, now that the SSRIs are available, I rarely use this group of medications for PMS, since they produce many more side effects including appetite stimulation, weight gain, significant dry mouth, constipation, "racing heart," and in older patients, problems with blood pressure regulation. A TCA may be indicated if you have a *co-existing mood disorder*; in this case, you should be evaluated by a psychiatrist knowledgeable in psychopharmacology. The TCA group of medications is *highly lethal* if taken in an overdose, accidentally or intentionally (not true of SSRIs, which makes them a safer choice).

9. LITHIUM. Lithium is very effective for bipolar (manic-depressive illness) to stabilize moods, and some physicians have used it to help PMS. I have not found it to be of much use, and since Lithium is a salt in the same family as sodium, it tends to aggravate fluid retention, and it also increases appetite, thereby contributing to weight gain. Lithium has a beneficial mood-stabilizing effect in unipolar depression as well as in bipolar disorders, but I think it should be given with the supervision of a knowledgeable psychiatrist and used when indicated for a major affective disorder. It also has potentially more severe side effects, and may contribute to hypothyroidism, which is already common in women in this age range. I do not recommend it as a PMS therapy.

Heading into the Future

PMS. Perimenopause. Depression. All have important implications for your health and well-being. Whatever name is given, each is treatable and each responds to a variety of mind-body approaches, including lifestyle changes and adding medication to rebalance brain chemistry, in addition to your "healthy living choices." The mid-life years may be a time of "hoppin' hormones" and other changes in the body, but this doesn't mean you should resign yourself to not feeling your best. Mid-life is a time to refocus, a time to pay attention to *ourselves* and take care of these wonderful gifts of our mind and body! No one else can do it for you. Ultimately, although I may help as a woman's professional medical "guide," *you* are your own best physician and your healing comes from within. The choices you make *now*, whatever your chronological age, have a major bearing on your health for the future. The name of the (health) game is, first and foremost, ***Prevention!***

CHAPTER 8

Is It Chronic Fatigue, "Yeast," or Perimenopause?

Intriguing Parallels

Consider these four symptom clusters, which I have seen in several books recently:

I. fatigue, low energy level, joint pain, impaired reasoning, memory loss, depression, sleep disturbances, anxiety, irritability, muscle weakness, dizziness, balance problems, lethargy, difficulty concentrating, low sex drive, joint aches, insomnia, chronic infections, chronic sinusitis, vision changes, menstrual irregularities, menstrual cramps, vaginal itching, vaginal burning, mood swings, irritability, feeling foggy mentally, difficulty concentrating, short attention span, diarrhea and/or constipation, bloating, indigestion, chemical sensitivities, appetite changes, cravings for certain foods

---

II. fatigue, low energy level, joint aches and pains, insomnia, bladder irritations and infections, intermittent diarrhea, episodic constipation, bloating, indigestion, allergic reactions, chemical intolerance, skin eruptions, chronic sinusitis, menstrual irregularities, severe menstrual cramps, vaginal discharge, vaginal itching, low sex drive, painful intercourse, rectal itching, vision changes, dry eyes, depression, irritability, angry outbursts, mood swings, migraine headaches, mental fogging, inability to concentrate, loss of memory, loss of alertness, feeling of spaciness, short attention span, restless sleep, appetite changes, alcohol and sweet cravings, dry brittle hair, dry eyes, dry skin

---

III. menstrual irregularities, severe menstrual cramps, vision changes, dry eyes, chronic sinusitis, joint aches and pains, insomnia, bladder irritations and infections, intermittent diarrhea occurring along with episodic constipation, bloating, indigestion, allergic reactions, chemical intolerance, food cravings—especially sweets, skin eruptions, vaginal discharge, vaginal itching, low sex drive, painful intercourse, rectal itching, fatigue, depression, irritability, angry outbursts, mood swings, migraine headaches, mental fogging, inability to concentrate, loss of memory, loss of alertness, feeling spacey, short attention span, low energy, fragmented sleep

IV. mental fogging, inability to concentrate, loss of memory, loss of alertness, feeling spacey, short attention span, low energy, fatigue, depression, irritability, angry outbursts, mood swings, migraine headaches, bladder irritations and infections, intermittent diarrhea occurring along with episodic constipation, bloating, indigestion, allergic reactions, chemical intolerance, skin eruptions, vaginal discharge, vaginal itching, low sex drive, painful intercourse, rectal itching, menstrual irregularities, severe menstrual cramps, vision changes, dry eyes, chronic sinusitis, joint aches and pains, insomnia

Now, see if you can match the symptom cluster, I–IV, with the proper "diagnosis" from the list below:

A. Candida albicans ("Candidiasis")
B. Hypothyroidism
C. Menopausal Syndrome
D. Chronic Fatigue Syndrome (or Epstein-Barr Syndrome)
E. Anemia
F. Major Depressive Illness
G. None of these

Did you get them all correct? Not sure?
The correct answer is: *Any one of the clusters I through IV may occur with any of the illnesses, A through G!*

One of the reasons I wanted you to think about all of these different syndromes and the multiple symptoms which can be produced is that you are seeing the importance of the total picture, instead of just approaching "diagnoses" based upon a list of symptoms. Western-trained physicians, Chinese medicine practitioners, homeopaths, chiropractors, herbalists, naturopaths, and other alternative practitioners all have one practice in common: *they are trained to treat people based on a cluster of symptoms*, whether the treatment used is pharmaceutical medications, herbs, homeopathic remedies, manipulation, or any other modality.

Granted, symptom clusters are *extremely important* in leading one to a particular type of disorder to decide what treatment options will be helpful. We cannot use just symptoms alone, however, because a wide variety of illnesses and imbalances may produce similar kinds of physical and psychological changes. The problem is that when you are faced with *any illness* or major biological change affecting the brain and body, you will see a wide range of symptoms. This is due to the fact that many body systems that are affected by imbalances produced by various stimuli, or *stressors*.

The stressors can be hormonal change, viruses infecting the body, bacteria overgrowth, "yeast" overgrowth, environmental pollutants, medications, or herbs. I have had patients with the symptom list above who were toxic from multiple vitamin and herbal supplements. Another example I have encountered in my practice is chronic insecticide exposure: it may lead to a clinical picture indistinguishable from Chronic Fatigue Syndrome (CFS), hypothyroidism, or menopausal syndrome.

Our problem, particularly in women's health, is that both patients and physicians have been taught to look for A cause of AN illness based on A list of symptoms. That's not quite how our body works. The *"fight or flight"* stress response produces the same body reactions ("symptoms") whether you are faced with an oncoming grizzly bear, an oncoming car, fear about financial collapse, a rapid fall in blood sugar, or a rapid fall in estrogen before your period.

That's why I think it is crucial for women to have a hormonal evaluation as part of the diagnostic process when they are experiencing a group of diverse symptoms. If you are working with a non-M.D. health practitioner, I think it is important for you to have a good diagnostic evaluation by an M.D. or D.O. first, so you know more clearly *what* it is you are treating. I made sure I had my herniated discs treated with what Western medicine had to offer (in my case, surgery) *so I could walk again*, and then I used a whole range of complementary therapies to get well again.

The syndromes I listed at the beginning of this chapter are all examples of ones that are difficult to diagnose with certainty because they produce a variety of symptoms. The best treatment options for you will vary depending upon which condition is the primary one triggering the symptoms. Two that often come up in my work with mid-life women are **Chronic Fatigue Syndrome (CFS)** and **Candida albicans (Candida)**.

There are a number of good resources to read further about both CFS and Candida. There simply isn't room in this book for me to go into all that we know and don't know about these syndromes. However, before you jump to a conclusion that you have one of these problems based on symptoms alone, I strongly encourage you to have a thorough medical checkup to rule out other common problems such as subclinical hypothyroidism and declining ovarian hormone production, which can mimic these other two syndromes. Both of these hormonal factors are _usually overlooked_.

Whether the initial trigger is a viral infection, yeast overgrowth, hormone changes, or other stressors on the brain-body, there is strong evidence that the resulting debilitating syndromes happen primarily due to the **accumulation** of stressors, which have adversely impacted on the immune system and the neuromodulators that coordinate functions of the brain and body organ systems. A brain-mediated mechanism would explain the diversity of clinical symptoms, and the overlap we see in the way in which these disorders manifest in different individuals. I do think that if we look for _common patterns_ in all of these, instead of just listing symptoms, it will assist us develop integrated approaches to helping women feel well again.

We are now finding that serotonin-augmenting medications help reduce the symptoms of many of these disorders. I am sorry that these medications are called "antidepressants," because they are much broader in their beneficial effects than this term would suggest. I prefer to call them _"serotonin-boosters."_ In addition, many different modalities which boost endorphins and seratonin such as acupuncture, relaxation training, biofeedback, and massage therapy—are also helpful in alleviating some of the symptoms of CFS, Candida, Perimenopause, and Depression. These common threads provide further support to the theory of a brain-mediated mechanism creating a cascade of events triggering multiple effects in many body systems.

What Are Epstein-Barr Syndrome and CFS?

First described by Drs. Paul Cheney and Daniel Peterson of Incline Village, Nevada, in 1984, Chronic Fatigue Syndrome (CFS) was initially dismissed as "yuppie flu." Many physicians are skeptical that it is a "real" disorder, and the condition has been shrouded in controversy, since researchers have been unable to identify a cause, predict its course, or find very many effective treatments. It was initially thought to be due to a chronic infection with Epstein-Barr virus, a type of herpes virus that triggers mononucleosis ("the kissing disease") commonly seen in teenagers and young adults. In the past, CFS was thought to be a more chronic form of infectious mononucleosis. More recently, CFS has been attributed to a variety of viral causes—the herpes group (EBV, herpes simplex oral and genital), cytomegalovirus (CMV), as well as possibly Candida albicans, a yeast. There has not been any *one* cause that has been clearly demonstrated in the research to date. Other stressors to the body's immune system have also been implicated in CFS: environmental pollutants, toxic chemicals (some of the ones many people use around their own homes), and prolonged stressful situations. Illnesses like depression and generalized anxiety that stress the immune system have also been considered to play a role in CFS.

At present, CFS has been given a "working definition" by the Centers for Disease Control (CDC) as follows: "new onset persistent or relapsing, debilitating fatigue lasting at least six months in a person with no previous history of similar symptoms." Numerous other clinical conditions that could produce similar symptoms *must be excluded* before giving a diagnosis of CFS: malignancy; autoimmune diseases; bacterial, fungal, parasitic, or viral disease; chronic psychiatric disease (depression in particular); chronic inflammatory disease; neuromuscular disease; endocrine disease; drug abuse; side effects of chronic medication or other toxic agent. Simply ruling out all of these can in itself be expensive and exhausting. These are considered the Major Criteria, and must be met for the diagnosis of CFS.

The CDC has also included the following Minor Criteria for CFS, at least *eight* of which must be present: mild fever, sore throat, painful anterior or posterior cervical (neck) or axillary (underarm) lymph nodes, unexplained generalized muscle weakness, muscle discomfort (myalgia), generalized fatigue for at least twenty-four hours after previously tolerated exercise, generalized headaches unlike any previous pain, migratory arthralgia without joint swelling or redness, sleep disturbance, a main symptom complex arising within hours or days, presence of neuropsychologic symptoms (such as mood changes, forgetfulness, confusion, difficulty concentrating, depressed mood, and others). Many of these same findings occur as a result of declining ovary hormones in perimenopause, so it seems plausible to me to check this factor.

Hormonal Decline: An Unrecognized Cause of Fatigue

Seventy percent of patients with CFS are women. I think it is crucial to look at what hormonal changes could be playing a role in this enormous gender difference in incidence of CFS. In all the medical articles I have read on CFS, however, *I have not yet seen one address this issue.* In one recent study of the characteristics of CFS patients, 60 percent were female and the average age was 41.9 years—

Do you see possible clues here? Pre(peri)menopause changes can *begin* about a decade before menopause; shouldn't *this* be considered??? The amazing thing to me is that the two investigators for this study were *both female physicians* and there was **not one word about hormonal factors mentioned anywhere in this medical article!**

In the discussion summarizing these study results, there was not even a comment that checking hormonal factors was important in future research. I was shocked at the time, although when I think about it now, I probably shouldn't be . . . it seems everywhere in medicine, physicians and researchers have had blinders on when it comes to looking at hormones that make a woman's body different from a man's. The same researchers also studied patients with fibromyalgia: 90 percent were female, and the average age was 44.0 years. Do you see another clue here? Again, nothing mentioned about hormones. We have a **long** way to go!

Keep in mind a point I made in earlier chapters about the dramatic and profoundly disruptive effects on sleep caused by declining estrogen levels. The sleep changes may begin as much as eight to ten years *before* menses cease. Sleep deprivation causes suppression of the immune system, and more obviously, is a major factor in causing persistent *fatigue*. It seems so obvious to me, I don't understand why there aren't a wealth of articles on these connections in the medical literature. Menopause may not explain why CFS occurs in males, but if 60 to 70 percent of the patients with CFS are women, wouldn't it make sense to try and help the majority of sufferers who are female by checking for hormonal factors?

In the same vein, what if we looked into what's happening to *male* hormone levels in men with CFS? I haven't seen a formal study of that connection either. I bring this observation to your attention in the hope that you will ask your physician to look into these possible hormonal factors if you think you may have one of these syndromes. It is tragic, in my opinion, that we overlook something so obvious that can be addressed in some fairly straightforward therapeutic ways.

Hormone Effects on Energy Levels and Sleep Cycles

I had a physician colleague call and ask if I would do a consult for his wife. He was very worried about the changes he had seen in her over the previous few months. In his words, "She has always been such a cheerful, outgoing, high energy person. On the go, exercising every day, and normally *very* even in her moods. She's always been a pretty happy person. I don't know what has happened. She's only forty-three and she still has periods. She saw her gynecologist who started her on hormones, but she's continued to get more depressed and talks about how tired she is. She doesn't even have the energy to exercise, and that's *really* not like her." He was concerned that she had Chronic Fatigue Syndrome and wanted to be sure that I considered that diagnosis along with checking for possible side effects of the hormonal regimen she was taking.

When I met with his wife in the spring of 1994, she described experiencing severe depressive symptoms, mood swings with a lot of irritability, and sudden tearfulness for no apparent reason. She also reported decreased energy, hot flashes, insomnia, diffuse arthralgias, myalgias, marked fatigue (she said "this is really unusual for me; I'm such a high energy person. I feel like I've had a long bout with the flu"), difficulties having orgasm, and diminished libido ("and I used to really enjoy sex, but I just don't have any energy for it because I'm so tired all the time").

I'll give you just the highlights of a comprehensive evaluation, which in her situation did not have to involve extensive laboratory testing for reasons that will become clear as you read on. Her father, to whom she had been very close, had died a year and a half earlier. This had been a major loss for her, but she felt she had "come through the grief pretty well." She also had been having times of heavy menstrual bleeding, so her gynecologist had done a

D&C in the spring of 1993, and then started her on Loestrin to keep her periods lighter and reduce problems with cramps.

Loestrin is a brand of oral contraceptive with a higher progestin content relative to the amount of ethinyl estradiol estrogen. She had been on these for about a year by the time I saw her. This was one reason it was not necessary to check her hormone levels, since oral contraceptives (OC's) suppress the ovaries' hormone production. She said, "I did pretty well at first, and then I just started becoming more and more fatigued, depressed, and lethargic." She had noticed that her depressed mood, irritability and low energy had become significantly worse about two months before her husband called me.

After her evaluation was completed, I told her I thought that I did not think she had a true CFS syndrome, although I couldn't conclusively eliminate this because there are not any good diagnostic tests for CFS. I explained that I thought one important issue was the timing of her symptoms relative to beginning the particular OC (Loestrin), which was higher in progestin and low in estrogen, and I thought our first step should be to see how she did on an OC with the reverse ratio: higher estrogen and lower progestin. Then, if that didn't lead to improvement, we would consider an antidepressant to improve her sleep, mood, and energy level. She and her husband agreed that this "step-wise" approach made sense, so I changed her oral contraceptive to one I thought would do better for her. I started her on Ovcon 35 which has much less progestin than Loestrin, and slightly more of the estrogen component. I have to admit, however, that I thought she would likely also need an antidepressant, due to the severity of her symptoms.

At her first follow-up appointment two weeks later, she said the following:

> *I feel like I've come back from the cellar. I'm not crying, I don't feel depressed, I have my energy, I don't have the headaches, I feel like someone flipped a switch on me. It was remarkable to feel well again in such a short period of time. When I first talked with you, I felt like I knew why people committed suicide, I just knew I couldn't continue like I was feeling, even though suicide isn't an action I would take. This is amazing.*

Needless to say, both of us were pleased at how well she felt, and I did not think it was necessary to start an antidepressant.

At the next visit, about two months later, she said she felt "totally back to my old self" and had none of the previous problems. Her muscle aches had gone, and she was back to her usual exercise regimen, which included weight-lifting three times a week. The only thing she had noticed was some breast fullness and tenderness, but then said "that's a minor problem compared to how I felt before. I don't want you to change a thing!" A few weeks later, I got the following FAX from her, which pretty much says it all better than I could:

> Dr. Vliet:
> As per our conversation . . . these are the dramatic changes I have experienced with the change of hormone therapy (as prescribed by you): I no longer experience insomnia, swimming in the head, incredible unhappiness, hot flashes, night sweats, joint pain, palpitations at rest, utter fatigue, feelings of absolute hopelessness, unexplainable depression with thoughts of suicide, nonproductivity, low self esteem, lack of uncontrollable humor and playfulness, terrible witch-like mood swings, short temper, lack of sexual interest, difficulty in reaching orgasm, thoughts of my husband losing interest in me, indecisiveness, inability to concentrate, not being interested in exercising and not wanting to do anything with anybody for any reason . . . YUK.
>
> Now, I am incredibly back to normal. I feel strong and hopeful . . . I'm vibrant with color. It is difficult to believe I was viewing the world in black and white . . . Gray is such a nasty color. I lost all hope for everything.
>
> I'm back to exercising a couple hours a day, and weightlifting is back in my routine. I'm currently contemplating boxercise at home . . making calls to find out who has the best equipment.
>
> Before the change of hormones, life had very little meaning to me. Napping and unexplainable sobbing were two big menu choices for me.
>
> Excitement and thrills of a new day await me now. No person or thing can break my stride, and I am on the move. Thank you Dr. Vliet for your expertise in this area.
> > D.

This patient ended up having a total of three appointments with me, including the initial visit. I don't know why her usual physician did not consider trying a different OC formulation, but this patient's situation is an almost daily occurrence in my practice. It just makes sense to me to think through the alternatives and try a different approach if one birth control pill formula isn't working.

Hormonal balance is certainly not going to be the *only* answer for everyone with fatigue or depression, but for women in their forties, it certainly seems like a good place to start! In addition, whenever the symptom pattern begins in conjunction with starting new medication, I think it is always important to look to the medication as a possible cause of unwanted changes, as well as to evaluate other possibilities.

Other physicians, and some women, have said it is too expensive to check the hormone aspects. Now I ask you, which was more "expensive" for the woman above—continuing on the way she was going, or looking for resources to help get answers? What price do you put on *your* good health? What price do we put on women's health collectively? Don't you think these are issues which deserve attention?

Changing Hormone Balance: A Factor in "Yeast" Infections and Syndromes

Chronic Candida has been another of the "women's diseases" which is purported to cause over a hundred different symptoms in multiple body systems. It was popularized by the 1985 book *The Yeast Connection*, based on the work of Drs. Crook and Truss. The mainstream medical community remains skeptical of the existence of a true "chronic yeast syndrome," since there are no well-done studies to document it, and we all have Candida albicans and related organisms throughout the genital and intestinal tracts as part of the normal flora. On the other hand, the mainstream medical community has also remained skeptical of hormonal factors in women triggering syndromes like PMS and migraines! You can't find a connection if you don't look for it!

Dr. Truss was the originator of the "yeast theory," and Dr. Crook has developed these ideas further. I think there is merit to what they have presented, but I also think many people "over-diagnose" yeast syndromes, since the hormonal aspects that cause similar symptoms are rarely addressed. Somewhere between the extremes of over-enthusiasm and overskepticism, there lies the reality—we just don't yet know what it is. The advantage of what Dr. Crook is describing in his book is that most of what he recommends is based on dietary change, eliminating use of repeated cycles of antibiotics, and other basic measures which carry little risk and may be very helpful to women with recurrent vaginal yeast problems.

I will not go into more depth on the various symptoms and management approaches in my book, but I do want to explore the possible relationship to hormone changes. Once again, we are dealing with a possible "syndrome" that occurs *predominately* in women and more often in the *midlife* years. Like other disorders more common in women, might this one have a connection with the decreases in female hormones? Let's explore this issue.

Allergies, herpes outbreaks, yeast infections, sinusitis, and asthma; all of these health problems typically are aggravated premenstrually and have to do with some of the very significant physiological changes that occur with the hormonal shifts each month. Most physicians can tell you that they see a relationship, but there haven't been good studies to try and identify some of the specific reasons for it. Hormonal balance alters immune system function, with *more optimal* immune function in the first half (estrogen-dominant) phase of the menstrual cycle. Changing hormone levels also alter many other body chemistry balances, which may contribute to the increased frequency of allergies, yeast, and herpes outbreaks premenstrually.

One thing many women don't realize is that during their thirties and forties, the changes in ovary hormone production alter the pH balance of the tissue lining the vagina, which in turn upsets the bacterial balance of the "normal flora," a medical term to describe the healthy, "good" bacteria which keep excess yeast in check. The summary below shows other factors which change the pH and bacterial balance in the vagina and intestinal tract, **making Candida ("yeast infections") more likely to occur:**

- diet: high-carbohydrate diets, especially if the carbohydrate source is refined sugars
- progesterone excess, or high progestin birth control pills
- stress: alters levels of many different hormones that affect pH of mucosal linings in the mouth, vagina, and intestinal tract
- excess alcohol consumption
- chronic or repeated use of antibiotics
- regular use of corticosteroids, such as cortisone, prednisone, etc.
- cigarette smoking
- stimulant abuse: has effects similar to, *but greater than*, chronic stress (diet pills, cocaine, caffeine abuse, etc.)

Another aspect to the potential "vicious cycle" with Candida is that declining estrogen contributes to pH and other changes that make yeast infections more common, AND the presence of excessive Candida organisms further *decreases* available estrogen, making the entire problem worse. It has been hypothesized that Candida organisms may actually bind the estrogen and prevent it from plugging into the body's estrogen receptor sites, producing an additional estrogen deficit in the body. What an awful double whammy. It's like adding insult to injury. If you are taking progesterone supplements or using progesterone skin cream, the Candida problem can be made even worse because progesterone helps *increase the available blood glucose*, allowing the Candida to flourish even more. Another vicious cycle!

Obviously I have not given you here an exhaustive review of Candida syndromes. I just wanted to raise your "index of suspicion" about possible overlooked hormonal connections, which you may want to consider if you have been experiencing repeated vaginal yeast infections, or if you think you may have a broader problem with yeast. I find that the repeated vaginal yeast problems at least *improve*, if not resolve, once a more normal hormonal balance is reached. I think it is worth having checked before you take repeated courses of antibiotics or the more potent antifungal drugs.

If you are presently taking a high progestin birth control pill and are having recurring vaginal yeast problems, talk with your physician about changing to a lower progestin pill and see if this helps. If you are on a menopausal hormone regimen using a synthetic progestin, ask your doctor about reducing the dose or changing to natural progesterone instead and see if this helps. If you are using large amounts of progesterone supplements for PMS treatment, talk with your health provider about trying to achieve a more normal physiological balance with adequate estrogen. There are a number of safe and relatively simple hormonal changes which may provide some relief from such an annoying health problem.

Heading into the Future

As we think about health care reform and what women's health needs must be addressed, clearly heavily female-predominant problems such as CFS will become significant concerns from both *quality of life* and *economic* points of view. In Australia, where the health care system makes it much easier to collect data on cost issues, CFS represents a staggering **$59 million** cost to their society **annually.** *Each individual patient* incurs medical costs, on average, of **$9,429.** The potential burden on the health care system—both financially and for delivery of health care services—is potentially enormous from CFS alone. Now do you suppose it *might* make sense to look at the hormone factor here . . .?

CHAPTER 9

It Went Right out of My Head: Menopause and Memory

Women's Fears: Am I Getting Alzheimer's?

During my residency at Johns Hopkins, one of the specialty rotations was the Dementia Research Program. I remember being very struck upon learning that dementias of all kinds are about *four times more common in elderly women* compared to elderly men of the *same* age. At the time of my specialty training, no one had any explanation for this marked difference in dementia rates between women and men. I was bothered by this statistic, but like many diseases more common in women, there simply wasn't any research to try and uncover the causes. It now strikes me as odd that researchers were not thinking about studying female hormone effects on the brain, since the gender differences were so striking.

Based on current projections, a female born in 1994 has a *one in six chance* of developing Alzheimer's, if she lives to an average life expectancy of about eighty years. For women, this lifetime risk is greater than the lifetime risk of breast cancer! A male born in 1994, who lives to the average male life expectancy, has a *one in sixteen chance*. It's about time we begin to research the role of decline in estrogen after menopause as a possible factor in women's higher rates of dementia. Finally, this needed research is underway, particularly in Canada, Australia and Japan, and a few studies in the U.S.

Dementia is a term that means generalized loss of the brain's ability to retain, perceive, integrate, utilize, retrieve and act appropriately on information, called *cognitive function*. It is a group of brain diseases with *many* different causes. Some types of dementia are treatable and reversible if the cause is caught early. An example is hypothyroidism, which diminishes cognitive function if left untreated, but is reversible if treated with thyroid hormone replacement. Alzheimer's disease is another type of dementia that involves progressive, irreversible degeneration of global brain function. At present, we do not have any treatments that restore normal brain abilities in Alzheimer's patients. If the early studies hold true, and estrogen does turn out to have a major role in preventing some of the neuron loss in certain dementias, including Alzheimer's, it will be a major breakthrough in providing hope for those who have a high risk of these diseases.

Milder forms of memory changes that women describe during perimenopause *are generally <u>not</u> the more serious dementia syndromes*. Dementia is an *illness* which affects about 10 percent of the population on average. Menopause, of course, is a *normal transition* for all women who live long enough, and does NOT alone cause dementia. But if hormonal decline in women is *one contributing factor* that would help explain the gender differences, then we need to consider this is discussing therapeutic options for an individual woman.

Over the years, as I worked with hormonal effects on many parts of the body and the effects on brain-mediated phenomena, I began to wonder whether hormonal changes in women were more of a factor than we had thought. When women talked about memory changes, and I inquired about when these problems were worse, they typically said "before my period" or "during my flow." These menstrual cycle phases are times of declining or low estrogen. Women's descriptions have been *so uniform* in the way they have talked about what they notice with memory related to these menstrual phases that I felt certain it was not all due to life stress or women being oversensitive to body-mind changes. I became convinced that there is an important effect of estrogen on memory. Fortunately, in the last several years, there are a number of new research studies in animals and humans that show some of the ways estrogen works in the brain to maintain normal memory function. I will describe these later in this chapter. But first, listen to the "voices" of these women.

In My Office: Women's Stories

I remember the poignant first appointment with Ann, a forty-six year old homemaker and community leader, who sat in my consult room in tears as she admitted her most terrifying fear:

My mother died of Alzheimer's and it began when she was in her early fifties. I'm beginning to have memory problems, and I'm so embarrassed. I'm afraid someone will notice, and deep inside I'm really afraid it's the beginning of Alzheimer's for me too. I can't seem to focus on my lists like I used to, I forget names, I go to say a word I know and suddenly it's not there and I feel stupid. I can't seem to add like I used to, and my mind wanders a lot. I'm really frightened. I just don't want to end up like my mother. What's happening to me?

I do everything right, and I really try to take care of my health, there's just nothing in my lifestyle to cause this memory problem. That's why I'm sure it must be the beginning of Alzheimer's. What can I do?

Her mother had an earlier menopause at about age forty-six and then was told she had Alzheimer's dementia at age fifty-five. Her sister's menopause was at age forty-seven. Ann had a hysterectomy four years earlier at age forty-three, but had not had her ovaries removed. She was in good health, was not overweight, did not smoke cigarettes, rarely drank alcohol, exercised aerobically four to five days a week, and also followed a weight-training program. She even made sure she took all the vitamins that were supposed to help memory! She really was "doing everything right."

Kay, a fifty-one year old writer, was disturbed by her growing awareness of difficulty finding the right words for her articles, as well as having trouble keeping her attention focused on getting a story finished on deadline. She described her observations:

My thoughts are fragmented, and I get distracted so easily. I never used to be like that. I was always one of the most focused people I know. My husband said I could tune out a freight train coming through the room. Now I feel like the slightest thing distracts me. I feel like my mind is flying in a million directions. What is happening to me? I'm really worried that I'm developing something like Alzheimer's. What can I do? I don't want to talk with my other doctors about this. They will just think I'm crazy, or tell me I'm under too much stress. But I've always lived with stress, and I used to thrive under the pressure of a deadline. That's when I did my best writing. I just don't understand this, and I'm frightened. This isn't me.

Kay had not yet gone through menopause, although she had noticed her time of bleeding getting shorter each month, and the flow had decreased significantly. She had less bloating and breast tenderness before her periods now but said her irritability and difficulty concentrating were clearly getting worse and seemed to be much more noticeable the few days before her period and the days she was having her menstrual flow. In the past, the week of bleeding had been a week she typically felt better. She had also noticed a marked loss of interest in sex, and said she felt more tired than usual for her. She had not noticed any hot flashes, but said she had "these funny tingly feelings, like something crawling on my arms, and they come and go." She thought she slept "pretty well." She did not smoke and drank wine occasionally when out to dinner. She had no other health problems, but did not exercise and was about ten pounds over her desired weight. Her mother went through menopause at fifty-four, and never took any hormones. About twelve years later in life, Kay said her mother became "senile," but she did not know any further information about what her mother's memory problems had been. Her mother died at seventy-one of a heart attack.

Both Ann and Kay had a common finding on their evaluations: each one had high FSH levels and *low* estradiol levels, typical of menopause. Both Ann and Kay had not thought they were menopausal. Kay was still menstruating (although her periods had gotten lighter, a clue that her estrogen was decreasing), and Ann's doctor had told her she was too young to be menopausal. Kay's doctor told her that since she was still menstruating her problems couldn't be due to menopause. And since neither woman had experienced any of the usual symptoms, such as hot flashes, they had not considered the idea of menopause. All of Ann's other laboratory studies were normal, but she did have a significant degree of bone loss for her age, in spite of her excellent health habits and exercise program. Kay's evaluation revealed no other health problems except a high cholesterol with a lower than desirable level of HDL.

Although it was the memory problems that brought each woman to see me, the bone loss for Ann and the cholesterol changes for Kay, along with the high FSH, were indications that each woman's estrogen had been declining for longer than either one was aware. After individually reviewing all of their evaluation data and talking in depth about their respective options, possible side effects, risks, potential benefits, and their specific desires, both Ann and Kay decided to try estrogen therapy. Ann wanted to be sure she took steps that would help prevent further bone loss, and Kay thought her risk of heart disease was high, given her own cholesterol picture and her mother's death from a heart attack.

I talked with each one about what we know about the effects of estradiol on brain centers governing memory. I explained that in my clinical work with women, I had seen noticeable improvements in memory if the estradiol levels were restored to the normal levels of the first half of usual menstrual cycles.

This was two years ago. Ann called a month after starting the estradiol, and in an upbeat voice, said *"it's better, I feel like I've got my own mind back again!"* By the time she had been on the estradiol for six months, she reported that all of the previous negative changes in her intellectual ability had now resolved.

I'm back to my normal self. I feel great. I didn't realize just how scared I had been than I might be getting Alzheimer's like my mother. I am so relieved to know that what was happening was just the hormone changes of menopause and it could be helped.

Kay also had a positive outcome: her cholesterol profile improved, and she described feeling that:

My ability to focus on my writing has dramatically improved. I didn't realize until I felt better just how much I had been slipping in my concentration. I can keep on track, the problem with words has gone, and I seem to do fine with organizing my thoughts again. I had no idea hormone drops at menopause could create such mental changes. Why doesn't anyone talk about this?

I think one reason not many physicians address these issues is that, in general, they have not been taught to think about the brain as a target organ of hormone changes. The focus has been on reproductive organs and the breast for the most part, with more recent attention turned to heart and bone health after estrogen declines. Frequently, when women ask health professionals about things like menory symptoms, the explanation is that memory and concentration changes are due to the stresses that women experience in this phase of life. As one woman succinctly put it, however,

Stress is ubiquitous throughout most women's lives, and the memory changes don't seem to be a problem in earlier years, so why *now*? It has to have some connection with hormone changes.

Consequently, since the questions and connections women think are important get written off, many are reluctant to talk any more about it, fearing they really are "going crazy" or developing some type of dementia. Often, they don't even want to admit to friends that these subtle changes are happening, so they end up experiencing their uncertainty and fear alone.

There was B.J., a fifty-one year old woman who wrote me a note after one of my seminars:

> I had not been told that memory problems could be related to menopause. No one explained about memory problems, libido changes, insomnia, etc. I was mainly told about hot flashes. I really didn't have anyone to talk to. None of my friends said they had these problems. Thanks for a wealth of information. It makes me feel better, I had really thought I was beginning to get Alzheimer's and it had really bothered me. Now I have some ideas to talk with my doctor about.

May was fifty-three when I saw her for a consultation. She had gone through menopause at forty-nine, and had started estrogen therapy shortly thereafter to help her severe hot flashes. She was also concerned about osteoporosis, since her mother had lost 2 inches in height in the years after menopause and had died of complications following a hip fracture in her late sixties. May had been on conjugated equine estrogens, 0.625 mg for twenty-five days a month, with a progestin added on days 16 through 25 of the month, since age forty-nine. She felt the estrogen had really helped her hot flashes and energy level, but she was concerned about continuing problems with memory. She talked about having trouble remembering what she had gone into a room to do, frequently forgot a word she was getting ready to say, had to write down telephone numbers as soon as she looked them up, and said she felt her brain "had a cloud pulled down over it. I just feel foggy, and that's not like me, what's happening?"

May's evaluation was normal on all the tests for other possible causes of her memory problems. Significantly, her estradiol was low and her FSH was still in the menopausal high range even though she was on estrogen therapy. She was a tall woman and very physically active. I thought there were potentially two factors to consider in fine-tuning her hormone therapy: first, I thought she may need a different amount of estrogen, given her body build and level of physical activity; second, I thought she would see a better improvement in the brain symptoms she was experiencing if she were taking the native human estradiol instead of the conjugated equine estrogens that she had been on so long.

In my clinical experience, I find that women generally have a better response on brain function using the native human estradiol since it fits, like a key in a lock, at the specific brain receptor sites which help to regulate memory and information processing. I suggested she change to 17-beta estradiol with an adequate amount for her, which we determined both by how she felt and her blood levels. In about a month, she reported that her memory and concentration were "greatly improved, I feel like I have my full abilities back. *It's hard to explain, but I just feel like my mind is clearer somehow.*"

I do not intend to sound like I think estrogen is a "cure-all" for memory problems. It isn't. But it is, however, one of the most frequently *overlooked* factors affecting memory function for women. There are still many questions to be answered about exactly how estrogen works in the brain and what types of estrogen are needed for these brain pathways. There are many, many types of medical disorders and lifestyle habits that can affect the brain and cause memory changes. Most importantly, if you are having these kinds of symptoms, you need a careful and complete medical evaluation for the various types of problems, hormonal and otherwise, which can result in these mental and physical changes. While I think probably all of us could use more time and practice in *relaxing*, I do not think that's the whole answer. **Body physiology affects brain function, too. It's that basic.**

We *have to listen to women*, and take their experiences and concerns seriously. For those of you reading this who have had memory problems, at least be aware that checking the hormonal factor is something important to address along with other approaches you may be taking. You don't have to sit there and be frightened that something terrible is happening to you. There are ways to properly and thoroughly address your questions and ways of arriving at feeling better. Speak up, and be heard!

Meanwhile, here's the latest information on estrogen effects on memory from worldwide research. The brain is truly an exciting frontier of hormone interactions and effects.

You Are Not Imagining It!
Menopause Does Affect Memory!

First Some Memory "Basics." To better understand what has been discovered about estrogen effects on memory, you will need to know some of the names of the brain areas involved in memory function, shown in the diagram below. Collectively, these structures make up the area called the *limbic system*, the mood-regulating area of the brain (rich in estradiol receptors, remember?) I described in

Chapters 3 and 4. Next to each of the memory-regulating structures, I have given an example of a disease process that typically affects that area of the brain and may cause memory disruption. The *temporal lobes* of the brain are major sites of these memory regulating centers, so you may also see this term in discussions of memory.

The complex components of our memory system have only recently been mapped out. It used to be thought that memory traces were spread throughout the brain and could not be localized to any particular structures. More recent studies have shown the primary components of the memory system in the brain are the *hippocampus*, the *mammillary bodies*, the *septal region* of the limbic system, and part of the *thalamus*. There is a great deal that remains to be understood about how these various memory processes work in the human brain, but at present the memory system appears to consist of "storage centers," which are located symmetrically in both hemispheres of the brain, primarily in the hippocampus and mammillary bodies. These centers in several parts of the brain provide "back-up systems" to prevent memory from being damaged or lost.

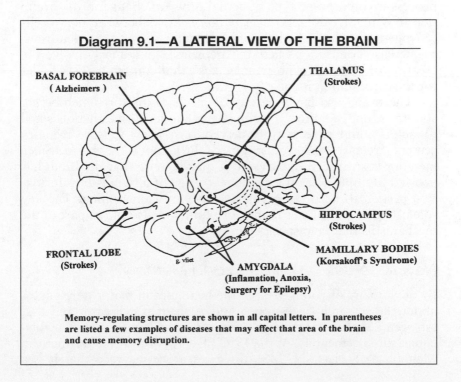

Diagram 9.1—A LATERAL VIEW OF THE BRAIN

BASAL FOREBRAIN
(Alzheimers)

THALAMUS
(Strokes)

HIPPOCAMPUS
(Strokes)

MAMILLARY BODIES
(Korsakoff's Syndrome)

FRONTAL LOBE
(Strokes)

g. vliet

AMYGDALA
(Inflamation, Anoxia,
Surgery for Epilepsy)

Memory-regulating structures are shown in all capital letters. In parentheses are listed a few examples of diseases that may affect that area of the brain and cause memory disruption.

If one hemisphere of the brain is damaged or injured, memory will remain intact as long as the other hemisphere has not been injured. If *both* hemispheres of the brain involving memory centers are injured severely enough, the person has lost the ability to learn new material and store it for future retrieval. Memory function, having multiple memory circuitry centers in various parts of the brain, is thereby different from other brain functions, which tend to have more specific locations in one or the other hemisphere.

There are several different types of memory, but to simplify this we can conceptualize memory as short term memory or long term memory. *Short term memory* comes into use in many day-to-day situations, for example when you hear a telephone number or a name and remember it just long enough to use it. When a name, number or other piece of information is something you wish to remember for a longer period of time, it is converted to *long-term memory*. The hippocampus and mammillary bodies, along with the anterior thalamus and septal region, appear to be the major centers involved in converting short-term to long-term memory. The research at present does tend to suggest that this conversion process involves some type of actual *physical* change in the brain, that may involve creation of *new connections* between nerve cells (estrogen stimulates growth of these new sprouts, or dendrites, to increase connections between neurons), or it may involve the creation of actual "memory molecules" that contain specific codes for the information involved.

The brain also has a variety of mechanisms for remembering specific sound (auditory), sight (visual) touch (kinesthetic), smell (olfactory), and other sensory perceptions. These sensory memory centers are also widely distributed throughout the brain. Since memory is so crucial to survival, it makes sense that the brain has evolved multiple areas for memory storage of all kinds of information needed to keep the organism alive and functioning. The key role of the sex hormones in memory function also fits as part of the mechanisms that help species survive.

New Research on Estrogen and Memory

By now, many of you have seen the headlines in major newspapers about the research on estrogen and Alzheimer's disease, and that estrogen deficiency may play an important role in causing, or worsening, some dementias. At the 1993 meeting of the North American Menopause Society (NAMS), three researchers agreed that it is a significant, and underrated, factor in some of these aging-related disorders. Dr. Stanley Birge and his associates from Washington University in St. Louis believe that the new research findings support the theory that estrogen loss at menopause contributes, along with genetic and environmental factors, to the deterioration of the central nervous system known as Alzheimer's disease and, potentially, other types of memory changes. Dr. Birge's studies have also found that women over seventy who take estrogen have an improved ability in a balancing exercise, "tandem stance," compared to women not on estrogen. He hypothesized that estrogen deficiency, through effects on postural reflexes and balance, may be a factor contributing to the unusually high rates of falls in elderly women.

Dr. Barbara Sherwin, at MacGill University in Canada, has spent a number of years researching estrogen effects on the brain and her studies have shown improvements specifically in *verbal* memory in healthy postmenopausal women on estrogen compared to those who are not. In a separate study, Dr. Sherwin prospectively evaluated surgically menopausal women and found that those treated with estrogen did significantly better on several measures of cognitive function than the women given a placebo. Yet another prospective study of surgically menopausal women showed that taking estradiol specifically enhanced short-term verbal memory. None of these women had any type of dementia; they were all healthy postmenopausal and would not have been considered *impaired* in their memory abilities. Yet, the improved performance in the women on estrogen therapy was statistically significant and also fits with the self-reports I have heard consistently from patients in my practice.

At the Baylor College of Medicine and VA Medical Center in Houston, Dr. Karl Mortel studied postmenopausal women who were either neurologically normal or had mild cerebrovascular disease (CVD), which had manifested as transient ischemic attacks (brief periods of decreased oxygen causing symptoms similar to a mild stroke). He found that among women with CVD, women on estrogen therapy showed improved blood flow to the brain and improved cognitive function compared to the women with CVD who were not on estrogen. He concluded that estrogen therapy may be an effective addition to the treatment of older women with impaired circulation. His work fits with other research that has shown estradiol to have a *relaxing effect* on arteries, leading to more dilation and better blood flow to all organs in the body.

Three years ago at the North American Menopause Society meeting, several researchers from Japan presented evidence of estrogen's ability to *improve* cognitive function in elderly women who already had developed Alzheimer's dementia. Dr. N. Hagino found that two-thirds of the fifteen study patients improved significantly in their communication with families, their ability for self care, memory for time and daily events. At the time, this research presentation did not get a lot of media attention. Since that meeting, we have seen a marked increase in the interest in, and attention given to, estrogen effects on brain function with additional studies now underway in the United States.

In an ongoing study of 8,879 female residents of Leisure World, a retirement community in California, researchers at University of Southern California (USC) studied the medical records of those who died during the period from 1982 to 1991, and found 127 women whose death certificates mentioned either Alzheimer's disease or dementia. These cases were then matched with those of the other women the same age who had *not* died of dementia. The resulting 635 cases were assigned to one of two groups: those women who had taken estrogen and those who had not. The researchers found that the estrogen users were 40 percent **less likely** to die of Alzheimer's disease or dementia than women who had not taken estrogen. Another way of looking at it, the women on estrogen ran only about 60 percent of the risk of getting Alzheimer's women had who did not take estrogen.

The USC investigators further found that the higher the maximum reported dose of the estrogen, the *lower* the risk of Alzheimer's. The risk of dementia also *decreased* with a longer duration of estrogen therapy. Women who had been on estrogen 7 years or more had *only 50 percent of the risk of dementia* seen in women who did not receive ERT. JoAnn McConnell, senior vice president for medical and scientific affairs of the Alzheimer's Association in Chicago, said "I think that these are very interesting results, and stronger than prior hints for an effect of estrogen." These results are preliminary but bring up potentially important additional considerations in weighing the decision about hormone therapy for women who have a family history of dementia.

How does estrogen work on the brain? A number of studies argue for a direct effect of estrogen on memory, specifically on verbal memory, and there appear to be a number of neurochemical and structural ways estrogen exerts its effect. The biochemical and nerve structure studies have been done in animals. While animal studies cannot always be extrapolated to humans, what we have learned about rat brains in other areas of research seems to also apply to human brains at the biochemical level. There is no practical way to measure these types of biochemical and nerve cell structural changes in people, so the animal research provides a working model of what to look for in humans in later clinical trials. Dr. Bruce McEwen, head of Rockefeller University Neuroendocrinology Laboratory in New York, has done extensive research on the effects of estrogen on brain tissue, and has found that:

- 17-beta-estradiol, the primary estrogen produced by the ovary, has specific receptor binding sites in many different areas of the brain, and these receptor sites appear to be quite *specific* for the native human form of the molecule. (All of my clinical work with patients strongly supports Dr. McEwen's findings in animal models.)

- estradiol promotes the growth of new dendrites between nerve cells (to make more synaptic connections), while progesterone breaks down the nerve cell connections. [Author's note: the more synapse connections, the more incoming signals the nerve cells can handle.]

- when estradiol declines, synapse density in the hippocampus (memory and learning center) decreases as well. [Denser synapses allow better cell-to-cell information flow.]

- estradiol enhances nerve cells' ability to take in *nerve growth factor (NGF)*. In animals without ovaries, those who did *not* receive estrogen had a marked (56 percent) decline in the number of nerve cells; the animals given estrogen had only a slight decrease in nerve cells.

- estrogens regulate cholinergic nerve cells in the *basal forebrain* of rodents. [This is one of the regions of the brain involved in cognitive function and one of the areas that degenerates in humans with Alzheimer's disease.]

- estrogens increase the production of choline acetyltransferase, an enzyme needed to make acetylcholine (ACh). Estrogen thereby prevents the marked loss of ACh found in patients with Alzheimer's. [ACh is the brain's most important chemical messenger for storing new memories in the brain, regulating memory retrieval and cognition. Loss of the cholinergic nerves and chemical messengers is the most marked of the brain changes in Alzheimer's disease.]

Dr. McEwen and other neuroendocrine researchers have concluded that the brain is an important target organ for estrogens and that effects on the brain functions, such as memory and cognition, must be considered in relation to the decline of estrogens in women after natural or surgical menopause. I agree. I think its time we looked at the brain as connected to the body and affected by the same kinds of changes that affect other parts of the body! Psychological symptoms, like memory changes, clearly may have *physical causes* as well as stress-related causes. Listen to the comments of these women who experienced the benefits on memory that came from making appropriate changes in their estrogen therapy:

> After a hysterectomy at age fifty-two, I took Premarin for nearly eight years. My memory began to deteriorate. Never one to be particularly concerned about getting old, I made fun of it at first. I reached a point, however, around age fifty-six when my memory loss was downright embarrassing. I felt I was in a mental fog. I couldn't remember common words, stumbled through sentences, lost my train of thought, had difficulty following complex conversations or instructions, and even skipped words when I wrote. My work suffered and I could tell my family and friends were being kind and patient with me. Loving and generous of them, but humiliating for me. Dr. Vliet suggested I use Estrace for my hormone replacement therapy. In a short time, I began to notice I was no longer constantly apologizing for lapses in speech and memory. The fog had lifted. Of course, my memory isn't what it was when I was twenty, but I have regained my pride and self-confidence. At last, I'm enjoying this stage of my life and all it has to offer.
>
> —A.F., age 62

I later received the following letter from this patient's mother, who is in her eighties, after she had seen the improvement in her daughter from the change in type of estrogen:

> I believe the first thing I noticed after changing from Premarin to Estrace was a cloud lifting from my skull (mind). Prior to that I seemed to be going around in a perpetual fog, never feeling as though I was thinking clearly. That was such a relief! I seemed to remember things much more clearly, not stumbling over names that I had known for years, once again being able to reconcile my bank accounts and being able to reply to questions that had previously left me with complete blanks. One of the things that had bothered me a lot was the shaking of my hands. There were days when I could hardly make out checks and when I finished, they looked like some person with palsy had written them and were almost illegible. Physically, I feel 100 percent better, and I am so grateful to you for recommending the Estrace to my daughter so I could ask my own doctor to make the change for me.
>
> —F.L., in her eighties

Don't suffer in silence. Know that help is available, and there are a number of such changes in hormone therapy which can improve your memory and clarity of thinking if you are having these problems.

Thyroid Changes and Memory

After about age forty, women have approximately *five to eight times* the incidence of thyroid disorders found in men of similar ages. We do not yet have a clear explanation for this gender difference either. Diminished thyroid function becomes more frequent in women as they age, and so has to be part of the proper evaluation of a women in the perimenopause and menopause years. One of the concerns is that brain symptoms of hypothyroidism such as memory loss, decreased concentration, difficulty organizing one's thoughts, and depressed mood are often so subtle that many women are not properly diagnosed until the disorder has progressed to produce the more obvious physical signs of dry skin, hair loss, weight gain, cold intolerance, slowed heart rate, decreased reflexes, high blood pressure, and high cholesterol to name a few.

The subtle brain symptoms *tend to occur first*, and memory loss is among the early changes when thyroid hormones are not adequately produced, or when their effect is blocked by antibody production as occurs in Hashimoto's thyroiditis. Since the changes found in thyroid disorders may overlap the symptoms women experience with menopause, it is particularly important that both hormonal systems be checked fully. If left untreated, hypothyroidism can progress to a dementia syndrome similar to Alzheimer's disease. I have also had quite a few patients who had been *misdiagnosed with Alzheimer's dementia*, but when proper tests were done were found to have a treatable hypothyroidism causing their memory impairment. The evaluation of thyroid function is significantly overlooked in women's health, particularly as women get older.

Of course, it is important not to *overtreat* thyroid disease and take *too much* thyroid hormone, since excessive amounts of thyroid hormone can cause heart damage and bone loss. These complications occur whether you take "natural" thyroid extracts or the medications made by pharmaceutical companies. Excessive amounts of thyroid cause your body's metabolic engines to be overly "revved up," with increased heart rate, jitteriness, irritability, excessive weight loss, and increased bone breakdown. Thyroid imbalances, either too high or too low, can produce marked effects on brain function, with resulting mood, behavioral, and cognitive changes. For optimal memory function, indeed all brain functions, *balance is the key*!

Sleep Deprivation and Memory

Tossing and turning, waking up wide-eyed, looking at the clock, going back to sleep, waking up, looking at the clock. This is a common scenario I hear from mid-life women. As estrogen levels drop before a period, after ovulation, or decline with menopause, the drop in estradiol triggers a firing of the "alerting" centers in the brain. These centers then discharge a burst of an adrenalin-type chemical messenger, which has an arousing effect and wakes you up. In addition, the burst of adrenalin hits the brain's heat-regulating center and triggers the "hot flash or flush," followed by sweating. These episodes of awakening at night may occur only a few times or may be quite frequent, leaving you feeling tired when you get up in the morning. Sleep disruption over an extended period of time is associated with daytime drowsiness, fatigue, feeling "foggy" mentally and also with disturbances in memory, concentration, focus, and even loss of libido. Prolonged sleep disruption can even be a cause of the biochemical changes which lead to a major (clinical) depressive episode. Getting a good night's sleep is more crucial to our health than most women realize.

I had always been a good sleeper until I hit age 39. I was much too young in my mind to even think about something like perimenopause! I couldn't figure what in the world was happening to me. My doctors just thought it was the stress of medical practice, (made sense to me, given how busy I was) and I acquiesced to that idea. A few years later, I realized, as many of my patients have also said, that I had been under a lot of stress at other times in my medical career and did not have the same problems sleeping. So what was this? It turned out, as you may recall from Chapter 4, that I really was in early ovarian decline. The loss of estrogen was causing the frequent waking up episodes. Extensive sleep research in recent years has helped us understand the many beneficial functions of sleep to maintain normal body restoration and repair each twenty-four hour cycle. The role of healthy sleep patterns in optimal memory function has not yet been fully defined, but researchers have identified a strong correlation between failing memory and abnormalities of the sleep cycle. Estrogen balance in women is important for regulation of both sleep and memory.

Of course, I recognize that there are many factors which cause disruption in sleep (see the chart below), and these must also be addressed. But, the one factor *frequently <u>overlooked</u> for women* is the effect of estrogen change in triggering fragmented sleep. I think women should have the endocrine factor *included in their medical assessment before sleeping pills are prescribed.*

SOME COMMON CAUSES OF INSOMNIA

- hormonal changes (ovary, thyroid, adrenal, pituitary, etc.)
- drug and alcohol abuse (acute effects and withdrawal), tobacco use
- excess caffeine, other stimulants (sodas, coffee, tea, chocolate, herbs with *ephedra*)
- medical illnesses (many types)
- medications (many types), especially allergy and cold ones with decongestants
- jet lag, shift work
- clinical depression, generalized anxiety
- life stress
- poor sleep habits (making your bed a second home office doesn't help you relax!)

Sleep architecture is the term used to describe the normal pattern of sleep stages (shown in the chart on page 194). Each of these is characterized by different electrical activity or "brain wave" patterns, measured on electroencephalogram (EEG) tracings, eye movement measures (EOM), and muscle activity (EMG). Non-REM sleep (NREM) are the four stages in which *dreaming does not occur*. REM sleep is the stage in which dreaming occurs, along with other physiological responses like penile erections in men. Sleep problems (apnea, narcolepsy, and others) can be evaluated in sleep laboratories to determine the specific type of disorder, which in turn directs the physician to the proper treatments.

As you sleep each night, you experience seventy to one-hundred-minute cycles of these stages, with more NREM sleep in the first half of the night, and more REM (dreaming) sleep in the second half toward morning. Sleep quality decreases with age in all of us, even in healthy individuals. The presence of medical problems, obesity, alcohol use, and cigarette smoking may all

NORMAL SLEEP ARCHITECTURE

	EEG Patterns	Eye Movement	Muscle Action
AWAKE	mainly alpha waves, some beta	depends on task	normal tone, voluntary movement
NREM—Stage 1	mixed theta, beta waves; alpha <50 percent	slow, rolling	relaxed, less tone
NREM—Stage 2	theta, bursts of sleep spindles, K complex	slow, rolling	relaxed, less tone
NREM—Stage 3	delta waves, 20–50 percent	slow	relaxed
NREM - Stage 4	delta (slow wave sleep), >50 percent	slow	relaxed
REM (dreaming)	**similar to waking**	symmetrical, rapid; jerky	none (atonia); penile erections occur

contribute to even more rapid deterioration in quality of sleep and may disrupt the normal sleep stages. If you become sleep deprived, the brain actively directs restoring the normal sleep patterns by lengthening total sleep time and the amount of slow wave sleep on the first recovery night. On following recovery nights, there is an increase (rebound) of REM sleep to compensate for lost REM during sleep deprivation. REM rebound causes *intense* dreaming for several nights or longer.

One of the reasons sleeping pills become a problem with prolonged use is that they interrupt the normal sleep patterns and the balance of the various stages. Stopping sleeping pills abruptly after more than two weeks of use will typically cause REM rebound, making it harder to sleep normally. Eventually, sleeping pill use makes it harder for the body and brain to function normally and will further impair energy, mood, and memory *independent* of the specific medication's effects on memory (more about this in the next section). This is another reason I do not like to see women have prescriptions for sleeping pills without looking carefully for the *underlying causes* of sleep problems, *including* hormone changes, and more serious kinds of sleep disorders, (e.g., sleep apnea), which could be dangerous in combination with sleeping pills.

For most women during the menopause transition, sleep disruption does *not* require sleeping pills. It can be managed with relaxation training; having a carbohydrate snack before bedtime to increase brain tryptophan which will then boost serotonin production (skim milk and cereal is good); a trial of herbal remedies, such as dong quai; or for some women with marked sleep disruption, a more natural approach than sleeping pills would be to consider small amounts of estrogen supplementation. I have some women who did not want to take a full therapeutic amount of estradiol who reported good results for sleep improvement with the weaker human estrogen, *estriol*. You should talk with your physician about these approaches to see what fits YOU best.

Sleeping Pills, Alcohol, and Other Memory Robbers

All of the sleeping pills on the market today, both prescription and over-the-counter ones, adversely affect your memory. The other "drug" that many people, particularly women, use to help them fall asleep is alcohol. It, too, impairs memory, along with its many other negative effects on health. Each class of medication acts by different means to decrease memory, but all of them contribute to memory loss over time. Fortunately, much of the memory loss produced by alcohol, sedative sleeping pills, and over-the-counter sleeping pills can be reversed if you stop using these substances. After prolonged overuse of alcohol, however, the nerve cells are permanently damaged, and memory loss does not return when a person stops drinking. The *progression* of further memory loss may be stopped by eliminating alcohol, but once tissue damage has occurred, normal memory function does not return. Another reason to limit alcohol to occasional, moderate intake! Let's look at what happens to the brain with each of these "memory robbers" to help you understand why memory changes occur.

Prescription sleeping pills are generally grouped under the term *sedative-hypnotic* medications and include the older *barbiturates* (Meprobamate, Seconal, and others), which are not used as much today due to their toxicity and addictiveness, and the *benzodiazepine group* (currently FDA-approved sleeping pills are Dalmane, Restoril, Halcion, Doral, ProSom; other benzodiazepines sometimes used for sleep include Valium, Libruim, Xanax, and Tranxene). All of the drugs in this category will initially improve sleep by inducing more rapid sleep onset and helping to maintain sleep. After about ten days to two weeks, these medications lose their effectiveness on sleep and also cause a disruption in the normal *stages* of sleep (mainly loss of stage 4 sleep). The sedative-hypnotics as a group *all cause memory loss* if used for an extended period of time, usually longer than two weeks. For some people, the memory impairment can come much more quickly than that. These drugs typically also cause a hangover effect of daytime drowsiness; this will be *worse* with long-acting ones (Dalmane, Valium, Librium) and less noticeable with shorter-acting ones such as Doral, Halcion, and Xanax.

The high potency, short-acting sleep medications, such as Halcion, produce much more memory impairment the next day and also tend to cause rebound anxiety when the drug wears off. I was concerned about the very short action of Halcion and its high potency; even when it first came out, I rarely prescribed it. With the subsequent publicity about the potential adverse reactions, I do not prescribe Halcion at all. I have personally treated many women who have had severe mood changes (anxiety, irritability, memory impairment, and other problems) from Halcion, and I do not recommend its use. The benzodiazepines have an *additive* effect on sedation and potential respiratory depression if you drink alcohol when taking them. All of the drugs in this category are potentially addictive and produce withdrawal syndromes if stopped abruptly after more than about seven days of use.

It can also be dangerous to use sedative-hypnotics if the person has sleep apnea, since these medications further suppress respiration. In my practice, it is uncommon for me to prescribe sedative-hypnotic medications. I much prefer to first see that the sleep problem is properly diagnosed and then to help the individual develop good sleep habits, use nutritional and other natural methods of improving sleep, consider hormonal options if appropriate and desired by the woman, and as a last resort use low dose serotonin-augmenting medications, such as Desyrel or Buspar for brief periods. These last two are not addictive, and if used in low doses, have very few side effects.

Another group of prescription medications is the "sedating" antidepressants, such as Elavil (amitriptyline), Desyrel (trazodone), Tofranil (imipramine), and Sinequan (doxepin). These all have mild to moderate antihistamine effects, enhance serotonin activity, and produce drowsiness at low doses. At higher doses used for treating depression, they decrease nocturnal awakenings, increase non-REM sleep, decrease REM sleep, and normalize the disturbed sleep which is characteristic of biological depression. I think these medications are safe and quite helpful, but there may be interactions with other medications you are taking, so your physician will have to discuss these with you.

The serotonin-boosting antidepressants are especially valuable in improving sleep in people with chronic pain syndromes. You may want to read more in the chapter on fibromyalgia about how these drugs work to reduce pain. The antidepressant group of drugs are *nonaddictive*, but if stopped abruptly, you may experience "REM rebound" which results in several days to a week of intense dreaming and irritability. If you are taking these medications, even in a low dose, it is best to taper them off gradually.

Over-the-counter (OTC) aids, such as Sleep-Eze, Nytol, or Sominex, usually contain antihistamine compounds (diphenhydramine is a common one) that are central nervous system depressants and produce drowsiness and sedation. Daytime sleepiness and difficulty with memory and concentration is common. You should let your physician know if you use these OTC sleep aids, because they all can potentially interact with other medications you may be taking. This group has an *additive* effect on sedation if you also drink alcohol. I have also found that many of my patients have the *opposite reaction* to antihistamines and become anxious and agitated rather than sleepy. Be cautious if you use these sleep aids, communicate with your physician and do not use them for an extended period of time without having your sleep problems fully evaluated medically.

There are many herbal remedies that have been used to promote sleep. Some of these can be helpful, and others may trigger allergic reactions in sensitive individuals. If you would like to use these approaches on a short-term basis, I suggest you consult with a knowledgeable herbalist rather than just taking the advice of a salesperson in a health food store. If you are someone with a lot of allergies to trees, grasses, and other plants, remember that these herbal remedies are derived from *plants* and have the potential to aggravate allergies. It was surprising to me how many people usually do not associate their allergies to plants with the possibility of a reaction to an herbal product.

Vitamins and Memory

A number of vitamins are crucial co-factors, or "helpers" for the brain to make important chemical messengers involved in normal memory function. Several of these, especially B_{12} and folate, have been known for decades to play a role in maintaining normal brain function, in particular memory and mood regulation. More recently, research in a number of countries had continued to identify the role of various vitamins and minerals in memory processes. Iris Bell, M.D., Ph.D., Director of the Geriatric Psychiatry Program at the University of Arizona, has significant research documenting the effects of vitamins B_1, B_2, and B_6 in improving both depressive symptoms and cognitive function in elderly patients. Dr. Bell has found that thiamin (B_1) deficiency impairs brain glucose metabolism and also contributes to high levels of homocysteine, a risk factor for cardiovascular and cerebrovascular disease, which can then lead to memory loss. It appears from a number of studies that significant numbers of patients may have laboratory values of these B vitamins which appear to be in the "normal" range, but may not be adequate for optimal nerve cell function in the brain.

Another area of research into factors affecting memory is the role of *antioxidant* vitamins in prevention of plaque formation in arteries, thereby improving blood flow to the brain. Oxidation, or "free-radical damage," is the process of cell damage and death associated with aging, environmental pollutants, poor nutrition, tobacco smoke, radiation, and other causes. What are free-radicals? These are "crippled" oxygen atoms which have lost electrons in the chemical reactions of our body's natural metabolic processes, or as a result of trying to make up for poor nutrition, environmental pollution, and other causes. These free radicals roam the body trying to replace their lost electrons by combining with electrons from healthy cells. This causes damage to the membranes and structures inside healthy cells, much like rust damage to your car.

What are antioxidants? These are molecules, such as vitamins E, C, beta-carotene, and selenium, (estradiol has also been found to act as an antioxidant) which have the capability of losing electrons to free radicals without initiating a damaging chain reaction of electron robbing! Antioxidants serve as "scavengers" to clean up these damaging free radicals and help prevent some of the damage to DNA and cell death. Brain neurons and nerve fibers are particularly vulnerable to damage and death from free radicals; the antioxidants reduce much of this oxidative damage and help keep brain cells working properly. The effect is to produce modest improvements in memory. Antioxidants, as I will describe in later chapters, also play a role in helping decrease the risk of certain cancers.

Unfortunately, as most of you now know, nutrition has only received brief mention in most medical school curricula. The critical role of vitamins and minerals in brain function is rarely addressed as an important clinical issue. Consequently, most physicians think that a balanced diet is enough and hardly anyone needs vitamin supplements. I must admit that this was my notion, too, when I first started medical practice. Over the years, with more collaborative work with dietitians interested in preventive medicine, and my own study of nutritional factors affecting mood, energy, memory, and a host of other problems, I have come to clearly see that probably *most of us* would benefit from vitamin supplements. That's quite a turn-around from where I was when I graduated from medical school! I am now diligent about taking my own vitamin-mineral supplements daily.

Very few Americans really eat a balanced diet to begin with and even fewer women have enough caloric intake and food variety on a daily basis to provide even the RDA for many vitamins and minerals. A classic example is magnesium. The average American woman has a daily intake of about 100 mg. The RDA is 400 to 600 mg a day. Magnesium is critical for nerve and muscle function, mood and memory processes, and bone development among many other roles in the body. Several years ago, I was struck by a nutritional study done by Angelica Cantlon, R.D. She calculated the amount of calories and variety of food that would be required for the average woman to get her RDA of all the basic vitamins and minerals. She found that daily calories needed to be 1400, and the food groups needed were far more diverse than any patient's food diary I have seen in my entire career in medicine! I was shocked, and so were the women in my seminars when I showed them the results of this study. An average woman who is chronically dieting to lose weight, and this is certainly more common in the premenopausal years when *everyone* seems obsessed with losing weight, has a daily calorie intake of 800 to 1000 calories, followed by marked increases on the weekends at social functions! No wonder there seem to be more memory problems in mid-life: not only are important estrogen levels changing, but also women are not eating well enough to sustain the brain's activity at optimal function. Fueling the brain with healthy, quality "fuel" is the best way to have better memory!

Start with a basic healthy meal plan, but consider that a good multivitamin with additional calcium, magnesium, beta carotene, and vitamin E and vitamin C will give you an added measure of benefit. For best absorption, try a liquid formula of the multivitamin you select. Magnesium and vitamin E (at antioxidant levels) are both difficult to obtain in a typical American diet. I don't endorse *mega*vitamin supplements, since I think these are frequently more expensive than necessary and may cause potential side effects and subtle toxicity syndromes.

"Smart Drugs": Marketing Ploy or Real Help?

A variety of these products are being promoted as "brain enhancers." I continue to be surprised at the amount of money patients spend on these supplements and how many they typically take. It is difficult to make any comments about the effectiveness of these products, since it is often difficult to know exactly what is in the product, and there so far is not a great deal of sound research to document positive results with their use. Deprenyl is one drug in this group that has been shown to be of help in reducing the nerve deterioration characteristic of Parkinson's disease. It has been used in Europe as an anti-aging drug and a memory enhancer. I have had a few patients who have been on it for preventing the progression of Parkinson symptoms, but I have not seen dramatic changes in memory or other of its purported actions. It has the potential to cause high blood pressure reactions when taken along with the amino acids tyrosine and phenylalanine, as well as tyramine in certain foods. Since these amino acids are also found in foods, persons on Deprenyl have to watch dietary sources as well as supplements. I do not encourage its use simply as a cognitive enhancer, but if you take it, I urge you to notify your physician. I have worked with a number of women experiencing anxiety symptoms, only to find out later that they were taking *ephedra* supplements or Deprenyl, and this was causing the anxiety problems! Please communicate with all of your health care providers about *everything* you take.

Emerging work on the plant extract, *Gingko biloba* (GBE), is showing promising results to improve brain blood flow, memory and cognition. Researchers at the Department of Geriatric Medicine at Whittington Hospital in London studied the effects of *Gingko biloba* on thirty-one elderly patients with mild-to-moderate memory impairment and found a statistically significant beneficial effect over placebo. Their study is significant in that it was a double-blind, placebo controlled protocol over six months, and also included EEG brain wave results. Another European study of seventy-one outpatients with cerebral insufficiency at three test centers were randomized into a double-blind placebo controlled protocol for 24 weeks. Statistically significant improvements in short-term memory and learning rate were found in the patients taking the gingko extract (EGb 761), but not in the placebo group.

European research over the past thirty years suggests that *Gingko biloba* extract acts as a vasodilator, improves oxygen and glucose uptake, and also acts to help decrease platelet clumping (a factor in arterial plaque formation). At present, there is no regulation of Gingko products, and they are proliferating rapidly (along with rising prices) as word spreads about these research findings. Most of the studies have been done on the original extract, EGb 761), and others may or may not contain the same percentage and compositions of the active compounds. This is another example where you need to use some common sense, and if you chose to try GBE, look for reputable sources of information and observe your body responses before you buy a year's supply!

I do not have the space to go into all the other "smart drugs" currently being touted as wonder agents to prevent changes in brain function with aging. If you are interested in this subject, I encourage you to seek sound information before adding numerous supplements to your daily routine. The best memory enhancers are still the basics listed below, along with a good multivitamin and the antioxidants. There is NO QUICK FIX!

What Can You Do to Improve Memory?

Practice using it! That's right, think of your brain as a "mental muscle" and *exercise it*! Research has shown that stimulating your brain with new learning actually helps increase the number of neuron connections. Take a class in an entirely different field, learn a foreign language, do crossword puzzles, practice solving brain teasers. When you want to remember something new, focus on it, repeat it several times, and perhaps write it down and look at it as well. Some simple principles of paying attention to basic health habits also improve brain function and memory:

- stop smoking (which deprives the brain of oxygen)
- stop using sleeping pills (talk with your doctor about how to do this safely, since these medications must usually be decreased gradually)
- eat smaller meals at regular intervals (keeps steady "fuel" to the brain)
- reduce fat in your diet. It contributes to plaque deposits in the arteries and blocks blood flow to the brain.
- exercise aerobically several times a week
- take a good basic multivitamin along with antioxidants
- eliminate or reduce alcohol
- practice relaxation exercises or meditation
- get enough sleep
- USE IT OR LOSE IT—Stimulate your brain with new ideas, and practice!

CHAPTER 10

Migraines in Women: Hormonal Links Women Know and Doctors Ignore

MIGRAINE

Even the name conjures up images of that throbbing, head-splitting pain; nausea that makes you ill just to *think* about moving around; vision problems that make you think you may be going blind; and wanting to crawl off to the darkest room you can find, and tell the world to "Leave me alone!"

For all of you migraine sufferers out there, have you ever asked a physician the question *"Could it be related to my hormones? The headaches seem to come (or get worse) right before my period?"* And how many of you have been told categorically, "No, there's no connection?" Well, it shouldn't take a rocket scientist to figure out that if the following observations have been true down through the centuries of recorded medical observations:

- migraines are 2 to 3 times more common in women than in men
- the gender difference begins at *puberty* and ends at *menopause*

then there just *might* be a hormonal connection to the problem in women! Again, most women know that. You have lived it. You have told me over the years of my practice that your migraines (1) almost always come a day or two before your period, or the first day or two of your period or (2) have a number of different triggers but are frequently worse right around your period. I couldn't accept that all these women who kept saying the same thing were wrong, or just "neurotic," which is what we often hear about women who try to offer a possible explanation or connection for their symptoms.

Like many health problems that affect women in greater numbers than men, migraine was relatively neglected by medical researchers until fairly recently. When studies were done, they were more often *done in men*. I will never forget the article I came across in Journal of the American Medical Assoiation (JAMA) in 1991, which was a study of aspirin prophylaxis in migraine. In the first two paragraphs, the authors described migraine being more common in women, yet the study they had just done *did not include a single female patient*. They concluded in the article that aspirin on a daily basis could be helpful to reduce migraine frequency *in men*, but *they didn't know whether it would work in women*. How could they if women weren't included in the study?!

Since migraine was typically found in women, and included many unusual symptoms, it was all too frequently dismissed and discounted by labeling the disorder hysterical or psychological. I can remember being taught this stereotype in medical school. Yet, you would think *because* migraines occur more often in women and have a relationship to the menstrual cycle in the majority of sufferers, that clinicians and researchers would have regarded hormonal influences as major clues to study in migraine headaches. It is hard for me to understand why such obvious connections in women's health have been ignored for so long.

The ancient Greeks, in the writings of Hippocrates, knew about menstrual cycle influences on the course of such problems as asthma, allergies, epilepsy, and *migraine*. But as an example of the magnitude of the current problem of overlooking women's hormonal changes as important variables, I found that a seven-hundred-page textbook, published in 1987, **there was not a single index reference to estrogen, even as a subheading under hormones!** This text was solely devoted to the topic of MIGRAINE, and edited by international medical authorities in research and treatment of migraine.

Fortunately, we have made some *slight* progress since 1987 in getting attention focused on the menstrual cycle hormonal changes as headache triggers in women. Due to the pioneering studies of Dr. B.W. Somerville, we now know that a common trigger for the hormonally related migraine headaches is the *drop in estradiol* (remember, that's the primary type of estrogen made by the ovary). Guess when the estradiol level drops the most quickly? You got it, right before your period. The estradiol level (along with progesterone and beta-endorphin levels) begins decreasing rather dramatically about day 22 to 24 of your cycle, and reaches its lowest point of the month on Day 1 of bleeding. The estradiol level also remains low for the first few days of your bleeding, and this is a reason for the increase in migraines during the early days of menstrual flow. There is another time in the menstrual cycle when estradiol levels drop and may cause a migraine: right after ovulation. So, for some women, there are two times in the menstrual cycle when they are vulnerable to having a migraine headache due to the drop in estrogen production. When might be some other times that women are more likely to be affected by hormonal headache triggers? You're right if you thought of (1) the week women stop birth control pills to have a period, (2) women who take ERT after menopause and stop their estrogen for days 25 to 30 of the month, 3) the few days after delivery (postpartum phase) when estrogen, progesterone, and endorphin levels drop about 100-fold over 24 to 48 hours.

If you add to this the usual migraine triggers: certain foods, alcohol, caffeine, **chocolate**, barometric pressure weather changes, stress, "rebound" from pain medication, and all the other classic ones—you have a whole host of potential interactions and headache causes. Most doctors, and most migraine sufferers (called "migraineurs" for short), know about and pay attention to the classic triggers I have listed above. *But the overlooked, hidden estrogen trigger, which can be addressed in some fairly simple ways, is ignored in almost 99 percent of women who have migraines.*

Not only does this overlooked connection cause a lot of unnecessary suffering, it also adds dramatically to the cost of caring for patients with migraines, which can include *expensive* and often unnecessary pain medication, expensive trips to the emergency room for injections of narcotics and other potent pain medications when the other methods fail, and even hospital admissions for managing "refractory" (or difficult to control) migraines. There *are* hormonal connections, and there are also some *hormonal treatment options,* which work extremely well for many patients. Here are some stories from women who have asked that I share their experiences so that others many benefit.

Listening to Women

Dee's Story

"Dee" came to see me two years ago for a consultation with the following concerns: "I have tried every estrogen there is, and they all cause migraines. How do I find something to take so I can feel better? And I'm worried about osteoporosis if I can't take any estrogen." She was forty-seven at the time, and at age forty-five she had undergone a total hysterectomy due to severe bleeding and multiple fibroids. She also had her ovaries removed at the same time. This woman described feeling "desperate" to find some relief for the migraines, for her loss of energy and libido, the fragmented sleep with nocturnal hot flashes, and the mood changes, which consisted primarily of depressed mood and irritability.

She did not have a major depressive disorder, although she did see a psychiatrist for psychotherapy dealing with the adjustments to a new marriage. Her psychiatrist had tried several antidepressants that have been useful for treatment of migraines but had been unable to find a regimen that eliminated her headaches. She had not experienced migraine headaches prior to her hysterectomy, although she had experienced occasional milder vascular headaches prior to her menstrual periods off and on during her thirties and early forties.

About a week following her surgery, she was started on her initial estrogen therapy with Premarin 0.625 mg daily. Within the first week of treatment, she developed bloating, breast tenderness, and severe migraine headaches with classic symptoms: prodromal aura, stabbing pain in the right eye with visual scotomata, nausea, and light sensitivity. She was directed to stop the Premarin and was then started on Estraderm patch 0.05 mg twice a week. Her migraines continued to occur several times a week and were so severe that they interfered with her going to work. Estraderm was stopped and she was started on Estrace 2 mg orally at bedtime. Her sleep improved and the nocturnal hot flashes resolved, but she again had severe migraines, which began midday on the third day of treatment and became daily.

Her physician told her to stop Estrace and informed her that she would not be able to take estrogen due to the migraines. She was then treated symptomatically with a variety of medications to decrease the migraine pain when it occurred: beta blockers, NSAIDS, DHE, and serotonin-augmenting antidepressants. None of these were completely effective for her migraines, and she also continued to have severe menopausal symptoms. She had remarried about a year before her hysterectomy, and she was particularly upset by her loss of libido and difficulty with sexual arousal. She said her husband was "very supportive and concerned, but he's getting at the end of his patience, too. I'm worried this is going to affect my marriage as well as how I feel." "Dee" initially called for a consultation after a friend had told her of the work

I was doing with hormonal connections in migraines. After our initial telephone consultation about her problems, she decided to come to Tucson for a more in-depth evaluation and to have me work with her in person to find a hormone regimen appropriate for her.

Dee had been in good health and exercised regularly. She did not smoke cigarettes. Before her surgery, she drank wine occasionally with a special dinner but otherwise did not drink alcohol. She had been unable to tolerate even a glass of wine since the onset of her migraine problem, and at the time I saw her, she had not had any alcohol in about two years. Her two pregnancies in her twenties had been uneventful, and she had not had any problems with postpartum depression or migraines. She had her mammograms regularly, and these had always been normal.

Her family history was important, since her mother had lost an inch of height in her later years and was also on medication for elevated cholesterol. Her mother had gone through a natural menopause in her late forties and had never taken hormones. Her father had high blood pressure and angina and was on medication for this. Dee also had a brother in his early forties who had high blood pressure, high cholesterol, and was already on medication.

When I examined her, she was at a healthy body weight for her build, had a blood pressure of 118/78, and no physical abnormalities. Her blood tests were quite significant in view of her symptoms and helped her to see quite clearly the hormonal connections: her FSH 132.7, LH 125.5 were very high as expected after a surgical menopause with no hormone therapy; her testosterone was low at 15 ng/dl and was a factor in her loss of libido; her estradiol was 32.8 pg/ml, also quite low and a cause of her menopausal symptoms. Her total cholesterol was high at 274 but since her HDL was 74, she still had a normal ratio of 3.7. Her LDL was too high at 182 and she was moving into a higher risk group for cardiovascular disease. She and I discussed that her regular exercise regimen was likely what had helped her keep a higher HDL and lower CVD risk than her family history would predict. Her thyroid tests, including the TSH of 1.32, were all normal.

Dee's bone density report showed a reason for more concern. In spite of her calcium intake and her exercise, both of which she had been doing for many years, she already had a significant degree of bone loss (osteopenia) at the hip. Her bone density showed the femoral neck to be 0.72 g/cm2, which was almost two standard deviations below the normal expected peak bone mass. Dee was worried about being able to find a way of taking estrogen that did not cause the severe migraines, but she saw from the results of her complete evaluation that she was clearly someone who had a number of reasons for being on an optimal estrogen replacement program: the relatively young age of her hysterectomy and removal of the ovaries; her present abnormal degree of bone loss and family history of probable osteoporosis; her present abnormal cholesterol profile and family history of heart disease; and her loss of libido and ability to have orgasm, which was caused by the low hormone levels, not the surgery itself.

From what Dee had told me, I realized that a key part of the problem she had been having with her headaches had been the fluctuating levels of estradiol with the previous schedules and types of estrogen. I explained to her that I thought she was sensitive to a *falling* estradiol level in between doses as the trigger for the migraine onset. She and I discussed my rationale for a trial on a regimen of smaller doses at more frequent intervals. She said "you know, that intuitively feels right. I think you are right about what was happening before." I thought she would likely need to reach a dose of estradiol about 1 mg to 2 mg a day, but I knew that we could not start at that amount all at once without having her headaches return. I recommended she start with 1/4 mg tablets, taking them three times a day for the first few days. Her headache came back about 6 hours after the first two doses, and we realized she would need to take it even more frequently. At least this pattern was helping us to work together to confirm the suspicion that the drop in estradiol was the trigger for her migraine. She was headache-free on a schedule of four times a day, with about 6 hours in between each dose of estradiol. She still had milder menopausal symptoms with her total daily dose at only 1 mg. To reach the point where she felt her best, and her symptoms *plus* headaches were gone, she was gradually increased to 2 mg daily. This amount fits with her age, the suddenness of her surgical menopause, and reaching a point where she felt *really well and energetic* without any unwanted side effects.

Her blood levels of estradiol were now in the desirable range of 100 to 150 pg/ml, consistent with the levels found in the first half of the menstrual cycle before menopause. After the first two months on Estrace, her sexual difficulties had improved significantly, but she still experienced a diminished libido. Since she had a low bone density along with the libido changes, and no longer had the ovaries to produce her own testosterone, I suggested she try a small amount of micronized natural testosterone. She responded well to 2.5 mg micronized testosterone daily. I had also recommended magnesium 250 mg twice a day as an additional supplement to help her bone density.

At her six month follow-up, FSH was 30 (now down to the range expected for a woman on the right amount of estradiol replacement), estradiol 145 pg/ml, testosterone 40 ng/dl, fasting total cholesterol 225 with HDL of 78, ratio 2.8. She had no adverse side effects from the testosterone and had remained migraine-free *as long as she took her 17-beta-estradiol on the regular schedule.* She tried to decrease her frequency to three times a day but found that she began to have the onset of the migraine prodrome when she increased the interval between doses. She commented that although it was "a nuisance" to have to take the estradiol four times a day, she was so glad to be free of the migraines and feeling better over-all, "it's worth it." Her husband was thrilled that she felt so much better and was no longer having migraines, and they both described feeling reassured that the sexual problems had been due to the low hormone levels, not a relationship problem! He said "everything's going really well, our sex life is the way we had been when we first got married, it's wonderful to have my wife back."

Reba's Story

Reba is now thirty-five, and began having migraines in her twenties after she stopped using birth control pills. She had identified a number of "triggers" for her headaches: red wine, chocolate, "low-pressure" days when the weather changed and became cloudy and rainy, certain cheeses, the onset of her period each month, and the "let-down" days after times of stressful situations at work or with her family. She had tried a number of medications, with varying degrees of success on these types of migraines, and she had also learned how to use biofeedback to help decrease her headaches.

Over the years, she had been able to eliminate most of the triggers she had identified, except, she laughingly pointed out "I haven't been able to control the weather, or eliminate all the stress from my life for those times, I just have to use the drugs I've found that will work. The sumatriptan shots have been a godsend, and that usually breaks the migraine right away. But the thing that really gets me is the *excruciating* migraines I get *right before my period*. The sumatriptan doesn't seem to work as well on those headaches, and sometimes I've ended up in the emergency room for Demerol shots. I have asked every doctor I've ever seen if it could be my hormones, and they all say no. And they all tell me I can't ever take the pill (birth control), but I wonder if that would help? I keep trying to tell my doctors that these headaches started after I stopped the pills, *but no one listens to what I have to say. I'm convinced that there is some hormonal factor, and I just want somebody to listen to me and try and help me figure this out."*

I talked with Reba about the connection I thought was a major factor for her: premenstrual estrogen decreases triggering migraines. We went over her headache diary which clearly showed the relationship between the time of her cycle when estradiol dropped and the onset of her migraine. I pointed out that her calendar showed that she frequently had a migraine at mid-cycle, corresponding with the estrogen drop at ovulation. She had not realized this pattern, and thought these were "stress-related." She had been using a diaphragm for contraception after several doctors had told her that her headaches would get worse if she used birth control pills.

I suggested that we consider trying a low-dose pill with steady hormone levels (monophasic pill) and keep the progestin content low since seems to be the primary culprit in birth control pills that may aggravate headaches. The low progestin pills I use most often in this situation are Ovcon 35, Modicon or Brevicon because I have found these work best with the fewest unwanted side effects. Modicon and Brevicon have a little more progestin and I use one of these if a woman has too much breakthrough spotting on the Ovcon 35. All three of these birth control pills have *half (or less)* of the amount of progestin found in other birth control pills.

Another factor in using birth control pills is the *drop in hormones* when the active hormone pills are stopped for seven days (the placebo pill days) each month to trigger the menses. I explained that she could try using the pills again, and stop the pills for only three days each month, instead of seven. This shorter time is enough to allow her period to start, but is not so long off hormones that it causes an estrogen-withdrawal migraine. She thought this made a lot of sense with what she had noticed, and wanted to try it. Even just three days off the pills was too long for her: the migraine hit again on the afternoon of the third day following the end of her first pill pack. At first she was a little discouraged and thought this meant she would not be able to continue with the pills. I reassured her and told her it just confirmed what we thought: one of her "triggers" was the drop in estrogen, and the next step would be to shorten the time between packs of active hormone pills to *two* days instead of three.

Voila! This worked. It has now been a year and a half since our first consult. Reba is happy on the birth control pills, glad to be free of the diaphragm and even more excited about finding a way to eliminate the trigger for her menstrual migraines. Since birth control pills also suppress ovulation to provide the contraceptive effect, being able to take the Ovcon eliminated the drop in estrogen at ovulation which had also set off Reba's migraines. She still has an occasional migraine when she's overstressed or the barometric pressure drops suddenly, and she has managed those headaches well with the Imitrex (sumatriptan) injections. An added plus for her has been having a lighter menstrual flow, no more bad menstrual cramps, and the elimination of her "PMS mood swings" now that the hormone levels are steady all month.

These are just two of the many women I have worked with to find creative options to reduce or eliminate the hormonal triggers for their migraines. Each women is different, and the challenge is to listen to her wisdom and insights about what she has noticed, track her headache pattern, and put it with what I know about the hormonal changes to come up with treatment approaches that make physiological sense. Yes, it takes time and patience, but isn't your health worth it?

New Understandings of Migraine Mechanisms

Migraine headaches occur in two primary patterns: those with an aura (previously called "classic migraine") and those without an aura (previously called "common migraine"). It had been thought that the phenomena that occurred in migraines—visual changes, sensitivity to light and sound, nausea, throbbing head pain—were due mainly to *circulation* changes: blood vessels becoming first constricted (vasoconstriction) and then dilated (vasodilatation). With more research, other aspects of the many biochemical, neural, and vascular changes in migraine are now better understood, and a unified theory has emerged.

Migraine is now best described as a state of central nervous system "hyperexcitability" that predisposes a person to episodes of spontaneous depolarization of the neurons, followed by suppression of neuron function, and then changes in regulation of blood flow. *A genetic predisposition* is now thought to be *underlying* the development of migraines upon exposure to a precipitating trigger. The majority of migraine sufferers have a family history of others with these headaches. A genetically susceptible individual has a *lowered* threshold in response to the external triggers and internal hormonal changes that can set off the migraine sequence. If a susceptible individual is exposed to the headache triggers, the threshold is exceeded and nerve cells in the brain stem are fired off, activating the exaggerated release of serotonin, norepinephrine, dopamine, Substance P, and other chemical messengers. These changes in turn set off reactions in blood vessels, and there you are in the vicious cycle again.

The aura of migraine is usually fifteen to twenty minutes before the headache pain starts and is itself painless. It is caused primarily by sudden vasoconstriction of arteries called the "intracerebral" arteries which serve the brain. When blood supply to brain areas is suddenly reduced, the loss of oxygen causes the varied neurological sensations that commonly occur during the aura: the characteristic visual phenomena—flashing or sparkling lights before the eyes, blurred or distorted vision, tunnel vision, blind spots, or lightening-like flashes. Other patients experience numbness and tingling in the face, weakness in an arm, smelling pungent or unpleasant odors that aren't really there, sudden mood changes with irritability or tearfulness for no apparent reason, and sometimes rhythmic contractions of the abdominal muscles.

The throbbing *pain* of migraine is caused by the distension and vasodilatation of arteries outside the skull, called "extracerebral" arteries. Vasodilatation occurs as a compensatory response to the diminished oxygen supply when the intracerebral arteries become constricted. Pain results when nerve endings are pulled by the artery distension and also with the decreases in pain-modulating chemical messengers like serotonin and the endorphins.

What sets off the cascade of events leading to vasoconstriction and vasodilatation to produce the migraine attack? Many different *initial* triggers have been identified as culprits (alcohol, tyramine-containing foods, chocolate, nitrites, MSG, histamine, bright flashing lights, loud noises, stress, barometric pressure changes, altitude changes and others), but the final common pathway in all of these appears to be through alterations in the release of norepinephrine (NE), serotonin (5-HT), and dopamine (DA), along with other chemicals such as endorphins, Substance P, and prostaglandins.

A great deal of research has implicated serotonin pathways in migraines, and it now appears that there are very specific serotonin receptors in the blood vessels of cranial circulation that contribute to the pain of migraine headaches. These are the 5-HT_1 receptors, the ones that are selectively activated by the new drug, sumatriptan, to abort an acute migraine. Drugs that *activate* the receptor are called **agonists**. Both 5-HT_{1A} and 5-HT_{1D} subtypes play a role in the relief of acute migraine attacks. Other agonist drugs are ergotamine and dihydroergotamine (DHE), which have been used for many years to *abort* migraine attacks. Medications which act as **antagonists** at the 5-HT$_2$ receptors seem to help *prevent* migraines: serotonin-reuptake inhibitor antidepressants, tricyclic antidepressants, cyproheptadine, and methysergide. **It is quite interesting to find that estrogen modulates both the 5-HT$_1$ and 5-HT$_2$ receptors.**

Excessive production of prostaglandins (PG) by the lining of the uterus, especially PG-F$_2$, is known to trigger both migraines and uterine cramps. Plasma taken from menstruating women and then given back at another point in the cycle will cause migraine headaches and uterine cramping. This suggests that there is a prostaglandin-generating factor in the plasma, which sets off these symptoms associated with menstruation. One hypothesis is that menstrual migraine may be the result of estrogen withdrawal, which decreases serotonin activity and also affects levels of PG-F$_2$ and possibly other prostaglandins (PG). Medications that inhibit PG production and action are the well-known pain relievers: aspirin, Motrin, Anaprox, and others belonging to the class of *non-steroidal anti-inflammatory medications* (NSAIDs). As most of you know, the NSAIDs are used to relieve menstrual cramps and also for treating acute headaches and helping to reduce the frequency of migraines.

Whole textbooks have been devoted to this subject! I can just give you an overview of important connections here. I have included a diagram to illustrate the migraine process and triggers as we now understand it. I hope this will help you identify ways to develop healthier habits, which will help decrease the headaches as well as provide a basis for understanding the hormonal and medication effects I will be describing.

Estrogen and Progesterone Effects on Headache

The high frequency of migraines occurring around the onset of menses has been observed for several thousand years, but it wasn't until the mid-1970s that Dr. B.W. Somerville did a series of studies, published in 1975, which clearly demonstrated the differing role of estrogen and progesterone: the migraine attack was actually triggered by the premenstrual drop in estradiol, not progesterone. Injections of estradiol in the study subjects produced a delay in migraine onset, but did not delay onset of menstruation.

When subjects were given injections of progesterone, the menses onset was delayed, but the migraine came at the expected time, when the estrogen level dropped naturally.

In the few articles that address women's reports of their migraine experiences, the observations of *when* women have most of their migraines in the menstrual cycle also support estrogen withdrawal as a key trigger, since all of the times of increased headache activity across the menstrual cycle are times of falling estrogen levels: at ovulation, premenstrual, and postpartum. One of the things I have found frustrating in trying to help patients all these years is this: if we have known *for the last twenty years at least* that estrogen withdrawal is a very common potential trigger for women with migraines, *why haven't we taken this into account in our management approaches for relieving headaches? And why haven't more women been validated in their observations that there is a hormonal connection? Why haven't physicians listened to women who tell us so eloquently what the pieces of the puzzle may be?*

I look at the publication dates of some of these articles and realize that these understandings were coming out when I was in medical school. Why weren't we taught some of the male-female differences and taught ways to treat patients according to individual approaches suitable for men and for women? And, why is it that women with migraines who have seen a hormonal pattern are *still* "screaming to be heard" about these connections? I think it makes more sense to *consider* a trial of keeping hormone levels steady, and see if this helps an individual woman, instead of insisting "there's no connection" and having the patient make repeated trips to the emergency room in excruciating pain.

In a woman with a genetic susceptibility to migraine, the headache is the end result of these various biochemical, neuronal, and vascular changes resulting from the rise and fall in estrogen. If a woman suseptible to migraines is at the vulnerable point in her menstrual cycle, and has environmental triggers (alcohol, weather, foods, etc) acting on top of the hormonal shifts, it is easy to see how the vicious cycle of headaches of can be intensified.

The Role of Progesterone and Progestins

In a number of studies on the role of hormones in migraines, a common pattern noted was the increased frequency and severity of migraine, vascular and muscle-tension headaches in women on

---

Mechanisms for Estrogen Effects on Headaches

- Estrogen increases serotonin production; falling estrogen decreases the amount of available serotonin, as well as the number of certain 5-HT receptors, that are important in decreasing migraine pain. The drop in serotonin levels causes cranial blood vessels to spasm painfully.

- Falling estrogen causes a decrease in the pain-relieving beta-endorphins in the brain, spinal cord, and body tissues.

- Estrogen withdrawal (either naturally in the cycle or by stopping hormone-containing medication) causes a rebound in dopamine, which may intensify pain.

- Estrogen decline causes vasoconstriction by contraction of the muscles in the artery walls.

- Dropping estrogen levels cause a burst of norepinephrine release in the brain's locus ceruleus, which increases vasoconstriction and diminishes blood flow to the area of the brain involved in vision, thus producing the aura. NE release further intensifies pain.

- A decrease in estrogen *lowers* the pain threshold, making the individual more sensitive to painful stimuli.

---

synthetic progestins, with the **worst offender being the progestin-only contraceptive pill.** The higher the progestin content, the more likely the headaches of all types. For this reason, if I use an oral contraceptive in a woman with migraines, I always try to stay with the lowest progestin pill. I also caution against using the long-acting injectable or implant progestin-only contraceptives (Norplant, Depo-Provera) for the same reason: they have a high frequency of aggravating migraines and producing daily tension-type headaches.

The role of natural progesterone in headache syndromes is a little more difficult to determine. In general, progesterone exerts an inhibitory effect on the brain and may produce a depressant effect. It also at the GABA receptor like the benzodiazepine tranquilizers (Xanax, Valium, Ativa, Klonopin, and others). If progesterone is given to *males or females,* it produces *slowing* effects, like the benzodiazepines, on blood pressure, heart rate (evident on the electrocardiogram), brain waves (seen on EEG) and respiratory rate. At high doses, progesterone acts like an anesthetic, but in some women, high doses of progesterone may cause marked depression. When progesterone has been given in therapeutic doses for several days or weeks and then stopped, it produces withdrawal symptoms just like ones seen with benzodiazepines, barbiturates, and alcohol. The progesterone withdrawal effects can include **throbbing headaches**, which can be mistaken for migraines.

Progesterone affects the interaction of estradiol at the serotonin (5-HT) receptors and stimulates the production of prostaglandins, which is thought to be one mechanism of triggering migraine. At this time, there is no clear answer to whether progesterone has a positive effect or a negative effect on migraines; I approach its use like I do other therapies and pay attention to what the individual women tells me about her headache pattern relative to hormone cycles, and then work with her to see what works. I have not found that giving progesterone helps women with migraines.

Pregnancy Effects on Migraine

The dramatic hormonal shifts in pregnancy—more than 100-fold increase over menstrual cycle levels—affect migraine headache patterns: some women develop migraines for the first time during pregnancy, others report *relief* of prepregnancy migraines. In fact, up to 70 percent of women who have migraines without aura experience relief of their headaches during pregnancy; and still others find that pregnancy *intensifies* migraines—a pattern seen more commonly in migraineurs with aura. The pattern is highly variable and depends, to some extent, upon the phase of pregnancy.

In women who experience relief of their migraines, the improvement is most often seen after the first trimester, when progesterone levels have dropped and estrogen levels are higher. Worsening of migraines typically occurs in the first trimester when both estrogen and progesterone are rising rapidly as the placenta begins making hormones independent of the ovaries. Migraines are also typically worse again a few hours after delivery, when estrogen, endorphin, and serotonin levels all drop abruptly.

Women very commonly describe enhanced feelings of well-being in pregnancy, and this is now thought to be related to the mood-elevating effects of the high estrogen levels in pregnancy. The absence of a cyclic hormonal "up-and-down" pattern and the increased production of endorphins are considered the primary reasons migraines tend to get better in pregnancy. Researchers in England have used the estradiol transdermal gel and patch, with dramatic results, in the immediate postpartum period as a way of keeping estradiol levels from falling so rapidly and precipitating migraines. Since this is the native human form of the hormone, giving this "boost" postpartum is not considered to be a problem for nursing mothers.

Oral Contraceptives and Migraine: New Findings

Until recently, it had been thought that women with migraine headaches who used birth control pills had a slight increase in risk of stroke at younger ages than we normally see strokes occurring in women. Earlier studies,which had found this connection, were done in women on the older, high dose oral contraceptives rather than today's low dose pills. In addition, earlier studies had not identified *cigarette smoking* as an *independent* risk factor for stroke in these women.

The Collaborative Group for the Study of Stroke in Young Women definitively reported that their analysis of the data did not confirm earlier reports suggesting that migraine headaches might increase the risk of stroke in young women using oral contraceptives. Although there are still physicians who think that women with migraine headaches should not use oral contraceptives, this caution has not been borne out by recent and more comprehensive evaluations. For women with migraines, *cigarette smoking* is the most significant risk for vascular disease of all types, and this risk may be further increased by taking oral contraceptives. **Conventional** teaching has also said that OC use will aggravate migraines, so women with migraines should never take birth control pills. This too turns out to be incorrect as a generalization.

Many women may actually achieve relief of their migraines with the right oral contraceptive to stabilize hormonal fluctuations, but it has a great deal to do with hormone ratios in the pill and *how* the pill is taken. As in many women's health studies, researchers did not take into account normal hormone physiology in interpreting the study data. Earlier studies, which concluded that OC use *increased migraines*, did not look carefully at the issue of *when* in the pill cycle the headaches occurred; for example, did the headache occur while *on* the active hormone-containing pills (which would likely mean the pill did worsen the headaches), or did headaches occur in the placebo days of the pill cycle (which would indicate *hormone-withdrawal* as the culprit). About forty to sixty percent of women who have migraines while taking the oral contraceptives experience their headaches *in the last seven days of the pill pack*, when on the placebo pills. This pattern supports the role of *falling* estradiol levels in triggering the headache. In *four* double-blind placebo controlled studies, there were *no differences in headache frequency* in women *on* the OC pills compared to women *on placebo*.

Current investigation of oral contraceptive effects on migraine reveal that headache patterns may change in one of several ways when women take OCs: (1) the headaches may increase, more often seen with triphasic pills, high progestin pills, or progestin-only pills; (2) migraine headaches may be eliminated or significantly decreased, which is seen more with monophasic constant dose pills. Some studies have found as much as a sixty to seventy percent improvement in migraines when women were started on oral contraceptives; (3) different types of aura and other symptoms may occur (this type of change is potentially serious and should be discussed immediately with your physician); and (4) in women with a family history of migraine, OC use may contribute to migraine appearing for the first time. I think this illustrates just how variable the OC effects can be and once again indicates that *individualization* of therapy is crucial, especially since multiple studies have found that in many women, use of the OC pills can *decrease* headaches.

Dr. Stephen Silberstein said in an interview published in *Neurology*, March 1992: "Estrogens and OCs are not contraindicated in migraine patients. In fact, they may actually be indicated for certain women. One needs to work closely with specialists to make the best use of the various chemical compositions now available." Listen to the patient, and use the approaches with the most likelihood of benefit with the least adverse effects. In women, that certainly has to include taking at look at the "hormone factor!"

Innovative Hormonal Approaches

For women who have a pattern of migraine headaches when hormone levels are changing or *dropping*, there are several options that can help stabilize the estradiol blood levels and help diminish the likelihood of hormone changes triggering migraines. If you want to try one of these options, you will need to work with a physician who will (1) evaluate you and see if hormone approaches could be used for you, (2) prescribe the hormone option that might work best in your particular situation, and (3) monitor your response and make adjustments as needed. If you have difficulty locating someone in your area, you may want to contact one of the resources at the end of this chapter or consider a consultation at our center, *HER Place™* in Tucson or Ft. Worth, to get started on an individualized program.

The first step is always a careful history of the migraine pattern and review of a headache diary, which I want a woman to keep for at least two, and preferably three or more ovarian cycles before I see her. Most women have already seen a number of doctors and have done a detailed headache diary by the time they ask for a consult with me. I think the diary is so crucial that I insist that my patients do one to help us work together effectively as a "detective" team to solve the problem.

If a woman still has ovaries producing the hormone rise and fall (whether or not the uterus is present), my initial goal is to find a safe and effective way to achieve suppression of ovarian cycling to determine whether this will indeed reduce the migraine frequency and severity. I have found the approaches I used with Reba to be helpful for a large number of women, especially women with new onset hormonally related migraines developing during the decade of the "roller-coaster" forties prior to menopause. These are examples of options I consider, based on an individual woman's medical evaluation and her preferences; you may wish to discuss these approaches with your physician:

1. **Low-dose oral contraceptives** (only if you are a *non-smoker* and there are no other risk factors that would preclude using OCs). Taking monophasic (constant dose) OCs will provide hormonal stability. A woman may take the active pills continuously for three to six months and observe the effects on her migraines. The estrogen content will protect her against bone loss and increasing CVD risks, as well as reduce or eliminate any premenopausal symptoms. The progestin content will suppress ovarian cycling and ovulation and reduce the hormonal fluctuations that we think are triggering her headaches. As I described with Reba, I first try shortening the time off hormone-containing pills each cycle to two or three days. If headaches occur during the days off active pills, then I may suggest *continuous treatment* with active pills to eliminate the fall of hormone levels in between pills packs. There aren't any known risks of taking the birth control pills this way for a short time, and it does help determine whether it is the drop in hormone level or some other factor that sets off the headache.

If a woman has a history of depression not on hormone therapy, or a history of feeling depressed on birth control pills, it is important to avoid an OC with more than 0.4 to 0.5 mg of norethindrone or progestin equivalent. The only oral contraceptives on the market in the U.S. that I would recommend are **Ovcon 35** (35 mcg ethinyl estradiol and 0.4 mg norethindrone), **Modicon or Brevicon** (35 mcg ethinyl estradiol and 0.5 mg norethindrone). When I began working with these issues, I figured out what balance of estrogen and progestin would be needed in a birth control pill to cause the least problems with depression side effects. I had to look up all the various ones sold in the U.S. and figure out the Estrogen:Progesterone (E:P) ratios, because everyone I asked about this just said "Oh, they are all pretty much alike, it doesn't really make much difference which one you use." Well, I knew that wasn't true based on my patients' descriptions about how they felt. I just trusted my own instinct and the insights from my patients, ignored conventional teaching that all the pills were similar, and started working with what I thought might work best!

Over time, it has become increasingly clear that there are marked differences in the way individuals respond to the various pill formulations. Even changing progestin *only 1/10th (0.1) milligram (mg)* can make a difference in side effects, especially depressive symptoms. Ovcon 35 has the least progestin of any pills available in the U.S. and is least likely to aggravate depression. If you try this one and experience depression as a side effect, it is *not likely* there are any *other* ones in the U.S. to try, since all of the others have so much more progestin. You may want to explore some of the other options I describe later in the chapter.

Nausea at the beginning of treatment with birth control pills is usually minimized if you take the pills at bedtime. Temporary side effects—nausea, breast fullness, bloating, slight weight gain, lethargy, and depressed mood—are generally related to the amount of progestin and tend to resolve by the second or third pill pack (if they occur at all).

2. Estraderm patch. If a woman does not want to try the birth control pill, or cannot take it for medical reasons, I have tried keeping the estradiol levels steady before menses and at ovulation by using the transdermal estradiol patch. This has eliminated the sharp drop in estradiol before bleeding starts, and, in many patients, has been quite effective at eliminating an identified hormone trigger for migraines. I have suggested that my patients put the patch on the buttock sometime between cycle day 24 and 28, change the patch two or three days later, and wear another one until about day 3 or 4 of the next cycle. This helps offset the body drop in estradiol, keeps blood levels steady, and can prevent the menstrual migraine in many women. In women with premenstrual migraine, I see the typical pattern of day 27-28 or Day 1 estradiol levels dropping to 20 to 40 pg/ml corresponding with their headache onset. I aim to keep estradiol levels between 70 and 90 pg/ml during these days, because this range seems to provide the best response in decreasing headache frequency. Since the patch is only being used for a few days each month, it does not add much additional estrogen, and doesn't interrupt your normal menstrual cycle flow and pattern. This would not be considered taking "unopposed estrogen" because (1) it's just a few days of boosting estradiol levels rather than continuous therapy, and (2) if you are still menstruating in a regular pattern with your normal flow, you are probably producing your own body progesterone.

3. GnRH ovarian suppression with estradiol replacement. This group of medications act on the brain's releasing hormones which govern the ovary production of estrogen and progesterone. GnRH agonist drugs such as Synarel or Lupron inhibit the brain's production of FSH and LH which stimulate follicle formation and ovulation; as a result, the cyclic ovarian production of estradiol and progesterone is also inhibited. Replacing *only* estradiol, *at a steady daily level*, enables stabilization of this hormonal component and ideally, elimination of the rise and fall as a migraine trigger. Adding back estradiol alone protects against further bone loss, and reverses menopausal symptoms and adverse lipid changes.

The goal of this therapy is again to use a medical means of eliminating ovarian cycling, which provides clues to the role of estradiol fluctuations as migraine triggers and also provides a therapeutic benefit in decreasing migraine activity. This approach is one I have only used as a last resort in patients who had been unable to find relief with any other means. It has a number of significant drawbacks: the medicine costs several hundred dollars a month, it requires daily injections (at least for the first month), it tends to cause irregular menses at the outset, and since it induces a sudden menopausal state, the risk of osteoporosis can be increased if GnRH drugs are used for a long period of time without adding back estradiol.

If you have to use this approach, make sure you work with a physician experienced in using GnRH agonist medications and providing hormone replacement, since the procedures can be complicated and require a significant amount of fine-tuning. One woman I saw for a consultation had been on Lupron injections for several months, but her physician had not realized that he had to add back estrogen at a constant level. She experienced severe menopausal symptoms, marked hair loss, and other problems. I do not usually recommend this approach except in difficult situations where literally *nothing else* has helped.

4. Migraine Headaches with ERT after Menopause. I have worked with a number of women who had migraines before menopause, which appeared to worsen with hormone therapy, as well as women who *first* developed migraines after starting on estrogen therapy after menopause. The most frequent cause is the starting and stopping ERT schedule: twenty-five days on estrogen and five days off each month. Again, the sudden withdrawal of estrogen seems to be the trigger for the biochemical and vascular changes that initiate the headache. A solution is often to change to taking the estrogen component *every day* to keep blood levels steady. Menopause specialists now recommend this mode of ERT instead of the older 25-day schedule for all of the other benefits of estrogen, so if you are on the 25-day regimen and are having headaches in the 5 days off, talk with your physician about changing to the daily ERT.

Dr. Stephen D. Silberstein, Director of the Comprehensive Headache Center at Germantown Hospital and Medical Center in Philadelphia has published several excellent review articles on management approaches for menopausal women with hormone-related migraines. Approaches he has found helpful are similar to the hormonal modifications I have also found effective with my patients. Another headache specialist, Dr. Lee Kudrow, Director of the California Medical Clinic for Headache in Encino, has also been a strong advocate of paying close attention to subtleties of hormonal changes to alleviate migraines in women on ERT. Collectively, some of the options I have found to help post-menopausal women with headaches aggravated by ERT are

- changing to a pure 17-beta-estradiol instead of the mixed conjugated equine estrogens
- dividing your total daily dose into smaller amounts taken morning and evening to keep estrogen levels from fluctuating widely during the 24 hours. I often find this works when other approaches have not.
- changing from an oral form of estrogen to a transdermal, vaginal, or sublingual one. Bypassing the liver metabolism may help keep estradiol levels more stable and reduce the swings that can trigger headaches. I do not use estrogen injections in migraine patients because the shots produce *erratic* blood levels, which tend to aggravate headaches even more.

- changing from a synthetic progestin (which also aggravates headaches) to natural micronized progesterone (if you have a uterus and need to take a progestin), which I find is much less likely to induce a headache compared to synthetic progestins.
- adding androgens (testosterone) may help decrease headaches in some women.

The Serotonin Boosters

Some exciting new developments have occurred in the last few years with new medications designed to act selectively on serotonin mechanisms to help both **abort** and **prevent** migraine attacks. As I described above, the serotonin system is one of the primary pathways that is involved in the cascade of neurochemical-vascular events in a migraine.

Sumatriptan (brand name: Imitrex) was approved by the FDA in late 1992 as an agent to interrupt the acute migraine attack and decrease pain. It acts specifically on $5\text{-}HT_1$ receptors in certain cranial arteries as an agonist to enhance the serotonin activity at these receptor sites. It is a potent vasoconstrictor of the arteries involved in causing pain and helps to rapidly decrease the throbbing vascular pain typical of migraines. It is very effective in the majority of patients and often enables the sufferer to return to normal activity in a few hours. It may be given as an injection, or as oral tablets, which have just been released in the U.S. (they have been available in Canada and Europe for a few years). In my experience, most patients find that the instruction kit for sumatriptan is easy to follow and, after the first injection with physician supervision, most women seem to do fine giving themselves the injection. Typically, sumatriptan causes few side effects, and these are usually brief flushing or tingling sensations and throat or chest tightness. It can, however, induce vasospasm of the coronary arteries and high blood pressure in patients with cardiovascular disease, so you need to assess this risk before using it. Sumatriptan is not recommended for use in pregnancy.

Ergotamine (Cafergot and others) and dihydroergotamine (DHE) are two older drugs in this group of abortive agents. These last two medications have many more side effects than does sumatriptan because they act at *multiple* 5-HT receptors: for example, both ergotamine and DHE also affect the 5-HT receptors that inhibit vomiting, so these drugs have the undesirable effect of aggravating the nausea and vomiting that can occur as part of the migraine episode. Sumatriptan, unlike DHE and ergotamine, *only* activates the 5-HT$_1$ receptors and does not typically cause nausea and vomiting. Drugs, such as Phenergan or Reglan, are usually given prior to DHE or Cafergot to decrease nausea and vomiting.

Drugs which enhance the activity of 5-HT$_2$ receptors can prevent migraines and are used for *prophylaxis* (the medical term for "preventive" therapy): newer ones in this category are fluoxetine (Prozac) and paroxetine (Paxil). At this time, neither of these medications is approved by the FDA for use in migraine prophylaxis, although many headache specialists find both Prozac and Paxil to be helpful for migraine patients without causing many of the side effects which occur with the older tricyclic antidepressants. Again, it is a difference in specificity at the receptors: Prozac and Paxil are specific for the 5-HT$_2$ receptors that reduce migraine activity; the other antidepressants (shown below in the chart) act on many different receptors, including serotonin, norepinephrine, and acetylcholine and thereby produce a wide variety of both desirable and undesirable effects.

Methysergide (Sansert) and cyproheptadine (Periactin) are 5-HT$_2$ antagonists that have been used for years to help prevent migraines, but both of these older medications have more bothersome, and potentially serious, side effects. I rarely suggest them since I think there are better options available today with the other serotonin-augmenting medications.

Medications for Migraine: A Summary of Options

The medications that are most effective for actually aborting an acute migraine attack are described above in the section on Serotonin Boosters. If you are someone with migraines, I encourage you to talk with your physician about some of these approaches instead of relying on narcotic pain medication. Narcotics blunt the pain but do not actually abort the migraine attack like sumatriptan and DHE do. In addition, if you determine that there is a strong correlation between hormone changes and your headaches, you may want to discuss with your doctor a trial on one or more of the hormonal options I have found effective.

Non-steroidal anti-inflammatory drugs (NSAIDS) are useful to relieve the pain of migraines and are considered *symptomatic* therapy rather than abortive or prophylactic. NSAIDS act by both antiplatelet aggregating effects and antiprostaglandin effects, which reduce inflammation and pain. All of these drugs can be effective, but individuals respond differently to the various ones in this group. If one doesn't work, you may respond to another. One of the most common errors in using these is *not using enough medication and not keeping adequate blood levels* by taking the NSAIDS regularly throughout the day during headache times. If you use the over-the-counter NSAIDS, remember that these are *only one-third* the dose of the same medication in prescription form, so you should talk with your doctor about the appropriate amount of over-the-counter pain relievers to substitute for prescription-strength ones. The list below does not show all of the NSAIDS available in the U.S., just some of the more commonly used ones. Remember, lack of response to one *does not mean another one won't do the trick!*

Common NSAIDS for Migraine

- ibuprofen (Motrin, Advil)
- naproxen (Naprosyn, Anaprox)
- ketorolac (Toradol)
- indomethacin (Indocin)
- oxaprozin (DayPro)
- mefenamic acid (Ponstel)
- flurbiprofen (Ansaid)
- piroxicam (Feldene)
- ketoprofen (Orudis)
- fenoprofen (Nalfon)
- etodolac (Lodine)

Other classes of medications that act by different mechanisms to prevent migraine attacks are shown in the next table. **I prefer to avoid beta-blockers if possible** because of their potential to produce depression, lethargy, fatigue, and problems with weight gain and impaired insulin secretion. Propanolol (but not other beta-blockers) inhibits the conversion of thyroid hormone T4 to T3, which may be one of the mechanisms by which propanolol contributes to depression in patients taking it regularly.

Another concern I have encountered in women on long-term beta-blockers for headaches is finding greater than expected bone loss in women who have no other risk factors. To my knowledge, there has not been any research on the possible connection between beta-blockers and bone loss, so the question of long-term safety *in women* for the beta-blockers, in my opinion, has not been adequately addressed. If you can find other medications to provide reduction in your headache frequency, I think that would be a more prudent course of action. As a group, I think the calcium-channel blockers are safer and have far fewer side effects than the beta-blockers.

You and your physician may have to experiment to find a choice that will give you the best response, since each person reacts differently. Be sure you keep a diary of how you feel and descriptions of your headache frequency and severity with each medication you try, so that you can better assist your physician in arriving at an optimal solution for you. I have tried to list some of the more common side effects of each class of medication, but keep in mind this is not the complete list. You must review with your physician the appropriateness of any medication based on your individual health problems and sensitivities.

Rebound Headache: Getting Off Painkillers

When I was Associate Medical Director of the Maryview Pain Management Program in Virginia, one of the most common problems I encountered in helping women with headache syndromes (especially migraine!) was that of "rebound" headaches due to the multiple analgesics and ergot medications women were taking on a daily basis. As many of these medicines wear off, the headache pain cycle starts again, so you take more medicine, pain is relieved for awhile, then it comes back, and the cycle continues. It often becomes a problem to even determine which is the migraine and which is the withdrawal headache!

We now know that daily use of ergots and analgesics, even ones like Aspirin and Tylenol, can *cause* headaches to become chronic and can also interfere with the effectiveness of medications used to prevent migraines. When you are caught in this vicious cycle of rebounding, whether it is from opiates, barbiturates (as in Fiorinal, Fioricet and others), NSAIDS, or ergotamine, practically speaking, *nothing else* works to prevent your migraines. The first step is to be properly tapered off the offending medications causing the withdrawal headaches, and then be started on a suitable *preventive* regimen. Dr. Joel Saper, founder and director of the Michigan Headache and Neurological Institute in Ann Arbor, Michigan, published the first paper about ergot dependency in 1986, which characterized the increasing severity of headaches due to ergot withdrawal. In contrast to typical migraines, patients with ergot withdrawal headaches have more diffuse and severe head

Medicines to Prevent Migraines			
Name Of Drug	**Typical Dose**	**Side Effects**	**Comments**
Beta-blockers			
• Propanolol • Timolol • Atenolol • Nadalol	40–240 mg/day 10–30 mg/day 50–120 mg/day 40–240 mg/day	weight gain, low blood pressure, lethargy, mood changes, sexual problems, depression, and others	Do not stop abruptly, may cause rebound high blood pressure
Anticonvulsants			
• Phenytoin (Dilantin) • Valproate (Depakote) • Carbamazepine (Tegretol)	200–400 mg/day 500–3000 mg/day 200–1200 mg/day	rashes, blood cell problems, drowsiness, and many others	Need careful monitoring of blood levels, CBC, liver enzymes, and side effects
Calcium-channel Blockers			
• Verapamil • Nifedipine • Diltiazem • Nimodipine	160–720 mg/day 30–180 mg/day 120–360 mg/day 30–120 mg/day	dizziness, low blood pressure, drowsiness, hair loss, constipation, lethargy, and many others	Watch for low blood pressure, slowed heart rate
Serotonin-enhancing Antidepressants			
• Fluoxetine (Prozac) • Paroxetine (Paxil)	20–80 mg/day 10–100 mg/day	mild nausea, gastro-intestinal upset, diarrhea, anxiety, decrease in sexual desire	Do not use with MAO inhibitors; may cause *more agitation in some*
TCA Antidepressants			
• Nortriptyline • Doxepin • Imipramine • Amitriptyline	10–80 mg/day 10–200 mg/day 25–150 mg/day 10–250 mg/day	weight gain, constipation, dry mouth, reduced orgasm, blurred vision, dry eyes	May cause rapid heart rate, blood pressure changes, many drug interactions

pain, more severe vomiting, and are likely to have headaches persisting three to five days during which time they often become dehydrated due to the vomiting. Ergot dependency also contributes to an increased frequency of headaches.

Migraines in their usual form occur at most once or twice a week, and more commonly, only once every two or three weeks. If the headaches are happening as often as three to five times a week in a person on ergotamine, then it is more likely that the headache is being driven by ergot dependency and withdrawal. The same pattern is seen in narcotic withdrawal and barbiturate withdrawal headaches: headaches show an increasing intensity the longer one is without the medication, a crescendo effect not seen in the same pattern with migraines; the headaches are quickly relieved by restarting the offending drug and typically are *not* relieved by any other medications; and the headaches become more frequent, with timing that relates to half-life of the particular drug.

If you see yourself described in these pages, you might consider a comprehensive pain management program for integrated treatment. You may look into resources at one of the headache centers listed in Appendix 2, or contact the National Headache Foundation (800-843-2256) for the names of specialists in your area.

Alternative Therapies: Acupuncture, Biofeedback, Hypnotherapy, Massage, and Others

Many studies in recent years have shown that biofeedback can be remarkably effective in reducing migraine headache pain. Acupuncture also can be highly effective and appears to work through a number of the neurochemical pathways I discussed earlier in this chapter. Both of these techniques have provided help to women who have side effects with medications or who simply prefer alternative approaches. I often recommend a trial of either or both options. The primary drawback is that you have to find a skilled therapist to teach you to use biofeedback or to administer acupuncture and both require a series of treatments for optimal effectiveness. You have to be motivated to practice the technique daily in order for biofeedback to be effective. Acupuncture and biofeedback may not have the long term preventive effects, which can be achieved with some of the newer medications, but these modalities certainly can be beneficial to decrease pain and reduce medication use. Acupuncture and biofeedback are helpful as stress-reduction strategies, which can be another way of decreasing headache frequency.

Speaking of stress, remember that eating regularly and well helps reduce the stress response which can trigger migraines and also helps prevent low blood sugar (hypoglycemia), another migraine trigger. Watching your alcohol and caffeine intake particularly at vulnerable times of the menstrual cycle helps avoid known headache triggers. Migraines in some women may also be precipitated by milk and other dairy products. Some people feel that vitamin B_6 and diuretics are useful for migraines although I have not found that either of these approaches is effective. Diuretics typically do not improve premenstrual migraine headaches and may actually make them worse by altering electrolyte balance. Vitamin B_6 has been reported to help some women with PMS, but it has not been found to help relieve menstrual migraines and large doses can cause neurological symptoms of numbness, tingling, and sensory abnormalities. If you suffer with migraines, you probably already have a pretty good idea of the triggers that affect you, so pay attention and avoid these at times in your menstrual cycle when you are particularly susceptible to attacks.

Aerobic exercise on a regular basis improves circulation, boosts endorphins and helps get rid of excess adrenalin, which accumulates with our typical stres-s-s-s-filled days! All of these benefits help to further decrease migraine headache frequency. A number of bodywork modalities help reduce the pain and spasm which may occur in neck and jaw muscles and add to headache pain or cause the chronic tension-type headaches. I have referred patients to physical therapists for myofascial release, to massage therapists for cranio-sacral, shiatsu and other massage modalities (very helpful to diminish headaches), and I have also recommended osteopathic manipulation as an effective technique to decrease pain. I think more headaches management programs should include these methods, since they are beneficial and have few side effects. Scheduling yourself for a massage therapy session at potentially vulnerable times for headaches is not only a great idea for stress reduction, but also it can provide generalized relaxation and decrease muscle tension that aggravates headache pain.

I encourage you to take charge of your headache problems and begin putting all these pieces together along with an understanding of the hormonal influences on migraine. This approach should help give you a better awareness of factors that are within your control and those you can discuss with your physician. It takes patience, persistence, practice, and partnership with a physician who listens and works with you but it's worth it in the long run. Migraines can be helped!

CHAPTER 11

Fibromyalgia, Aches, and Pains: The Estrogen Factor

If someone told you that there was a medical disorder in which 80 percent of the patients were women, and the average age of onset was thirty to fifty years of age, what connections do you think might be obvious to study? It seems pretty important to look at a factor, or factors, that make women different from men in that age range, wouldn't you agree? I have done a great deal of work with chronic pain patients since my residency at Johns Hopkins in the early 1980s. I have been struck by the fact that almost all of the *fibromyalgia* patients I saw were women, typically over forty, and frequently with a history of hysterectomy or early menopause. The obvious gender difference in this common medical disorder made me consider two important points:

1. the age range of thirty to fifty is a time of significant hormonal changes for women, but not typically a time of marked hormonal change for men, and

2. women's pain symptoms typically flared up at certain times of their menstrual cycle and subsided at other times in the cycle. I thought there might be a connection with changes in estrogen and progesterone and how these hormones affected brain chemistry in the pain-regulating centers of the nervous system.

The more I began looking into these connections in evaluating my patients, the more I was stunned to find marked degrees of hormonal loss, which clearly could be of clinical significance in addressing the chronic pain problems. I realize that with something as complex as fibromyalgia and chronic pain, there are *multiple* causative and contributing factors. It is too simplistic to say that these medical problems are *due to*, or *only* caused by, declining estrogen and other female hormones. My question, however, is why haven't physicians and researchers in the field of chronic pain even considered female hormonal factors *when the majority of patients with fibromyalgia are female?* The collective lack of awareness of women's physiological differences is astounding.

Listen to one woman's voice (one of many I hear on this subject and, like most women I see who have these problems, she had made the connections with her menstrual cycle and menopausal hormonal changes):

> I am forty-five, and I've felt for a long time, about ten years, that there were problems with my hormones. Around the time of my period, the pain seems to increase markedly. As I have been getting closer to menopause, I feel like my fibromyalgia has increased a lot. When I have asked these questions of my doctors, I have been told there is absolutely (!) no hormonal connection in fibromyalgia. I've been made to feel I'm stupid for even asking such a dumb question. When I have asked what can help my pain, I have felt talked down to. The only thing offered me was to exercise more. No one is really listening to me.

In addition to overlooking the role of female hormones in fibromyalgia, we have also been too slow in looking at some of the brain hormones and chemical messengers (serotonin, dopamine, epinephrine, substance P, and others) in approaching chronic pain as a problem very different from *acute* pain. It was almost fifteen years ago that I completed my specialty training at Johns Hopkins, and we were using serotonin-modulating medications at that time to help patients with chronic pain. But use of these types of medications in fibromyalgia is just now beginning to gain more widespread use. Management options for *chronic* pain are still largely in the dark ages with negative stereotypes of patients (the majority of whom are women, remember?) as "neurotic," "drug-seekers," addictive personalities," and so on. I hope this chapter will help you see that new hope, help, and treatment approaches are available if you have been struggling with the chronic pain of fibromyalgia.

Fibromyalgia:
The Mysterious, Elusive Medical Condition

"Fibromyalgia Syndrome" (abbreviated FMS) is the name for *persistent, diffuse, aching pain* affecting the muscles and connective (fibrous) tissues of the body (tendons and ligaments). It is a condition that has been described in the medical writings for hundreds of years and has been called a number of different names: *myofascial pain syndrome, myositis, fibrositis, fibromyositis, mylagia.* FMS is difficult to diagnose on objective physical findings. There are no consistent lab abnormalities such as objective measures of inflammation or actual damage to the muscles. Patients do not have a specific, easily identifiable lesion of the body. I have only once seen a medical article mention checking blood levels of ovary hormones in women with fibromyalgia.

For all of these reasons, FMS is a particularly frustrating condition, both for patients who suffer with it, and doctors who want to offer their patients some help and relief. Since FMS has been difficult to pin down, it was long viewed by medical people with skepticism and disparagement. Doctors saw it as something vague and psychosomatic because its symptoms came and went, the pain was hard to localize, and there were no objective changes in the body when the person experienced pain. Add to all this what I have already described about the negative stereotypes given to women patients, and you can begin to see how a problem that was a vague, ill-defined syndrome was often labeled a psychogenic illness.

We now use the guidelines in the chart below to make a diagnosis of FMS. Finally in 1990, FMS was recognized as a legitimate disorder and was given standard diagnostic criteria based upon (1) the presence of persistent pain or achiness at multiple body sites, and (2) the presence of positive painful "trigger points" at eleven of the eighteen classic sites shown in Diagram 11.1 on the next page.

Hallmark Features of Fibromyalgia

- generalized stiffness and soreness, often worse in A.M.
- increased pain in neck, trunk and hips
- restless, fragmented sleep
- exquisite tender points where muscles and tendons meet
- numbness, burning or cold sensations in muscles and/or extremities
- diminished energy, marked fatigue
- may be associated with mood changes: irritability, lability, depression
- may be associated with alterations in memory and concentration

A trigger point is defined as *positive* when pressure applied to the area during physical examination causes a localized sensation of increased tenderness and pain. It is possible to have other types of chronic pain syndromes without having all eleven painful trigger points. FMS is often confused with *arthritis*, a group of inflammatory disorders that lead to *joint* deterioration and pain. **Unlike** the various types of arthritis (inflammation of the joints) and arthralgias (soreness, aching of the joints), *fibromyalgia* does not affect the joints directly. It affects the *muscles, tendons, and ligaments,* which affect the way joints function; that's why you might think that fibromyalgia is in your joints. FMS does not cause deformities or permanent crippling as may happen with arthritis, but it can certainly interfere with quality of life and ability to function optimally.

Diagram 11.1—TRIGGER POINT SITES

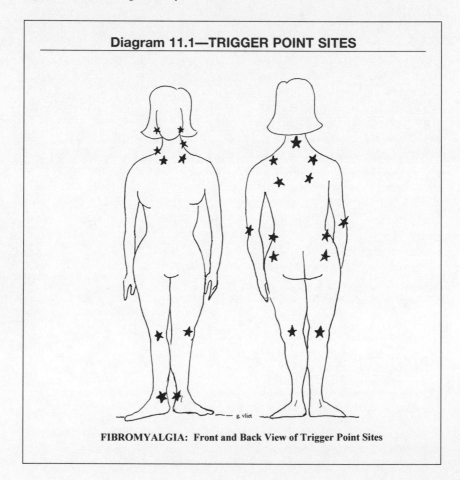

FIBROMYALGIA: Front and Back View of Trigger Point Sites

Female Hormonal Connections

As I noted, when we look at who gets FMS, some glaring trends pop out: **eighty percent of patients are women between the ages of thirty and fifty.** Yes, FMS does occur in men, and can begin in adolescence in both males and females, but it is much less common in these groups. When I took careful histories of *when* the onset of FMS symptoms occurred, another glaring trend appeared: for the majority of my patients, the FMS began insidiously following some event that typically is associated with a *significant decrease* in ovarian hormone levels.

I have summarized my hypothesis about the most likely times in women's lives when FMS may insidiously begin; all of these times are when estrogen is low. I think this hormonal connection is crucially significant. **I am not being sexist. There simply isn't anything else which so <u>clearly</u> differentiates male and female bodies!** I think many women with FMS find it helpful and hopeful that I discuss these connections. Very commonly, they have already been asking these kinds of questions and have been frustrated with the lack of validation and acceptance of their observations about these connections. *These potential hormonal connections simply have not been explored.*

COMMON TIMES OF ONSET FOR FMS IN WOMEN

- postpartum (particularly if the pregnancy was after the age of 35)

- perimenopause, associated with sleep changes

- postmenopause, particularly if not on ERT or on suboptimal ERT

- 3 to 5 years after tubal ligation

- 2 to 3 years after hysterectomy (even if the ovaries were not removed in the surgery)

- a period of sustained major stresses or illnesses which interrupt menses for several months

- younger women with chronic anorexic-type dieting, which suppresses ovary hormones

---

Scattered in the recent medical literature are other clues to the existence of these ovary hormone connections beyond just my clinical experience. In one study of 100 patients cited by Jon Russell, M.D., Ph.D. of the University of Texas Health Science

Center, San Antonio, the average age at which Fibromyalgia was diagnosed was 48, a common age of menopausal hormone decline. Dr. Russell described clinical observations that in women who developed FMS between the ages of 25 and 40, fully 40 to 50 percent of them were *menopausal prior to the onset of FMS*— either by surgical menopause or a premature natural menopause.

I think if we actually *measured* blood tests of female hormone levels, we would see an even *higher percentage* of menopausal women in such studies. Instead, the questions about menopause are rarely asked, and most physicians tend to just depend on the patient's chronological age or her own knowledge of whether she is menopausal. This was one of the striking findings I noted when I did the thorough history and medical evaluation of the women admitted to our pain management program.

When I actually measured hormone levels in these patients (FSH, estradiol, testosterone, and sometimes progesterone if the woman still had her ovaries), I was quite struck by how low the levels of estradiol and testosterone were compared to the expected normal range for a woman in her twenties through early forties. One of the treatment approaches I used, in combination with the other therapies we incorporated in our overall approach to pain management, was restoring the woman's hormonal balance to normal levels. I was pleasantly surprised to find that the improvements in FMS occurred much more rapidly with optimal hormonal therapy added to the overall therapeutic program.

I must caution that, at this time, there is simply no *controlled* study to determine whether there is a cause-and-effect relationship with female hormones and FMS or whether this observed connection is simply an *association* of the phenomena of *pain/FMS* and *menopausal hormone changes*. Even if there is only an association, it certainly is important enough to at least include in our medical assessments. If there are hormonal imbalances, these can be properly addressed in designing an individualized treatment plan. Helping women find an optimal hormonal balance, in my experience, has frequently meant they could reduce the amount of pain medication.

Ria's Story

Ria is an example of what can happen in women with fibromyalgia when hormonal balance is addressed. She is now fifty-three, and had been injured in an automobile accident about eight years ago. Following the accident she developed a severe pain syndrome called Reflex Sympathetic Dystrophy (RSD), which produces a burning, excruciating pain difficult to relieve even with narcotic medication. She has undergone extensive evaluation and treatment by physicians very experienced in managing RSD. Two years later, when she went through menopause, she was started on a standard cyclic hormone therapy with conjugated equine estrogen (Premarin) therapy and progestin (Provera). Her menopausal hot flashes stopped, and she was sleeping better. She felt better getting these concerns addressed, even though the RSD continued to cause pain.

Over the past five years, however, she developed a *new and different type of pain*, which she described as clearly distinct from the *burning* pain of RSD. She described the new pain as dull, aching pain in the muscles of her arms, hands, legs, and back associated with intermittent sharper pains along with stiffness in her joints. This pain had gotten so much worse over the last year that she now had difficulty walking and had to begin using a cane. Understandably, she was becoming more and more discouraged about her health. She had observed that this new pain developed when she began hormone therapy after menopause. It seemed a reasonable question to ask her doctors if there could be a possible hormonal connection to produce this new type of pain. She asked several of her doctors whether it was possible to check hormone levels to see if she was taking the right amount. Each time she asked, she was told that it couldn't have anything to do with her hormones. She was told that she had fibromyalgia. She met the criteria I described above for FMS, so this seemed a reasonable diagnosis. She was further told that there was no way to do any tests for hormone levels, and the hormone dose was fine because she wasn't having any more hot flashes. Her doctors recommended physical therapy and anti-inflammatory medication added to the pain medicine she had been taking for the RSD. She continued to have more and more difficulty with both the RSD and this new pain problem.

Ria's friend told her about the work I was doing with women with FMS. Ria scheduled an appointment and had her hormone levels checked along with the other blood tests I think are important. In addition to the new pain syndrome, Ria was also having problems with weight gain, loss of energy, diminished libido, restless sleep, and said she just didn't feel "like my old self." Ria and I spent an hour going over all that she had been through, her lab results, and the options I thought could help her. Even though she was taking estrogen, her FSH was still too high in the menopausal range, and her estradiol level was markedly low (less than 30 pg/ml). Her hormone therapy was clearly not giving adequate levels of the estrogen she needed replenished.

Since she had experienced breast enlargement on the conjugated equine estrogen, I did not want to increase the dose and suggested she change to the native human form of estradiol. I recommended that she dissolve the estradiol under her tongue (instead of swallowing the oral tablet). I knew this would give a better ratio of estradiol (E2) to estrone (E1). I thought this would help reduce the breast enlargement and weight gain she had experienced, and still provide optimal levels of estradiol to help diminish her symptoms. At this time, there is only one commercial tablet form of estradiol which can be dissolved under the tongue, and that is the brand Estrace. I had explained the rationale above and she decided to try it. I did not give her any particular suggestions about the change other than to say I thought this estrogen may help her feel better, improve her sleep more effectively, and *perhaps* help with the overall pain she had been experiencing.

At her first follow-up visit about two months later, she said she felt more energetic, was sleeping well again, and had gone down a bra size. She reported that she did not feel as bloated, her joints were not as swollen and painful, and she felt she had a better range of movement. She was surprised to see that over the two months, her overall pain seemed less intense. She asked if I thought that could be related to the hormones, and I told her that this was the response I had seen in most of my patients, and I thought it did have an important hormonal connection. We agreed that she would continue the same amount of Estrace, and she would come back in another two months to be rechecked.

Four months later she returned for follow-up, and I hardly recognized her when she walked in the door. She looked happy and cheerful, walked more quickly and fluidly, did not need her cane to lean on (although she still carried it) and had more normal overall body movements. I commented that I had not seen her in such a long while, I had begun to wonder if she had given up on the hormonal approaches we were trying. She laughed and said,

No, I was just feeling so much better, I forgot to call and make an appointment! About two weeks after my last appointment, I got up one morning and realized that *my joint and muscle pain was completely gone.* At first, I was afraid to believe it, but after a few more weeks, I realized the resolution of that part of my pain was very real,

and it has not come back. The RSD pain is still there, but I can cope
with that now that I don't have my joints and muscles hurting so bad
all the time. I am even using less pain medicine for the RSD now.

Ria's whole countenance just radiated her newfound release
from the joint pain and her happiness that she felt so much better
and could do more things she enjoyed. Even I was surprised by the
marked change in her appearance and movements since her last
appointment. She talked about how angry she felt that other
physicians had not taken her seriously when she asked questions
about her pain possibly being triggered or aggravated by hormonal changes. She was angry about the years she had spent in
additional pain, while her ideas and insights ignored. That's one
of the reasons she readily agreed for me to have her story told in
this book. She said through her own tears of anger and frustration: **"Maybe other women who read this won't have to go
through what I did."** I hope her story *will* help someone else find
ideas for possible options to help with chronic pain.

The normal premenopausal balance of estradiol in a woman's
body has a number of effects on nerves and chemical messengers
to reduce pain sensations, particularly chronic pain. Other underlying triggering mechanisms in fibromyalgia can be metabolic,
neuroendocrine changes. These chemical changes in the brain and
body would then affect the way peripheral nerve fibers function
and trigger increases in the painful spasms that set up the vicious
cycle of fibromyalgia. An example of this mechanism is the way
declining female hormones, particularly estradiol from the ovary,
cause *heightened sensitivity of nerve endings to pain* and other
stimuli. Decreases in estradiol also cause decreases in serotonin
production, so there are several possible ways for hormone change
to trigger the variety of pain and aching with FMS. In this way,
FMS may be dysfunction of the nerve fibers, with changes or
abnormalities occurring in the way nerves to the body transmit
pain signals. The stress of chronic pain on the body can also cause
further decline ovarian production of hormones, so situation
aggravates the other.

The estradiol receptors heavily concentrated in the limbic system areas of the brain provide another connecting link between
the chronic pain of FMS and the hormonal changes leading up to
menopause. The nerve pathways carrying *chronic pain* stimuli
from the body to the brain travel *through* the limbic system centers, which regulate mood and sleep. You can imagine how the
constant day to day presence of pain signals can then disrupt nor-

mal sleep regulation and contribute to depressed, irritable moods through effects on the limbic system. Remember that I talked in Chapter 4 about the way in which decreases in estradiol can disrupt the limbic system pathways and cause irritable mood and fragmented sleep. Now we see that *both* chronic pain stimuli and decreases in estrogen have similar effects on the same brain centers. *Acute pain* pathways *bypass* the limbic system as they travel from the body to the higher brain centers, so when you experience an *acute* injury producing pain, it is not likely to cause the same types of sleep and mood upsets that we see in people who have a chronic pain syndrome.

If you have FMS, what could you do check these connections for yourself? I suggest asking your physician to check hormone levels, so you can then determine whether adding the hormones might be helpful for you. I discuss these connections with my patients, and then measure FSH, estradiol, and testosterone blood levels. If the results show low estradiol levels, and she wants to try it, I prescribe estradiol alone or possibly with low-dose natural testosterone. If she has a uterus and needs to use a progestin, I *do not* use a synthetic progestin (such as Provera, Cyrin, Amen or Aygestin). I have found the synthetic progestins seem to make fibromyalgia pain *worse*. One possible explanation for this observation is that the synthetic progestins actually block estrogen binding at the estradiol receptors in the brain, which will then reduce estrogen's beneficial effects on pain. I have also found that synthetic estrogens and the mixed animal-derived estrogens (such as Premarin, Ogen, and Estrovis) also appear to aggravate FMS symptoms. For women with FMS who may benefit from hormone therapy, I *only use the native human compounds* and make certain they reach optimal estradiol blood levels of estradiol. If you are having difficulty getting someone to check your hormone levels, you may want to schedule a consultation at a women's center like ours, where the hormone issues will be addressed as part of a comprehensive evaluation.

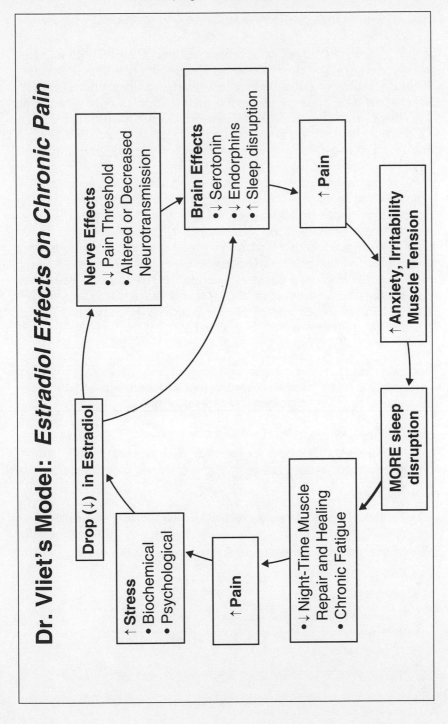

Dr. Vliet's Model: *Estradiol Effects on Chronic Pain*

Serotonin and Other Neurohormonal Connections

There is a great deal of overlap in the chemical messengers involved in fibromyalgia and those affected by the decline in ovary hormones during perimenopause and due to stressors (surgical, life situations, or lifestyle habits) that suppress ovary function. I do not find in the medical literature much mention of these *overlapping effects* on pain-modulation pathways and neurotransmitters. I think there is much to explore in understanding these interconnecting pathways and functions.

The list below shows the most important of the known neurotransmitters involved in regulating pain. Since there are so many of these, you can begin to see how many different disorders can contribute to making FMS pain worse. I have already mentioned that hypothyroidism is *many times* more common in women than men, and this hormonal disturbance may be another overlooked factor in FMS. In FMS patients, I think it is particularly important to also check antithyroid antibody levels, since autoimmune thyroid disorders which contribute to muscle pain may be found in their early stages even if TSH is normal.

Key Neurotransmitters and Hormones Involved in FMS and Pain

- Serotonin (pain-relieving chemical messenger)
- Tryptophan (building block for serotonin found in many foods)
- Norepinephrine (NE) and Epinephrine (EPI)
- Dopamine
- Substance P (pain-inducing chemical found in higher than normal levels in FMS)
- Monoamine Oxidase (enzyme that breaks down dopamine, NE, EPI)
- Endorphins
- Thyroid Hormone
- Ovarian Hormones (some researchers say this is still open to question)
- Adrenal Steroids

Although medical researchers and physicians don't know the exact causes of fibromyalgia, they have recognized a number of different conditions and biological changes in the brain and body that are associated with it. In order to properly help patients with FMS, we must look at these pieces of the puzzle and look at how changes in one group of neurotransmitters or hormones can have a cascade effect on other tissues throughout the body—including the muscles affected by FMS.

It was originally thought that the symptoms of fibromyalgia were caused by stress and worry, which caused additional muscle tension. Although recent studies of people with fibromyalgia do not prove that stress itself causes FMS, stress, anxiety, and fatigue can make the pain worse. In fact, chronic pain and fatigue often cause stress and anxiety, which in turn can increase the pain and fatigue. Do you see a vicious cycle happening?

Many times people who are caught in this tension-pain cycle turn to readily available drugs for relief: alcohol, nicotine, caffeine, pain killers, and the like. We are so accustomed to having these substances around that we often do not think of them as the drugs they are. Each one of these substances has many adverse effects on the brain chemical messengers, which collectively result in intensified pain.

I urge my patients with FMS to reduce or eliminate intake of alcohol, caffeine, nicotine, and other drugs, which may make chronic pain worse. Take a look at the next diagram, which shows how some of the many different factors are related to one another and typically create this vicious cycle effect. This may give you some ideas of ways you can begin to make healthy habit changes, which will contribute to reducing the chronic pain. At the same, time, if you begin to take into account the hormonal factors that are involved in altering pain sensations, you can begin to see how all these pieces of the puzzle are connected through similar effects on serotonin, endorphins, and other body messenger systems.

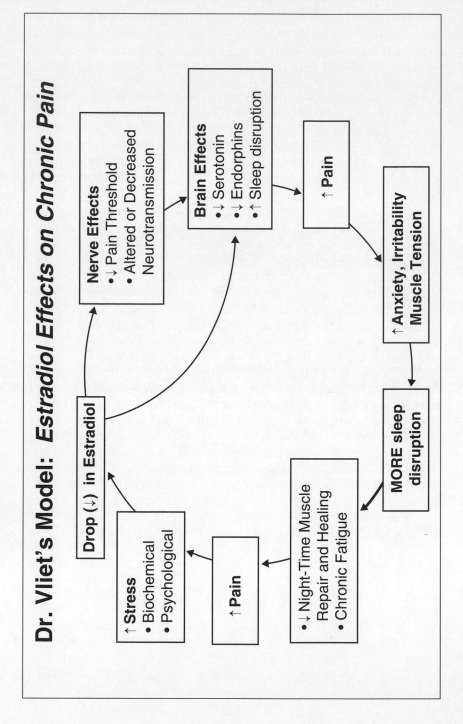

Dr. Vliet's Model: *Estradiol Effects on Chronic Pain*

Fibromyalgia may also be precipitated by some type of trauma, whether a car accident with whiplash injuries, a severe jarring type of fall, or a surgery followed by prolonged inactivity. The anatomic and biochemical changes that occur with such traumas then set the foundation for the chronic pain cycle to begin. Since there are so many factors involved in aggravating and perpetuating fibromyalgia, it takes a comprehensive and *integrated* approach to achieve optimal reduction in pain and improvement in well-being. Taking pain killers alone will not provide for long-term relief and return to normal activity. Let's look at some of the conditions which are found to be present with fibromyalgia.

Conditions Associated With FMS

- physically unfit muscles

- an associated sleep disorder

- metabolic abnormalities

- immunologic abnormalities

- vascular changes (example: Raynaud's Syndrome)

- neuroendocrine changes (decreased Somatomedin-C, increased cortisol, etc.)

- situational stressors (which affect all of the above)

- whiplash and fall-type injuries (common precipitants)

Unfit Muscles

While it is not yet known whether *unfit muscles* are the cause or the result of FMS, there is increasing evidence that people with fibromyalgia have unfit or poorly developed muscles. Women also typically lose muscle mass as they age, so there is less reserve muscle tissue than in earlier years. As the cycle of pain contributes to more inactivity, the muscles become even more unfit and atrophied, which makes them more likely to be injured or damaged with to exercise. This is a vicious cycle: more pain causes more inactivity causes more loss of muscle causes more pain causes more inactivity causes more loss of muscle. I think you get the picture. Over time, underuse of your muscles leads to a negative, detraining effect, which results in even more unfit muscles which are more likely to become injured or damaged from exercise. This sort of muscle damage is commonly called "microtrauma," and it causes delayed muscle pain and fatigue that may not appear until a day or two after exercising and may last six to seven days. The pain and fatigue makes us postpone further physical activity until they are gone and our energy has been restored, thereby again contributing to the vicious cycle.

It is common for anyone to experience the effects of microtrauma after too much physical activity. That's the kind of pain a weekend athlete will experience on Monday or Tuesday. Yet for people who have unfit muscles, these problems may develop after even slight exertion, such as routine day-to-day activities. Microtrauma may also result from other kinds of muscle overuse or injury: poor posture, sitting hunched over at a computer or a desk all day; damage caused by a blow or a fall; or the kind of torsion damage which occurs in a whiplash injury. In the normal person, muscles repair and restore themselves from microtrauma during stage IV sleep each night. But in FMS patients, (and in women who have decreasing ovarian estrogen) the deep stages of sleep are disrupted, so normal muscle growth and repair during sleep does not occur.

In addition, there is an important chemical for muscle growth and repair, called Somatomedin-C, released by the liver when the liver is stimulated by growth hormone (GH). Eighty percent of our daily amount of GH is secreted during the deep stages of sleep, which, in FMS patients, are markedly diminished or missing altogether. It may well be, then, that the tendency toward muscle fatigue and weakness may be due to the loss of deep sleep stages, which in turn decreases the normal production of GH. Also keep in mind what I have said about the role of serotonin: this important chemical messenger in the brain is one of the crucial regulators of sleep, and serotonin production is typically also low in FMS patients.

If you think about what I have said about the role of unfit muscles in causing and/or maintaining FMS, you will see why beginning an exercise program under the supervision of a physical therapist is one of the cornerstones of effective treatment. It is crucial to break out of this vicious cycle and retrain your muscles. Patients who diligently follow a graded exercise program have a significantly better, and more rapid, recovery, because they are rebuilding and strengthening muscle tissue. A gradual increase in aerobic exercise also provides better blood flow to the muscles, which brings new oxygen and fuel and takes away the waste products (particularly lactic acid), which otherwise would build up and contribute to more pain.

Sleep Disorders and FMS

Almost all patients with fibromyalgia have a major sleep disturbance as part of the clinical findings. It is not yet known whether the sleep disorder *causes* FMS or whether the sleep disruption is produced by the chronic pain. At the point a person has FMS, sleep is disturbed, causing a worsening of the FMS and pain. I prefer to view it as an *integrated* problem and try to identify ways of constructively breaking the cycle. The clue to the sleep disorder connection in FMS has been determined from sleep laboratory studies in which patients sleep in a "bedroom" laboratory, with monitors keeping track of brain wave patterns, muscle activity, eye movements, heart rate, breathing rate, oxygen concentration in the blood, and a number of other objective measures of the quantity and quality of sleep.

Patients with fibromyalgia typically show a marked degree of fragmented sleep. The deepest or most restful stage of sleep (stage IV) is repeatedly disturbed or interrupted, and there are more waking episodes at night. This abnormal pattern is called "alpha intrusion of stage IV sleep." Remember that I have also talked about the sleep disturbances that are caused by declining estrogen levels affecting the brain centers that regulate sleep. Here we see another hormonal connection that may aggravate, or help to set up the conditions for FMS: **decreased estrogen makes nerve endings more susceptible to pain and disrupts sleep; the pain of fibromyalgia disrupts sleep; the stress to the body of continued sleep loss causes more pain and more decrease in ovary hormone production.** See how it all fits together?

Sleep disturbances may be a significant the reason that women with FMS describe having such low energy levels and feelings of marked fatigue. A decline in hormone such as estrogen and particularly testosterone may be another reason for the low energy levels. There is also evidence that **both** sleep problems and decreased ovarian hormones can lead to increased muscle pain. When normal, healthy volunteers were stressed by artificial disturbance of their stage IV sleep, they developed pain and soreness in their muscles, which were very similar to that of fibromyalgia.

This combination of pain and fatigue then often limits physical activity and endurance. The resulting lack of physical exercise can contribute to the unfit muscles which are more susceptible to further pain, and the FMS symptoms continue to get worse. As I mentioned above, stage IV sleep is important in repairing tissue damage and feeling physically and psychologically rested when you wake up. So if stage IV sleep is reduced, it can contribute to many of the other symptoms of FMS.

If you have trouble going to sleep, you may find yourself turning to alcohol thinking it will help you sleep better. The problem with using alcohol, especially for FMS patients, is that alcohol contributes to *more* fragmentation in sleep and *more loss* of stage IV sleep.

Alcohol used on a regular basis has several other effects that make FMS worse: (1) alcohol depresses the central nervous system and aggravates the biological depression which occurs in about 90 percent of patients with FMS; (2) heavy alcohol use further suppresses ovarian function; (3) alcohol diminishes production of endorphins, the body's natural painkillers; (4) when alcohol is wearing off, it creates an adrenalin rebound which leads to increased muscle tension and pain; (5) alcohol is also toxic to muscle fibers.

For these reasons, I urge you to avoid drinking alcohol on a regular basis if you have FMS. Nicotine (cigarettes) and caffeine (coffee, tea, soda beverages, etc.) are other common substances that stimulate the adrenalin system, add to muscle tension and pain, and cause further fragmented sleep and reduced stage IV sleep. I encourage you to cut down on both nicotine and caffeine.

Neuroendocrine, Vascular and Metabolic Changes Associated with FMS

Many people with fibromyalgia have other problems, which often confuse their doctors. These include: Raynaud's Phenomenon (poor circulation to the hands or toes), tension headaches, migraine headaches, dizziness, tingling and numbness, an irritable bowel (abdominal bloating with alternating diarrhea and constipation), muscle tremors, bladder spasms, and blurred vision. You have read in earlier chapters that **estrogen loss or decline** *may also* **cause most of these same symptoms.**

In Chapter 13, I will describe several different mechanisms for how estrogen acts to preserve normal blood vessel elasticity and to regulate dilation of blood vessels, which improves circulation. As estrogen decreases in mid-life, there are subtle effects on blood vessels, which can then aggravate the tendency to have Raynaud's and other vascular problems. Changes in blood flow also affect muscle tissue's ability to clear metabolic wastes produced by daily activity. There are a number of ways, both direct and indirect, that decline in ovarian hormone can instigate or aggravate FMS. The estrogen factor certainly is not the only cause of FMS, yet I think hormonal changes may have *more* of a role in triggering or aggravating FMS than anyone has realized. Meanwhile, until we have clearer answers from research, if you have FMS you may find it helpful to have a comprehensive neuroendocrine evaluation to see whether hormone factors are part of the problem for you. If an unrecognized decline in your own body estrogen is causing a number of the triggers that we know will make FMS worse, you may feel better by adding appropriate hormone therapy to your overall FMS treatment.

Immunologic Changes

There's been a great deal of recent interest in the "chronic fatigue syndrome" (CFS), which had been thought to be due to a persistent infection with the Epstein-Barr virus (EBV, the cause of infectious mononucleosis). The EBV *causal* link in CFS has not held up under the scrutiny of further research. We have found, however, that many people who had previously been diagnosed as having "chronic fatigue syndrome" have been found to have FMS and their fatigue appears to be the result of the chronic sleep deprivation. Fatigue is sometimes the most debilitating aspect of fibromyalgia; it is experienced by some as a lack of muscle endurance, while others describe the fatigue as an overall lack of energy. But it does not appear that there is a *causal* link between EBV or CFS and FMS.

There are other potential links with the immune system, however, which could contribute to FMS patients having a greater tendency to have more frequent infections of all types. Sleep deprivation suppresses immune system function, and so does a decline in estrogen and testosterone. Persistent overstimulation of the fight or flight response, for example by ongoing pain stimuli, leads to suppression of the immune system. Chronic pain is a stressor of the body, which also causes excessive production of cortisol, the stress hormone. Increased production of cortisol adds to the reduction in the body's immune response. Remember that cortisol production is *also increasing* in response to decline in estrogen. Once again, do you see how the many pieces of the puzzle fit together with women's hormonal changes and the high frequency of FMS in women?

Problems with Pain Medications

There are a variety of medications useful in alleviating the symptoms of FMS, including some hormonal therapies. Many of the pain medications we use for *acute* pain treatment can actually be detrimental when working with *chronic* pain. Acute and chronic pain are very different, both in their nerve pathways as I mentioned earlier, and in the biochemical and psychological changes they produce. The best way I can explain the difference between acute and chronic pain is to use the analogy of a loud fire alarm in a building. The fire alarm goes off, gets your attention, and you move out of the building rapidly to avoid harm. Acute pain is the body's alarm that something has gone seriously wrong and needs your attention now. Acute pain triggers bursts of adrenalin, the pain-relieving endorphins, and other chemical messengers to prepare you to deal with the emergency. Narcotics and other potent analgesics are very helpful in relieving acute pain by a number of different mechanisms.

Chronic pain, on the other hand, is like a fire alarm *without* a cut-off switch. The persistent jarring sound of a fire alarm that won't stop is one of the most intrusive and penetrating sounds I have encountered. I once had to handle a patient emergency with the hospital fire alarm persistently ringing in the background. They couldn't get the fire alarm turned off, and I thought the sound would literally drive me nuts! This is also very much what your mind-body-spirit goes through with chronic pain: pain alarms go off continually without stopping and intrude on every dimension of one's being. The spirit feels beaten down, the mind is overwhelmed, and the body feels like it *hurts everywhere*.

In chronic pain, the excessive activity of the "alarm system" contributes to an imbalance in the adrenalin system (too much) and the serotonin-endorphin system (too little). Your brain and body actually become depleted of the pain-relieving endorphins, which then *reduces* the effectiveness of the medications we use for acute pain (such as those listed below). Sedatives, or sleeping pills, taken longer than about two weeks will cause disruption in the deep stages III and IV sleep, and alter REM sleep. These adverse effects on the sleep cycle end up making FMS sleep disorder and pain *worse*.

If medication is needed to help improve sleep for women with FMS, I prefer to use a *serotonin-boosting* one such as Zoloft, Prozac, Paxil, Desyrel (trazodone), or Buspar. The serotonin-boosting medications are not sleeping pills. They do not depress the brain as sleeping pills do, so they are safer, do not cause addiction, and have fewer side effects. These medications are more specific for the deficiency of serotonin, which is thought to be a major underlying factor in FMS. While none of these (except trazodone) are *directly* sedating, each works *indirectly* to restore sleep stages back to normal and to also decrease pain by enhancing the activity of serotonin and improving the serotonin-norepinephrine balance. Improving the quality of your sleep is a major part of effective treatment for FMS.

A different class of medication, cyclobenzaprine (Flexeril), is also helpful for some patients. It appears to help relax tense muscles and, for many people, also improves sleep. The older tricyclic antidepressants like amitriptyline (Elavil), imipramine (Tofranil), doxepin (Sinequan and others) have been prescribed in the past to promote stage IV sleep. I do not use these older tricyclic medications any longer, because they have too many side effects, and we now have the more selective serotonin-augmenting options available. One common side effect of *all* the tricyclic antidepressants is that they cause weight gain in a large percentage of patients. Needless to say, this bothers women immensely.

If you are taking one of the tricyclic antidepressants and are having unpleasant side effects, talk with your physician about changing to one of the selective serotonin-boosting medications. Corticosteroids are sometimes used for pain relief in FMS, but they do not seem to be that effective for stiffness and fatigue. In addition, these drugs actually have marked weight gain effects and potentially serious side effects. I do not recommend using corti-

---

Pain Medications to Watch Out For

- narcotics (morphine, Demerol, Vicodin, Tylox, codeine, and others)

- excessive amounts of acetaminophen (Tylenol and generics): taken in large amounts on a regular basis, acetaminophen can lead to liver and kidney toxicity

- sleeping pills (examples: Restoril, Dalmane, Halcion; also Valium, Serax, and Ativan, which are not technically sedatives but are often used to help with sleep)

costeroids in FMS unless you have been carefully evaluated by a rheumatologist, and there is a specific *inflammatory* component that is being treated by the corticosteroids.

Mind-Body Approaches

Fibromyalgia is one of those conditions whose "treatment" is best described as helping patients *manage* their symptoms to achieve relief and improved body-mind function. There really isn't a cure for FMS in the sense that physicians could prescribe a medication or other form of treatment that would make all the symptoms and pain go away forever. It can best be compared to a disease like diabetes, in which the symptoms can be controlled and reduced with a "multiple modalities" approach. The disease progression can be halted dramatically by efforts the patient makes to minimize lifestyle factors that aggravate the pain. There are also *nonaddictive* medications that can be used safely for an extended period of time to rebalance body chemistry and help you maintain productivity and pursue fairly normal life activities.

It is really important that you plan to work with a team of health professionals over a period of time to decrease the symptoms of FMS. This is not a condition that can be treated quickly in three or four office visits with a physician. It is going to involve *your* active participation in a variety of therapeutic modalities and your commitment to a maintenance program of aerobic, strength, and flexibility exercises on a regular basis. I find that most patients with FMS respond best to a *combined* approach, which may include hormonal balance and medication along with **physical therapy, neuromuscular-massage therapy, acupuncture, biofeedback or relaxation training, supportive psychotherapy, stress management, regular exercise, and healthy eating habits.**

Recent studies have shown that regular aerobic exercise can improve energy, and decrease chronic pain to provide you with a sustained benefit in many aspects of your health. I find that many women with fibromyalgia are reluctant to exercise because they are afraid it will cause more pain. I suggest having a physical therapist or an exercise physiologist experienced in working with FMS evaluate you and design an exercise program that starts out slowly and gradually becomes more challenging as your strength and endurance increase. If the exercise regimen is gradual, and tailored to your individual needs, there is little risk of increased pain or muscle microtrauma. Your body will eventually be able to accept more vigorous exercise routines. Consult your physician before beginning any aerobic activities, and ask for a referral to a physical therapist who can teach you appropriate stretching exercises and help you get started on an exercise program.

I recommend *nonimpact* aerobic exercises for FMS patients to avoid aggravating pain or stiffness. These include brisk walking, swimming, water-walking, aqua-aerobics, and using a stationary bicycle or cross-country ski machine. I would suggest that you avoid activities such as jogging, aerobic dancing, "step" aerobics classes, and racquet sports until you have reached a good overall level of physical fitness and your physical therapist feels you are ready to graduate to more strenuous activities. It is especially helpful to do your exercise program in a pool, because this reduces the wear and tear on muscles weakened by FMS. A number of hospitals, YMCAs, Jewish Community Centers (JCC), and fitness clubs now have pool classes available.

Remember to gently stretch all your major muscle groups for about five minutes both before and after you exercise. Stretching helps reduce the chance of muscle injury, but make sure that you stay within your body's limits and don't overstretch, since this will cause more injury. Bouncing movements when you stretch also cause more muscle injury and are not recommended. An excellent book I have used for years to provide safe and effective stretching exercises is simply called *Stretching* by Bob Anderson.

The type of activities you do at home and at work may be additional factors in adding to the FMS pain. For example, if you sit slumped over a desk all day, by the end of the day the pain may have gotten worse because of bad posture. I think it can be very helpful to have a posture analysis and recommendations about proper body position for various activities. Your physical therapist is a good resource to help you with these aspects. Many of us are not aware of the abnormal body positions we use daily, which are often the result of compensating for pain. One physical therapist I frequently work with makes a videotape of the person's posture and movements prior to the session and then again after the treatment. This helps a woman to see clearly posture and movement differences so she is better able to maintain them at home.

Some physical therapists are able to help you assess your home and work environment for body positions that aggravate FMS. It may be helpful to change physical arrangements in your environment to reduce such pain triggers. You may be able to reduce pain by raising the height of your typewriter or computer table and by learning the acupressure points to use yourself to relieve muscle spasm. A more comfortable mattress may help relieve reduce morning stiffness. If driving is a problem, try using a backrest or changing the way you sit. I have found that certain makes of cars have seat back angles that I cannot use without aggravating my back problems, so I am particularly careful about which cars I rent when I travel. Being aware of these details can help improve FMS pain immensely.

Worries, fears, anger, and other intense emotions may also worsen pain and fatigue. Feelings are sometimes harder to identify than our physical symptoms, yet they may definitely intensify symptoms. Look for appropriate support resources to discuss stresses in your life. I am not saying that FMS is a psychogenic disorder. Everyone has stresses—including me—and everyone reacts to stress in different ways. Always keep in mind what I have been saying throughout this book:

> Your mind and brain and body are all connected; what affects one, affects all others!

Thoughts and feelings produce chemical changes in the pain-mood regulating chemicals, just like physical pain produces chemical changes in the body. You may benefit from psychotherapy to help you express uncomfortable or distressing feelings and to help you cope more effectively with situational stresses. Many psychiatrists and psychologists specialize in helping people with chronic pain and may also have experience in teaching self-hypnosis and relaxation skills which reduce stress and tension aggravating pain and fatigue. I teach patients techniques such as visual imagery, autogenic conditioning, and progressive muscle relaxation. You may also find it helpful to take a stress management class.

About 80 to 90 percent of patients with chronic pain will develop a biological depression *due to the persistent pain*. Recent studies have shown that chronic pain patients are not typically depressed people who express depression as physical pain; they have ongoing physical pain (even when the cause is unclear), which alters brain-body chemical messengers and produces the depression. In such situations, specific medications, such as the serotonin-boosting ones mentioned in earlier chapters, are needed to alleviate the depression. Psychotherapy can be helpful but is usually not enough to treat a biological depression. A psychiatrist is a physician trained in both medication use and psychotherapy, and he/she can be an excellent resource to evaluate your integrated needs for medication and/or psychotherapy. You may then decide to see a psychologist or therapist for ongoing individual or family sessions, but it is better to have your evaluation done by a psychiatrist who knows how to identify and treat biological depression and understands the physical connections between chronic pain and depression.

In order for any of these treatment approaches to be effective, **you must be an active partner in the process.** This includes becoming knowledgeable about fibromyalgia, which I hope I have helped you to do. You may find it valuable to attend educational lectures on FMS given by doctors and self-help groups in your community. It can be well worth your time and effort to find a physician who is knowledgeable about fibromyalgia and with whom you feel comfortable. Keep in mind that people respond differently to various treatments, so what works for your friend may or may not work for you. It usually takes a trial of several different kinds of treatment before you find an effective combination. I encourage you to be prepared to modify some aspects of your lifestyle, to expect flare-ups to occur from time to time, and to make time for exercise and practicing relaxation skills. If you invest the time, energy, and effort in carrying out your personalized pain management program, you will be more likely to achieve positive results.

Fibromyalgia syndrome is now the subject of carefully controlled research studies in many of the leading universities of North America. The leading question facing investigators is the metabolic-immune and other abnormalities that cause FMS. Another major focus of research clearly needs to be on the role of female hormonal decline in triggering and perpetuating the debilitating symptoms of FMS. The results of this research will have a major bearing on whether fibromyalgia can be controlled with new drugs and whether there will need to be more emphasis on assessing and adjusting hormone levels in women who suffer from FMS. Even with use of hormone and medication therapies, I think we will always need to include the complementary approaches I outlined for stress reduction, improved quality of sleep, reduced pain and maintenance of physical fitness as cornerstone strategies for coping with fibromyalgia. Don't give up hope. There are lots of helpful options available.

Interstitial Cystitis and Other Bladder Problems: Unrecognized Hormonal Connections

Odessa's Story

Forty-two years old, Odessa is a typical patient coping with **Interstitial Cystitis (IC)**. In excruciating pain, up off and on all night long to urinate, exhausted from lack of sleep and the chronic pain, having to urinate *forty to sixty* times a day, and tired of being told "there's nothing wrong, you're just stressed out," she was dismissed by the urologist in her HMO who told her she didn't need any more tests and said "you just need to stop drinking so much water." Odessa is one of the persistent women who did not give up. She finally found a urologist who knew something about interstitial cystitis, an acutely painful disorder is *found almost exclusively in women*. She began getting appropriate help through a combination of medications and lifestyle modifications.

I first saw her two years after her initial diagnosis of IC when she had a consultation to explore the possible hormone connections with IC. She came in with the question "I have interstitial cystitis, could it be estrogen-related? I think I may be starting menopause." I found that she indeed had both *symptoms* of low estrogen and objective *signs*: thinning of the vaginal lining, diminished breast size, decrease in pubic hair, and low blood levels of estradiol. Her bone mineral density had also decreased below normal for her age. She was a good candidate to begin a trial of low-dose estrogen therapy to help improve her health picture as well as to see what improvements could be achieved with her IC.

A year later, her sleep has improved, her energy and concentration is back to normal, her sex drive is back, and she reported that her frequency of urination had decreased by about 50 percent and the intensity of the bladder pain had also decreased. Her IC is certainly not gone, but it is better. Neither she nor I can say whether the improvement was due solely to the addition of estradiol, or to the combination of everything she was doing, but she said "it was encouraging to me to have my questions and insights taken seriously and included in my treatment." Since estrogen has so many direct effects on the bladder lining, nerves, blood vessels and muscles that govern urinary function, it made a great deal of sense to address this issue in her treatment.

Astoundingly, considering that IC is a *woman's* bladder disorder, there is almost nothing in the scientific literature about the possible effects of hormone change in triggering it, or on the use of hormones as a part of the treatment approach. Every single IC patient I have seen has asked me this question "Could it be related to hormone changes?" Seems a pretty logical question, doesn't it, if the problem is pretty much found only in females! I tell women that it makes *physiological* sense that there would be a connection, but there is simply no research on the question.

What Happens to the Bladder
When Estrogen Declines

Women are frequently embarrassed to tell me that they are having urinary problems, especially if they are experiencing *incontinence* or urinary "leaks." This is truly a problem no one wants to talk about, yet it affects more than *10 million* women! It is much more common in the years just before menopause and gets gradually worse in the decades after menopause. Is this just due to aging? What is the connection to hormone changes? Another ironic twist: I reviewed many of the current books on menopause to make recommendations to my own patients for reliable resource information, and guess how many had chapters addressing urinary problems? I was rather shocked to find only one! So this appears to be another overlooked, taboo topic even for women's menopause books!

Just like other organs and tissues in the body, the lining of the urinary bladder itself and the urethra have estrogen receptors. These lining cells are sensitive to the effects to rise and fall in estrogen levels during the monthly cycle, in pregnancy and at menopause. Changes in estrogen cause measurable changes in the characteristics of the cells (cytology), intensity of symptoms experienced, as well as measurable changes in the pressure of the bladder and urethra (urodynamic changes). When estrogen levels decline and remain low, the cells lining the bladder, urethra and vagina become fewer and thinner (atrophic) as well as more easily torn or damaged with friction ("friable"). The *smooth muscle* of the bladder, urethra and vagina also contains estrogen receptors. When estrogen declines, the smooth muscle gradually loses its tone and strength. Lack of estrogen contributes to a decrease in the urethral closure pressure, which allows for more "leakage" problems.

Nerve endings also contain estrogen receptors. With normal estrogen levels, the sensory threshold is *raised*. When estrogen levels decrease, the sensory threshold is *lowered*, and the nerve endings become *more* sensitive leading to an increase in pain perception.

As a result of these hormone-triggered changes in the lining tissues, women are much more susceptible to several problems:

EFFECTS OF ESTROGEN DECLINE

* vaginal dryness, itching, burning
* pain with intercourse (dyspareunia)
* recurrent bladder infections (cystitis)
* urethral infections (urethritis)
* recurrent vaginal infections (vaginitis)
* incontinence (loss of urine)
* painful urination (dysuria)
* urinary frequency
* urinary urgency

When you look at how common all of the various bladder problems are for women, and the increase in such problems just before and after menopause, it is appalling that in 1994, we still don't have more controlled studies looking at the hormonal effects on these problems. Dr. Vicki Ratner, physician founder of the Interstitial Cystitis Association, acknowledged that women's hormonal changes may play a role in this disorder but also says "there's just no research on this issue!" I have attended a number of medical continuing education meetings on women's health issues, and I have heard presentations on interstitial cystitis, but not one has mentioned possible hormonal factors, even when they describe the disorder as being "epithelial (cells lining the bladder) dysfunction" or "immune dysfunction" (both affected by changes in estrogen).

There are a few double-blind, placebo-controlled studies which have compared the effectiveness of estrogen therapy in treating urinary urgency, frequency, urge and stress incontinence. These studies have used several types of estrogen: estriol, 17-beta estradiol, and conjugated equine estrogens. To date, the results are mixed. There are several studies from Europe that have shown that *all* of the three types of estrogen above can improve symptoms of burning, urgency, and frequency; but estrogen therapy *alone* has not shown a consistent positive effect on stress incontinence.

In the studies I was able to locate, the authors commented that the doses of estriol used may have been too low to achieve optimal benefit. I also thought that the amount of estradiol used was low compared to what we typically recommend for heart and bone benefits. Until we have more definitive scientific data, it is clear that being *estrogen-complete* for our postmenopausal years *does* improve and enhance many functions of the urinary bladder, urethra, and vagina—even if estrogen doesn't solve all problems. This is a factor you should explore with your doctor. Don't be afraid to bring it up!

What Exactly Is "Incontinence?"

Continence is the ability to control urine flow, and hold urine in the bladder when you feel an urge to urinate. Once we are toilet-trained as children, most of us control urination urges unconsciously as we go about our daily activities. Accidental loss of urine, or difficulty controlling the urine flow, is called **incontinence**. A tragic aspect of incontinence problems is the degree to which women do not know it is a *treatable problem*. For example, it is a widespread *misconception* that urinary incontinence is an *inevitable* part of normal aging. This is not correct. The Alliance for Aging Research says it best:

> **You should never think of incontinence as something you have to put up with, or as just a part of growing old!**

And it's not just the issue of comfort that is at stake. Urinary incontinence has a devastating economic impact, individually and collectively, in this country. Americans spend more than *10 billion dollars* annually on products to either *hide the problem of incontinence*, or to help them cope with it, *without* looking for ways to *treat or eliminate the cause*! And older women are hit even harder. Did you know that loss of bladder control is one of the most frequent causes for nursing home admission? Once in a nursing home, patients are even less likely to have a thorough diagnostic evaluation; they are "managed" with catheters and repeated courses of antibiotics, both of which have potential adverse consequences.

With our current knowledge of the causes, and variety of diagnostic and treatment options (and definitely not always just using drugs and surgery) better than 50 percent of incontinence patients can be *cured*, another 35 percent markedly *improved*, and the remaining 15 percent made more *comfortable*. Please do NOT sit home and suffer in silence if you have this problem. See a knowledgeable, caring and competent physician, or call one of the resources at the end of this chapter to locate an appropriate professional near you.

There are different types of incontinence, and it helps to understand the characteristics and causes of each.

Stress Incontinence is one you hear often, and patients are frequently confused about what it means. I remember one woman in her seventies who came to see me, and when I asked her what was bothering her, she burst into tears and said "my doctor told me I had stress incontinence. I know it's real, and it's not just stress in my life." Ah, it pays us to ask our patients what they understand from what we say! Her doctor, I am sure, had no idea how upset this lady was by his use of a medical term that she misunderstood to mean something very different and she was too embarrassed to ask what her doctor had meant. "Stress incontinence" does NOT refer to *emotional factors* causing loss of urine. It means the loss of bladder control due to the *physical stress* of increased pressure in the abdomen from such activities as laughing, coughing, sneezing, sexual orgasm, jogging, or straining to have a bowel movement.

This type of incontinence is not caused by bladder spasms; it results from *weakness or loss of tone* in the bladder *muscles*, which is primarily due to *mechanical factors*, such as damage to the bladder muscles in childbirth, or ligaments and muscles weakened by age. It may also be may be due to hormonal decline contributing to loss of muscle tone. 35 to 40 per cent of women experience postpartum stress incontinence for as long as 6 to12 weeks after childbirth due to trauma to the bladder muscles, and perhaps the sudden drop in hormone levels after delivery. Stress incontinence is usually *not* associated with urinary frequency and urgency.

Urge (urgency) Incontinence is defined as the sudden urge to urinate and the inability to hold your urine long enough to reach the bathroom. It usually results from bladder spasms, and is associated with both *increased frequency and urgency*. It may be aggravated by habits that cause increased urine formation, such as excessive fluid intake, alcohol, use of diuretics ("water pills"), beverages with caffeine, and/or tobacco use. It is important to see a physician for a thorough evaluation, because bladder cancer is also a cause of urge incontinence which has to be ruled out before proper treatment is started.

It is not a good idea to keep taking antibiotics for urinary tract infections (UTI), a common cause of urge incontinence, without having a careful medical evaluation to find causes which may need different treatment approaches. It is also common for many cases of urge incontinence to occur without a clear-cut physical cause, and in these situations, the symptoms are often helped by behavioral re-conditioning and management of fluid intake.

COMMON CAUSES OF URGE INCONTINENCE

- urinary tract infections
- bladder inflammation
- estrogen deficiency
- spinal nerve-root disorders (e.g., disc disease)
- pelvic irritation
- chemotherapy
- spinal cord injury
- pressure from uterine fibroids
- emotional stress

Mrs. G. was a seventy-two year old professional woman in New York who still had a thriving business to run. She came to see me for a variety of health concerns, including bone loss and incontinence. She wanted to discuss the possibility of estrogen replacement therapy. She had been told by her doctor that her incontinence was "to be expected, it's what happens when you get older, just wear pads." Needless to say, this was a difficult idea to accept and a source of embarrassment and anguish for her. Gynecological urology is not my specialty, but I knew that she needed a complete evaluation of her incontinence and this had not been done by her own physician. I referred her to a specialty center in Baltimore, and after the proper diagnostic studies, she was found to have a very treatable type of urge incontinence. She was started on a medication regimen in addition to the hormone therapy I had prescribed. Six months later, her incontinence had dramatically improved to the point where she rarely had any more accidental episodes of urine loss.

Overflow Incontinence is the accidental loss of urine from a chronically full bladder. A common cause is a *cystocoele*, which is a vaginal hernia or bulge due to weakened vaginal muscles seen often in postmenopausal women. The bulge from the cystocoele makes a mechanical obstruction and *prevents* complete emptying of the bladder. A woman can then lose small quantities of urine when she stands, sits, or bends. Another cause of overflow incontinence is damage to the bladder nerves from diabetes, or from a herniated lumbar disc. This is what happened to me when I was *twenty-eight*, before I was correctly diagnosed with the lumbar disc. I can certainly relate to the embarrassment caused by episodes of incontinence and the frustration patients experience trying to get help. Overflow incontinence is treated by identifying and resolving the underlying cause. Pessaries may sometimes be used to lift the bladder away from an obstructed outlet, or bladder surgery may be needed to repair a cystocoele. In my situation, removal of the herniated disc, and getting the pressure off the spinal nerves, allowed normal nerve function to return and the incontinence resolved.

As you can see, it is important to distinguish which type of incontinence you have, because the effective treatments are different: for example, stress incontinence is often relieved by bladder surgery, but urge incontinence is not. Prompt diagnosis is crucial so that treatable problems get addressed in time. In my case, if the problem had gone unrecognized another few days, I would have permanently lost the nerve control of my bladder and been left with having to use a catheter the rest of my life in order to void.

Interstitial Cystitis: Bladder Pain that Doctors Overlook

Interstitial Cystitis. IC can be excruciatingly painful, and yet women often have to see *multiple* different doctors before being properly diagnosed. There are some staggering statistics with this disorder. Once thought to be relatively rare, current estimates from the National Institutes of Health put the number of sufferers at 500,000 women in the U.S. This comes out to 1 in every 260 women. About *half* of these women are so adversely affected that they cannot hold down a full-time job, and over 75 percent cannot have intercourse due to pain. Fully *one-third* of women with IC have been abandoned by a husband or lover as a result of their illness. Even more sobering and alarming, *fewer than 1 out of 5 sufferers have been properly diagnosed*. Women have seen an average of 8 to 10 physicians before they are diagnosed. Even if we don't focus on the *human suffering* involved in such an arduous search for help, what about the *financial* impact of individuals paying out of pocket and insurance companies paying for multiple doctors' visits, not to mention lost time from work and other responsibilities?

Now some startling additional connections that support my theory that loss of estrogen is an overlooked factor in the development of IC: in a study of 374 IC patients published in 1993, researchers at Scripps Institute found that the mean age of onset for IC is *42 years*, and *44 percent* of the patients *had hysterectomies prior to onset of IC.* What else happens in the decade of the forties? You got it, women are often beginning the climacteric time of hormone changes. What else is commonly associated with hysterectomies? You got it, women often begin an earlier ovarian decline of estrogen (even if the ovaries are left in place) due to the effects of surgery on blood flow to the ovaries. Other surveys of IC patients have found that flare-ups tend to occur *after ovulation* and just *before menses. Both* are both times when *estrogen levels are falling*! Why aren't these obvious hormonal connections put together and considered? Hormone changes are not the whole story; yet, I think it is a glaring omission to ignore the hormone issues altogether.

Symptoms

Part of the problem with IC is that many women suffer silently until the primary symptom, pain, becomes so severe that it interferes with normal activities. The characteristic symptoms of IC are, unfortunately, *nonspecific* and may occur in other kinds of bladder disorders: increased urination, sudden strong urges to void (urgency), intense pain becoming worse as the bladder fills up and often decreased by voiding (one woman called it "like passing fire"), pain with intercourse, having to urinate multiple times at night (nocturia).

Causes

A variety of possible causes are usually given, but at this time, we simply don't have a definite answer. One of the common findings in women with IC is a history of repeated UTIs and repeated use of antibiotics over an extended period of time (another reason I urge women to avoid indiscriminately taking antibiotics). It has also been suggested that IC is due to a "dysfunctional bladder epithelium" (what about hormone effects here?) or a manifestation of an autoimmune disorder, which are also many times more common in females than males (again, what about hormone effects?). I think I must sound like a broken record, but it just amazes me that these obvious *female* connections are overlooked). Other proposed theories are that a toxic substance in the urine, or a chronic persistent infectious agent, damages the bladder lining leading to the characteristic tiny hemorrhages in the bladder wall.

Treatments

A large percentage of women are given antibiotics in their primary care or gynecology settings, but most IC specialists agree that antibiotics *help this condition very little*. Yet many women, whose IC has not been properly recognized, have been told that they have recurrent bladder infections in the wall of the bladder and need to be on extended courses of antibiotics. In addition to the expense of unnecessary medication, these women often end up with difficult-to-treat yeast infections.

A variety of medications have been tried for IC, with varying degrees of success. Oral medications include:

1. Elmiron (sodium pentosanpolysulfate), a heparin-like compound that provides a protective "coating" of the bladder lining. The success rate with Elmiron is about 45 to 50 percent. This drug is used investigationally in the U.S. but has not yet received FDA approval;
2. anti-inflammatory medications (NSAIDS);
3. antihistamines, i.e., hydroxyzine (Atarax, Vistaril) shows promising results so far;
4. nalmefene;
5. amitriptyline (Elavil and others), a tricyclic antidepressant that also has good pain-relieving properties; it is also an antihistamine and its *anticholinergic* properties reduce frequency of bladder emptying.

Filling the bladder with medications, called intravesical therapy, is another approach used for more severe cases of IC. One regimen, with about a 35 to 50 percent success rate, uses DMSO (dimethyl sulfoxide) as an anti-inflammatory agent to decrease pain. Patients typically receive a treatment on a weekly or monthly basis for six to ten sessions, but one problem is that patients become progressively resistant to it over time. Other drugs inserted directly into the bladder, some of which cause pain and must be done under anesthesia, include silver nitrate, adriamycin, lidocaine, and chlorpactin WCS-90. Obviously, you should seek out a highly skilled urologist, with experience in treating IC patients, before you undergo these treatments.

Unusual Bladder Effects from Dyes, Medications, and Diet

Food Triggers

Certain foods are potent bladder irritants, and some experts recommend that the following culprits be eliminated or reduced: caffeine, alcohol, tobacco (nicotine), chocolate, spices and spicy foods, acidic foods (citrus fruits, tomatoes), NutraSweet, sharp cheeses, coffee, tea, carbonated beverages, and chemical preservatives (found in many foods and beverages). When you stop and think about the typical diet of many women "on the run" with busy schedules, you begin to realize just how many of these "triggers" most people consume every day. I continue to be surprised at how many of my patients obsess over an extra gram of fat, and then drink cola beverages all day that contain a wide variety of irritant chemicals, not to mention all the calories from sugar!

These foods may irritate the bladder lining, and increase the frequency and urges to void, which end up aggravating incontinence. They may also cause bladder spasms and pain in some women. Keeping a dietary diary, correlated with your bladder symptoms, often helps identify the food culprits so you can make the necessary modifications in what you eat and drink. If you are having bladder problems, it really helps to *clean up* your diet!

Dyes

It was during my specialty training at Johns Hopkins that I first became aware of how potentially serious, and bizarre, patients' reactions can be to something as seemingly innocuous as the coloring agents used in medicines (even vitamins and herbal products can have coloring agents that cause these problems). My mother had been researching the role of dyes in atypical allergic reactions at about the same time I had a patient with asthma admitted to our service. In the course of treating the patient's admitting illness (not his asthma) his asthma kept getting worse. We could not figure out what was happening, since his asthma medications were the same and blood levels were therapeutic. Based on the work my mother was doing, I raised the possibility that perhaps it might be the orange-colored tablets we started using to treat his other illness. We changed to a different brand of the orange medication (one with a *white* tablet), and within a short period of time, the asthma cleared! Since the patient was as curious as we were as to whether the culprit had indeed been the orange dye in the first tablet, he agreed to try taking it one more time. The wheezing returned rapidly. No more orange dye for this person. All of us learned an important lesson.

I started collecting whatever information I could on *tartrazine-based dyes* (a common one is FD&C yellow #5) in medications, foods, and beverages. I was able to find a few articles on allergic reactions to these compounds. The tartrazine-based dyes have a similar chemical effect in the body to that occurring with salicylate, the chemical name for aspirin. Many people who are allergic to aspirin may also react to tartrazine, but often don't know it. Since dyes like FD&C yellow #5 are found in so many common products, *even including medications used for asthma and allergies*, people may be getting a daily dose of a chemical they are allergic to and not realize it. Over the course of my medical career, I have found this to be a much more common problem than I had ever been taught, and so I have included these cautions in many of the educational programs I do for other physicians. I have seen reactions from rashes to wheezing to severe bladder spasms, all traceable to the dyes in a daily medication.

Janie was an energetic woman in her late forties who came for a consult about her bladder spasms, which had progressed to the point that she had to catheterize herself several times a day to urinate. She had been hospitalized on several occasions with such severe bladder spasms that she had been unable to void at all. She had been healthy, without any history of bladder problems, until about two months after she started estrogen therapy with Premarin. The estrogen effectively relieved her menopausal symptoms of hot flashes and sleeplessness, but she started developed the new symptoms of increased frequency of urination, sudden urges to void, and a burning pain in the area of her bladder. She had seen multiple doctors; had been treated with many courses of antibiotics, pain medications, tranquilizers and had been told she was obviously having emotional trouble over her children leaving home, so she should see a therapist. Meanwhile, nothing seemed to be helping, and Janie was having such frequent spasms and difficulty voiding, she had been taught to catheterize herself.

During her visit to our women's health program, she had planned to pursue biofeedback training and acupuncture to help decrease the spasm and pain. In our consultation, she said "You know, it sounds silly, but I keep wondering if this problem could have any connection to starting the Premarin. Before that, I never had anything like this. I've asked all my doctors this question, but they have all said there's no connection, or it's not possible." I told her in my experience, I had seen problems like this due, not so much to the drug or hormone, but to the dyes in the tablet. I explained that the simple way to test her idea would be to change her to a completely dye-free form of estrogen and see if it made any difference over the next few months. At that time, there were no commercial estrogens on the market in the U.S. which were free of dyes. That in itself is amazing and disconcerting to me, given the number of women with allergies, who may need estrogen. So I called the pharmacist in Colorado who had compounded individualized prescriptions of natural hormones for some of my patients and asked him if his tablets had any dyes. They did not, so I ordered the dye-free estradiol tablet for Janie to try.

She was so excited that someone thought she could be on to something that might help, she had it sent overnight mail! I had already told her not to get her hopes up, since this might not be the cause of her bladder problem, but I did think it was worth trying. I also told her that if the dye was an irritant to her bladder, it could still take *several weeks* for her to see any difference with the change in estrogen tablets. Three days later she called me, and practically yelled over the phone "It's GONE! I have actually been able to urinate on my own without the catheter! This is amazing!"

Even I was astonished at the rapid response. I have seen some pretty surprising turn-arounds over the last fifteen years of working with patients, but none this fast. It is now two years later, and the last follow-up I had was that her bladder spasms had resolved, and she had remained on the dye-free estrogen. Doctors should be willing to make a simple change like this to a different tablet *without dyes* and at least *see* what happens, rather than taking the arrogant stand that the patient couldn't possibly be right.

These same azo-tartrazine dyes are known carcinogens and skin irritants, and some have now been banned due to these effects. My suggestion to you is that if you have bladder sensitivities and an "irritable" bladder (or bowel!), it may be wise to watch for these types of chemicals in the foods, beverages, and medicines you consume.

Another common irritant for many women is the *propylene glycol* in various vaginal creams, including some of the estrogen vaginal creams which are used to help *treat* vaginal itching and burning. If you have persistent problems with these symptoms, talk with your physician or pharmacist to see if what you are using contains these dyes and other chemicals. The *Physicians Desk Reference* is now required to list these dyes and other inactive ingredients, so you can always ask your pharmacist if you are in doubt about a particular medicine. Many food manufacturers will send you a complete ingredient list of their products if you write to their consumer information office.

Chronic Bladder "Infections": Is It Really an Infection or My Hormones?

I really have a problem with women calling doctors' offices and getting repeated courses of antibiotics for "bladder infections". First of all, burning, frequency and urgency may have many causes. Not all causes are due to infections. Secondly, repeated use of antibiotics creates problems with resistant bacteria and with chronic yeast infections. So make sure you take the responsible course of action, and go see your doctor for a urinalysis and urine culture before you start on antibiotics.

I think it is important to have your hormone levels checked if you are having problems with burning, frequency, urgency, or leaking of urine. Many people still don't realize the degree to which loss of estrogen plays a role in causing these changes during and after menopause. Rather than continuing to think you have an infection and taking antibiotics, I think it is far more effective to assess the possible hormone causes and address this problem directly, perhaps first with a vaginal estrogen cream or by taking one of the hormone therapy regimens if your doctor feels that is appropriate for you.

If estradiol blood levels are below the 50 to 60 pg/ml range, it is highly likely that this is a major cause of the urinary problems. Occult diabetes is another very common cause of urinary problems in older women, especially if you are overweight. In its early stages, before the fasting glucose is significantly high, frequent yeast infections, burning on urination, increased frequency, and leaking of urine are common. If you have a family history of diabetes, or have noticed an increase in craving for sweets, you should talk with your doctor about checking more closely for diabetes. In patients I see for consultations, I find that these two endocrine changes are the *most frequent unrecognized causes* of persistent urinary problems.

In addition to the hormone levels, there are some other important tests which you should discuss with your doctor. Not every patient will need all of the tests, but you should at least ask whether any of these are needed to determine the cause of your problem if your doctor doesn't mention them. This is *not an exhaustive list*, since there are many medical problems which can cause urinary problems. But at least this list gives you an idea of some of the newer techniques that are available to aid in the diagnosis of urinary disorders.

COMPONENTS OF A DIAGNOSTIC
EVALUATION FOR INCONTINENCE

- detailed patient history

- food/beverage intake diary, and urinary voiding diary

- use of prescribed, and over-the-counter medications (and herbs, vitamins, minerals, etc.)

- physical examination

- blood chemistries, hormone levels

- urine culture

- urine cytology (rule out cancer)

- post-void residual urine volume (measures urine remaining in bladder after voiding, which can contribute to incontinence)

- ultrasound (assess kidney size, structure to look for tumors, etc.)

- urodynamic studies (checks for filling and emptying patterns)

- voiding cystourethrogram (checks urethra pressures)

Help for Bladder Problems: Hormonal Balance, Exercise, and Other Options

Hormones

If you are already on ERT or HRT and are still having problems with bladder symptoms like I have described, you may want to ask your doctor to actually check blood levels of FSH and estradiol to determine whether you are taking the *right amount* of estrogen for your body needs. I continue to find that what we thought was an adequate dose turns out to be less than what's needed for many women. If you are still bothered by symptoms, it is especially important to determine if you are on the right amount of estrogen because you may not be getting enough for estrogen's *other benefits* either! I typically aim for estradiol blood levels of over 100 pg/ml, which is what is typical for the first part of the menstrual cycle. If your ERT/HRT regimen provides estradiol blood levels over 100, the FSH will usually come back down to 35 or less. I find these objective measures very helpful in deciding about doses for individual women, especially if they are still having urinary problems.

Another option is to change the *type* of estrogen you are taking. Women have many individual differences in absorption and metabolism of foods, hormones, vitamins, and medications. We have to take this into account. The standard estrogen your doctor uses simply may not be well absorbed in *your* body, and you can ask to change to a different one to see if this helps your symptoms. You may find that a native human 17-beta estradiol works better than the mixed estrogens. In Chapters 3 and 5, I have information on the different 17-beta estradiol and the mixed-estrogen preparations available in this country. Selected pharmacies in the U.S. will also compound *estriol* tablets and creams, which your physician may consider adding to your ERT/HRT regimen if needed. I *do not recommend* taking estriol without your doctor's knowledge and without adequate monitoring of estrogen effect, since too much estrogen may lead to increased risk of uterine (endometrial) cancer.

Another pointer, which I have found helps some women: if you are taking estrogen and continue to have bladder irritation symptoms of burning, frequency, and urgency, you may find it helpful to ask your physician to prescribe an estrogen *without dyes in the tablet*. Many of the chemical dyes used in medications (and foods and beverages—see previous section) are irritating to the bladder lining. Looking for dye-free (usually white) tablets for your medications can reduce this source of additional irritation to the bladder. This is a fairly easy step to take, and it may give significant relief.

Exercises

You may ask "how on earth do I exercise my *bladder* muscles?" Dr. Arnold Kegel, in 1951, first described the method of muscle exercise to treat incontinence without drugs or surgery which were the means used by most physicians at that time. The pubo-coccygeus, or "PC" muscle for short, is the primary muscle of the pelvic floor which governs control of urinary flow and also contracts the vagina (which can intensify pleasurable sensations during intercourse). The PC muscle also supports the uterus, ure-thra, and rectum. Dr. Kegel was able to show, by means of a device he invented, that the PC muscle could be trained and strengthened with sets of rhythmic contraction-hold-release actions. When the PC muscle is strengthened, it lifts the organs of the pelvis back into their normal positions, and enables a woman to better con-trol her urinary flow. Dr. Kegel monitored the strength of muscle contraction with biofeedback so the woman could objectively see how she was doing and learn how to increase her contraction. By 1956, he reported an 86 percent success rate in 455 women with incontinence who had undergone muscle training exercises at his clinic.

Studies since that time have confirmed the marked effective-ness of these methods. The success rate increases significantly if biofeedback techniques are used at the outset to teach women how to isolate the proper muscles and to contract the muscles more effectively. Patricia Burns, R.N., found dramatic improve-ment in stress incontinence using biofeedback: she reported 50 to 99 percent *decrease* in episodes of urine loss. Her research project, conducted at the School of Nursing at the State University of New York at Buffalo, was the first *carefully controlled* study of behavioral treatments for stress incontinence to show their marked effectiveness.

In the biofeedback group, women watched a video screen dis-play of the strength of their pelvic muscle contractions while a nurse trained in the techniques measured those contractions using a vaginal sensor probe. Another technique to strengthen pelvic muscles uses low intensity electrical stimulation to contract the muscles and progressively strengthen them until the patient can learn how to do it herself. Combining the electrical stimulation with biofeedback has been particularly effective for patients who have not responded to Kegels or biofeedback alone.

Once the techniques are learned correctly, these exercises can be practiced anywhere. Not only that, the behavioral techniques are promising because they don't involve the risks of surgery or the possible side effects of medicine. You just need motivation, commitment, and practice! If you are having any of the symptoms I have talked about, bring this up with your doctor to find out what resources are available in your area. And before you rush into "bladder tuck" surgery, make sure you have explored the options for strengthening your pelvic muscles nonsurgically! As one woman in her early forties laughingly said "I practice my Kegels at business meetings, and driving home on the Jersey turnpike, and nobody but me knows what I'm doing! My sex life is great now, and all those embarrassing 'leaks' have stopped. And, this way, there's no expense and no side effects!" Talk about taking charge of your health and regaining your freedom!

Bladder Training

Another nonsurgical method of relieving urgency incontinence is to follow a timed schedule of voiding, with progressive lengthening of the time interval between urinations. For example, if you find that you are not able to go more than three hours without accidental loss of urine, you would be instructed to urinate every two hours, whether the urge to void is there or not. Each week, you would increase the time between voiding by 15 to 30 minutes until the bladder is trained to reach your goal for time between urinations. This simple method is also dramatically effective, but it does take your commitment to follow the training schedule. Again, it's free and there are no side effects.

Medications

In addition to the benefits of estrogen to improve urinary function, there are other medications that help reduce incontinence. Antispasmodics (such as probanthine, flavoxate, oxybutynin, and imipramine) help reduce bladder spasms which cause urge incontinence. Alpha-receptor stimulating medications, such as phenypropanolamine, help to improve the bladder sphincter muscle tone. All of these drugs must be prescribed and properly monitored by a physician to avoid undesirable side effects. Phenylpropanolamine in particular can cause serious high blood pressure emergencies if taken by someone with hypertension and not supervised carefully.

Surgery

If other methods are not successful, or if there is a specific mechanical repair needed, you may wish to have a consultation with a urologist experienced in the surgical advances for treating incontinence. There are a number of new approaches which can be considered, and the specific types of surgery need to be evaluated in the context of your individual needs. Some resources are given at the end of this chapter to help you locate a specialist in your area.

Annie's Response

Soon after finishing an early draft of this chapter, I happened to have a follow-up appointment with one of my patients who had experienced these difficulties with bladder problems and who had been through several surgeries over a number of years. No one had checked her hormone levels or suggested the newer approaches with biofeedback. After hearing my seminar, she came to me for a consult, had the hormone blood levels done and a hormone regimen designed for her. She had been doing very well, and at this follow-up appointment asked more questions about estrogen's effects on the bladder. I offered to let her read the draft of this chapter so she would have more information on what we now know. This is her letter, sent in response to reading this chapter.

December 20, 1994

Dear Dr. Vliet,

I really enjoyed reading your article on the bladder especially the part on incontinence. I do agree with your conclusion that estrogen loss affects incontinence. That has certainly been the case with me. I have lot more leakage when my estrogen level is down. I only wish I had been given this information years ago. It is wonderful that you are writing about this now. Hopefully it will help some women so that they do not have to go through what many others of us have.

My stress incontinence began when I was in my late thirties. I would leak when I laughed, coughed or sneezed. Ten years later it had become a significant problem. I had started to wear a pad every day. I had to leave the golf course on many occasions because I had not just leaked, but had completely wet through my pad and my clothes were soaked. This also happened several times when I had left a restaurant without going to the restroom first. On the way to the car I would leak through the pad and urine would be running down my legs.

I am sure during this ten year period my estrogen level had dropped tremendously. This thought had never crossed my mind nor was it ever mentioned to me by my gynecologist. All I was ever told was that my bladder had dropped and needed to be suspended. I finally made the decision to do this and two gynecologists told me it would not be effective unless I also had a hysterectomy. So I had both done. Worst mistake ever made! After the surgery I leaked constantly. I have never been given a good answer as to why. Some doctors have said I had a urethra problem not bladder one. I feel I must have had some muscle or nerve damage during the surgery. Also, after reading your article I wonder if I might have a cystocoele? My bladder just can't be very full without leaking. Since the first surgery I have had fat injections into the urethra by a doctor in New York. Then I had a sling operation by another surgeon. It did not work so I am now having collagen injections. They have helped, but it is temporary because it tends to break down. The estradiol therapy has helped diminish the leakage, at least. I will try to find someone here to do the biofeedback you suggested.

I hope this information can help other women from having to go through what I have been through. Needless to say, the quality of my life has not been good. It has been a very stressful situation as well as very expensive. I spend fifty dollars a month on Serenity Pads alone (by the way I do like them the best; they are less like a diaper).

Sorry this is so messy. I am strapped for time. Merry Christmas!

"Annie" (not her real name)

Changes in bladder function do occur as we grow older, but keep in mind, there are many ways to cure, or certainly improve, these problems. Don't let embarrassment keep you from asking for help, and don't suffer in silence. I really want to encourage all of you reading this book that there is hope, and help, out there in a variety of organizations, physicians, nurse-specialists, and support groups. I have listed a number of these resources in the Appendices at the end of the book. Don't let urinary problems keep you homebound when you have treatment options available.

CHAPTER 13

Estrogen and Your Heart:
An Update

Cardiovascular disease kills approximately 485,000 women per year in the age range 40 to 65, compared to 60,000 deaths annually for *all* reproductive cancers combined: breast, uterine, ovarian, cervical, and vaginal cancers. Over age 50, *heart disease account for **53 percent of the deaths in women.** Compare this with the **4 percent of deaths due to breast** cancer in women over 50.* Consider these recent findings:

- Women in their 40s, even though still menstruating, are beginning to show the early effects of from declining estrogen that predispose them to higher risk of heart disease after menopause: rising total cholesterol, dropping levels of HDL (the "good" kind), rising levels of LDL (the "bad" kind), and rising blood pressure. The hormonal factor is usually not checked until *after* menses cease, missing an important window of opportunity for reducing disease risk for later years.

- 50 percent of women who have had a hysterectomy, without removal of their ovaries, become **endocrinologically menopausal** by three years after surgery, regardless of age. Their heart disease risk increases when they become *menopausal*, **not** at the magic age of 51.

- Women who present to medical offices and emergency rooms with complaints of palpitations are *far more likely than men* to be given a diagnosis of "anxiety," a prescription for Valium or Xanax, and sent home. Tragic cases abound of women such as this then having a massive heart attack. Some have died as a result of misdiagnosis. I have had many women referred to my practice who had been labeled "anxious," only to find on further evaluation that they had significant early cardiovascular disorders which required *different* medications, or they had perimenopausal decline in estradiol which needed hormonal management.

- Commonly, women in their 40s and 50s who describe symptoms of palpitations, chest discomfort or pain, and other cardiovascular symptomatology are not given the same degree of comprehensive evaluations and treatment options that are offered men.

- Recent studies in the gender differences in health care patterns indicate that women are *less likely* than men to be offered angiography, angioplasty, and cardiac bypass surgery.

- Alcohol is known to have specific toxic effects on heart muscle fibers, and excessive alcohol consumption is increasing alarmingly in women. Yet women are less likely than men to be identified as alcohol abusers at early stages of the illness and are less often referred for alcohol treatment until later stages of abuse, when cardiac and other severe complications have occurred.

At mid-life, each of you have a unique opportunity *prior to menopause* to identify potential risk factors for cardiovascular disease (CVD) and to implement lifestyle changes at a time when preventive approaches can be the most meaningful for your long-term quality of life. But if you are not aware that heart disease can affect women so dramatically, you may not know to discuss these issues with your physician. And physicians, like all the rest of us, had been taught to think of heart disease as a *man's* disease, which did not affect women until sometime after age sixty-five. This misconception appears to be part of the reason that women with heart disease are sicker when the problems are recognized and have a higher death rate when they have a first heart attack compared to men with first attacks.

Several alarming trends in heart disease statistics have emerged in the last few years as I have just described, but women are typically more aware of and fearful about breast cancer than about heart disease. Part of this difference in awareness directly results from the greater publicity and media attention given to breast cancer in women. Far more women silently, and without much press attention, die of heart disease every year. You can do something to reduce your risk of these problems!

Risk Factors Affecting Women and Men

Unfortunately, it has only been in the last few years that women have been included in studies of heart disease risks, as well as clinical studies of new medications to treat heart disease. The information we have shows that women have similar risk factors as men, *except for estrogen!* This seems so blatantly obvious, it's appalling to consider that the role of estrogen in heart disease has only recently been studied. I will talk further about what we have come to understand about estrogen's specific role in reducing risk of heart disease. Since I am sure you have already read a great deal about the general risk factors for heart disease (listed below), I will not address those in depth in this chapter. There are a wealth of good books and pamphlets describing each of these risk factors and ways you can modify your lifestyle habits to reduce your risk. Let me say at the outset: Before you turn to hormones as a "magic bullet" for heart protection, I think it is critical to begin making the healthy lifestyle choices as your *first and most important step* you can take to help prevent diminished living capacity or premature death from heart disease. At least **eight** of the CVD risk factors below are either *modifiable* or can be *eliminated altogether* by making lifestyle changes alone. JUST DO IT, as the Nike ad says. Your health is your greatest *wealth*.

Putting risk factors in perspective for women shows the importance of studying gender differences: total cholesterol levels are better predictors of CVD risk for men, but not women; high levels of triglycerides are an *independent risk factor* for women, but not for men; *low* levels of "good" HDL are a greater risk factor for women, while high "bad" LDL levels are a greater risk factor for men. Among diabetics, when triglyceride levels increase above normal, cardiovascular risk increases about three-fold in men, but nearly *200-fold in women.* A person who has the "lipid triad" of high total cholesterol, low HDL and high LDL is *thirteen times* more likely to have an acute myocardial infarction (heart attack) in the next four years. What can you to improve your lipid triad? Stop smoking, start exercising, reduce dietary fat and sugars, and for women, consider estrogen therapy. The National Cholesterol Education Program (NCEP) has now advised that estrogen therapy should be considered for women to lower LDL and raise HDL *before using lipid-lowering drugs,* such as niacin, Mevacor, or Pravacol.

Cardiovascular Disease Risk Factors

- family history of cardiovascular disease
- growing older
- cigarette smoking
- high-fat diets
- lack of exercise
- obesity
- increased abdominal (truncal) body fat (waist-to-hip ratio greater than 0.85)
- hypertension (high blood pressure)
- elevated cholesterol and/or low HDL (for women, HDL is a better predictor of CVD risk than for men)
- elevated triglycerides (a greater risk factor for women than for men)
- diabetes or impaired glucose tolerance
- clotting abnormalities (coagulopathy)
- history of chest pain, or prior cardiac problems
- premature ovarian failure, or premenopausal removal of ovaries (oophorectomy)
- chronic use of prednisone or other corticosteroids

Cardiovascular Symptoms and Disease: Many Variations

Symptoms are the changes and sensations you experience, such as headaches, racing heart, clammy skin, pain, flushing, tingling, and a myriad of others. These changes may indicate a normal body response to an environmental stimulus or to even your own thoughts. These sensations may also be a potential warning of *disease*. Not all symptoms indicate disease, and not all diseases (at least in early stages) produce symptoms. Hypertension and osteoporosis are classic examples of diseases that do not produce symptoms until damage has already been done to the body by the disease process. One of my tasks in helping patients is to sort out what the symptoms may indicate, and what diseases could be present that are still silent and not yet producing symptoms.

Palpitations, those fluttering or pounding sensations in the chest, which can be quite disturbing and even frightening, are quite common as part of the endocrine effects of declining estrogen in the perimenopause and menopause. In numerous studies, palpitations occur in anywhere from 40 percent to 60 percent of women in the pre- and perimenopause transition. For about 15 percent to 20 percent of women, palpitations may be the *only* symptom serving as a clue to the hormonal changes. But the presence of palpitations does not necessarily mean you have cardiovascular disease.

Palpitations may occur as a heart response to the bursts of adrenalin in the brain that occur with drops in estrogen levels. This increase in heart rate is a normal part of the fight or flight reaction; the brain sends a signal to other body organs that something is changing rapidly and is out of balance. Palpitations may also occur in certain types of *benign* heart disease, such as mitral valve prolapse or in potentially serious types of heart disease such as *atrial fibrillation*. Hyperthyroidism may also produce palpitations through other mechanisms. Panic disorder is a biological condition of excess and erratic production of adrenalin-type compounds in the brain, which then may produce palpitations as I described for hormone changes. So palpitations as a symptom have *many* causes; some normal responses, some serious conditions, and some not-so-serious conditions. And for each cause, the best treatment may be different.

Yet, this symptom is not often viewed as a possible endocrine-based one: if women are evaluated medically for the problem of palpitations, they are most often seen by internal medicine or cardiology specialists who check for the possibility of heart disease with cholesterol blood tests, physical exam, electrocardiograms, and exercise (treadmill) electrocardiograms. If nothing abnormal is found, women are then likely to be told that the cause of their symptoms is stress or anxiety. The average woman is *not told* that her symptoms may be related to menopausal hormone changes, and she typically does not get evaluated with FSH and estradiol blood tests. Listen to CC describe her experience.

CC was thirty-nine years old when she came to see me. She described "terrible pounding sensations in my chest, and it feels like my heart is going to come right through my chest, it actually hurts it's beating so hard. Then it will go away for awhile, and all of sudden it will come back. It seems to be worse at night, and the funny thing is it doesn't bother me when I'm out jogging. My doctor did an EKG and tells me there's nothing wrong with my heart; he said I'm just too much of a Type A person and I need to relax.

But the stress isn't worse now, in fact my life is really pretty good except I want to know what this is because it hurts." She had no history of any health problems, did not smoke, only rarely had any alcohol, did not use any street drugs, and regularly participated in 5K "Fun Run" activities in the community in addition to her daily jogging. Over the past year, she had increased her jogging to between six and ten miles a day, usually six days a week. She reported a lactose intolerance and had cut out dairy products about ten years earlier. With her exercise, she did not think she needed to worry about calcium supplements. She appeared to be healthy and quite fit, and I could not elicit any other problems or symptoms in going through the usual medical "review of systems" checklist.

She was still menstruating, and at her recent gynecological checkup for her annual pelvic and Pap, she said she had been told "Everything's fine, you're normal." When I questioned her more about her menstruation, she said her periods had been a lot lighter and less frequent over the past two years, since she had been running more. I asked if her heart poundings had any relationship to her menstrual cycle. She said, "Well, now that you ask, I have noticed that it seems to always get *really bad* the day or two before my period starts, and it will last a couple of days and go away. Sometimes it seems to hit again mid-month, then go away again. Other times it will be there occasionally in an erratic way."

Her complete medical evaluation, including a thyroid and cholesterol profile along with a Holter monitor of her heart activity for twenty-four hours, were normal. On the first day of her period, when her heart poundings were the worst, her estradiol level was 23 and her FSH 2.0. The low FSH along with the low estradiol is fairly common when women have unwittingly suppressed their ovaries' hormonal function with significant increases in their exercise regimen. I was suspicious from her dietary history and her alterations in menstrual pattern and flow that she may have begun to have early bone loss, and I suggested she consider having a bone density test. She was shocked to find that she had a bone density, at age thirty-nine, one standard deviation *below* the bottom of normal for her age.

When we reviewed all of her information, I explained that the hormone levels were quite low, and I thought the drop in estradiol each month before her period likely triggered the brain burst of adrenalin that increased her heart rate. Since she also had these episodes at mid-cycle some months, I told her I thought she had the same heart response when her estradiol dropped after ovulation. From her history, I did not think she ovulated every month, which helped her understand why the palpitations did not seem to happen on a regular basis with her mid-cycle point. I thought her bone loss had developed gradually with her reduced calcium intake as well as the decline in estrogen when her exercise intensity altered her menstrual pattern and decreased her overall body fat percentage. She did not have any more serious underlying heart disease causing her palpitations.

After we reviewed all of her options and choices, she elected to take the low-dose oral contraceptives to improve her hormonal balance, maintain her bone mass, and help eliminate the estrogen drop that triggered her palpitations. Needless to say, I also urged her to take calcium and magnesium supplements to help keep from losing further bone. She has done extremely well since then and has not needed further medical visits, since her palpitations have resolved. Her gynecologist agreed with her being on the oral contraceptives and plans to manage that with her as part of her annual checkup. I have seen quite a lot of patients like CC in my practice, and find this rewarding because I feel that together, in a physician-patient partnership, we are arriving at options that result in *preventing* the progression of disease risks. In my approach, this is a great example of "A stitch in time saves nine."

Another difference in the way cardiovascular symptoms appear in men and women is in the pattern of chest pain called "angina." Men typically experience "crushing" chest pain, with pain that spreads down the left arm and up into the neck area. Women are more likely to have what is called "silent angina," which does not produce this crushing severe pain and does not radiate down the left arm and into the neck as we see in men. Women may just experience a "tightness" or "heaviness" in the chest, which can often be mistaken for anxiety if a health professional is not aware of these gender differences in the way angina can present.

This difference in how the pain is experienced may be due to differences in pain threshold, differences in pain pathways in women, or to other factors we have not yet identified. But it is clear that this difference in the pain symptoms for women are one of the reasons women with angina, or ischemic heart disease, do not get diagnosed early and then have more serious disease by the time it is found. If you are at high risk of heart disease and are experiencing this kind of chest pain, *be assertive* in pursuing an evaluation by your physician. Listen to what this woman went through.

Meg was forty-seven, and terrified of having heart disease. **Both her parents died of CVD. Her mother had a heart attack in** her late forties and then died in her early fifties. Meg's Cholesterol was 337, TG was 400, and the CHOL/HDL ratio was 5.5, much too high for a woman her age who had not had any menstrual irregularities. She was significantly overweight, had high fasting glucose, and high protein-bound glucose. She described physical sensations of angina (ischemia of the heart muscle) with even mild exertion. All of these risks placed her in the highest risk group for her age, yet her **HMO physician would not evaluate her further, even with her high risk of CVD.** Her husband even went in to see the doctor and try and talk with him. When he came home, he said to his wife, *"Meg, that man doesn't like you!"*

They finally talked with the head of customer service at their insurance company, who agreed to reimburse her for the cardiac treadmill stress test she had been requesting. I had prescribed it for her due to her many heart disease risk factors. This woman and her husband fought appropriately for what should have been done in her health care. Many patients, however, are more passive than this and simply do not realize that they need to speak up to the health insurance company about such matters. Remember, you are the customer, and you have the right as well as the responsibility to seek appropriate medical evaluation under your health coverage.

Women may be affected by many different types of disorders affecting the circulatory system. These are other common examples and terms, which your physician may use. Make certain to ask for patient education material to read if you are told you have one of these problems.

- **arrthymias** (heart rate, rhythm disturbances)
- **hypertension** (high blood pressure)
- **hyperlipidemia** (high cholesterol, low HDL, high triglycerides)
- **ischemic heart disease** (angina)
- **myocardial infarction** (heart attack)
- **strokes,** TIA (cerebrovascular disease)
- **peripheral vascular disease** (e.g., thrombophlebitis or "blood clots")
- **murmurs, heart valve problems** (example: mitral valve prolapse)

As a brief overview, the circulatory system is basically comprised of a **pump** (the heart, which is a muscle) pushing **fluid** (the blood) through a **series of tubes** of different sizes (arteries, capillaries, veins) to provide **nutrients** (e.g., oxygen, glucose) and remove waste products for all the cells, tissues, and organs of the body. This is boiling it down to its most essential aspects. In reality, the massive process of constantly circulating fluids to all parts of the body day and night is incredibly complex, with many different mechanisms for regulating it and keeping the critical balance of the many chemicals the body needs to work properly. I really cannot do this subject justice in the short space of this chapter, but I wanted you to have a brief description of the basics to help you better understand the many roles of our female hormones in this process.

There has to be a **force**, called **blood pressure (BP)**, that moves the blood fluid through the system. BP is measured by two numbers, which provide us with information about whether the heart is having to work harder to pump the blood (high blood pressure) or whether the pressure is too low to keep blood moving to the necessary organs (low blood pressure, which can cause fainting spells and lightheadedness). The top number is the *systolic pressure*; elevation of this number is usually less serious since it may be briefly elevated by stress, anxiety, and pain as well as by hypertension. The bottom number is the *diastolic pressure*; *sustained* elevation of the diastolic pressure greater than 90 mm Hg generally indicates hypertension.

An average blood pressure is considered to be 120/80 mm Hg, but most women (and many physicians) don't realize this number is *based on an average male*. If we had carefully evaluated gender differences, we would find that the average healthy younger *female* may have normal blood pressures in the range of 110/60 to 110/70. Thus, women who have a blood pressure of 120/80 may actually be *higher* than is normal for them.

What happens in the process leading to high blood pressure and arteriosclerosis (cardiovascular disease)? When cholesterol levels are abnormally high and levels of the good cholesterol (HDL) are low, the LDL cholesterol deposits more cholesterol molecules along the artery wall. Since there isn't as much HDL to clean up these deposits and take them back to the liver to be broken down and excreted, plaque builds up on the walls of the arteries. Plaque is a mixture of cholesterol-containing particles along with platelets and fibrin. These deposits cause a narrowing of the arteries, much like a wad of dirt partially plugging a garden hose. This means it takes more pressure for the blood to get through the arteries, which results in high blood pressure.

The narrowing of the arteries due to plaque leads to reduced blood flow to tissues, which then deprives cells of vital oxygen and nutrients (called ischemia). Loss of oxygen damages or destroys cells (called infarction). When the damaged cells belong to the heart muscle itself, this is called a *myocardial infarction*. When the damaged cells are in the brain, it is called a stroke. The entire process is quite complex, but this is a simple overview of the basics to help you understand the role estrogen plays in reducing risk of both cardiovascular disease and stroke.

The Cardiovascular Protection Role of Estrogen: Research Advances

Heart disease rates for women rise dramatically with the declining estrogen in the climacteric years and after menopause. Morbidity and premature deaths in post-menopausal women could be significantly reduced if women were given adequate information about the cardioprotective effects of estrogen replacement therapy and had an *individualized discussion* of their risks of various health problems.

Unfortunately, so many women, and their health care practitioners, have been frightened by the biased reporting of the breast cancer risks, that they are unwilling to consider taking estrogen after menopause. Primary care physicians, in particular gynecologists working with mid-life women, can play a major role in correcting the misinformation among consumers. This would help women make informed choices about postmenopausal estrogen therapy *based on their own individual needs*, rather than comparisons with what friends may have decided about hormones.

There has been a great deal of exciting research in the last few years that has helped us now understand the many ways that the normal female hormone, estradiol, exerts its protective effect on heart disease. You may have read about the way that estrogen reduces total cholesterol and increases the body's production of the good type of cholesterol, HDL. But have you seen some of the latest findings?

- *Estrogen decreases LDL, the plaque-forming kind of cholesterol by increasing liver breakdown of LDL so that it is eliminated from the circulation.* In a 1991 Harvard study of healthy postmenopausal women, oral estrogens reduced LDL an average of 15 percent, and *increased* HDL by 16 percent. Transdermal estradiol did not have the same effect on HDL and LDL, but does generally decrease triglyceride levels.

- *Estrogen stimulates the production of HDL*, the good cholesterol which carries plaque away from the artery wall and back to the liver to be broken down and excreted.

- *Estrogen stimulates the formation of LDL receptors in the liver and possibly the walls of arterial blood vessels.* These receptors bind the LDL, which removes LDL from the circulation and from its damaging effects in plaque production.

- *17-beta Estradiol acts as a calcium-channel blocker to relax artery walls, which helps dilate the arteries, improve blood flow throughout the brain and body, and helps to reduce blood pressure.* Calcium-channel blocking medications (many are on the market; some examples are Calan, Cardizem, DynaCirc, Isoptin, Procardia and others) are used medically to treat a number of disorders such as angina, hypertension, migraine headaches, and bipolar mood disorders among others. This mechanism of action on the blood vessels' calcium channels may be one way estradiol performs its normal function of keeping blood pressure lower in premenopausal women compared to men of the same age. After menopause, as estrogen goes down, we see rises in women's blood pressure more similar to the readings in men.

- Dr. Philip Sarrel of Yale University School of Medicine has shown that estradiol given sublingually improves coronary artery blood flow and exercise tolerance on treadmill testing in postmenopausal women with previously documented coronary artery disease (that had produced at least 70 percent occlusion of the arteries).

- *Estrogen stimulates the release of endothelium-derived relaxing factor (EDRF, thought to be nitric oxide) a chemical having an important role in dilating blood vessels to maintain normal pressure and flow.* In a two-year study of twenty-six postmenopausal women, levels of this blood vessel relaxing agent kept *rising in women on estrogen* and continued to increase the longer they took estrogen. Levels of the nitric oxide compound were not changed in women who were not receiving estrogen. Dr. Raghvendra Dubey, of the University of Pittsburgh, who headed this study, said that their results helped to explain another way in which estrogen protects against heart disease before menopause and why it may be important to consider as therapy for postmenopausal women at high risk of CVD.

- Estrogen maintains the normal balance of prostacycline and thromboxane, two chemicals that regulate clot formation. Prostacycline dilates blood vessels and prevents platelets from aggregating and forming plaque. Thromboxane has the opposite effect: it constricts blood vessels and stimulates platelet aggregation as a means of defending the body against hemorrhage. When thromboxane levels are high, blood pressure goes up and more "sticky" platelets aggregate to form plaque along the artery wall. Estrogen *increases* artery production of prostacycline, which *improves* blood flow and *reduces platelet aggregation* to form clots and plaque. This is also similar to the way that aspirin works to help prevent clots, which could give rise to strokes and heart attacks.

• In the PEPI studies, released in January 1995, fibrinogen levels rose by about 3 percent in women *not* on estrogen, but women who were taking estrogen showed no change in fibrinogen levels. A 3 percent *increase* in fibrinogen (a *clot-forming* factor) *doubled* the risk of heart attack in women in the Framingham Study.

• *Estrogen therapy* (to restore levels to premenopausal ranges) *also improved clot-dissolving ability*, based on recent analysis of the second generation of women in the Framingham Study. Premenopausal and postmenopausal women taking estrogen had significantly *lower* levels of *plasminogen activator inhibitor (PAI-1)*, than did women not on estrogen therapy. Since PAI-1 is a chemical which *interferes with* natural clot-dissolving ability, lower levels are desirable.

• Late in 1994, a study from Europe reported evidence of estrogen acting as a free-radical scavenger, helping to break down plaque similar to other compounds with antioxidant properties (vitamin E, vitamin C) that also have cardioprotective effects. I talk more about antioxidants and free-radicals in Chapter 9.

With what is now definitively known about estrogen's protection for women in the heart disease process, I think it is tragic that we still see headlines from alternative therapy newsletters that describe estrogen as "lethal" and the natural progesterone they

---

SUMMARY OF ESTROGEN BENEFITS ON CVD RISK

• lowers blood pressure
• increases HDL cholesterol
• decreases total cholesterol and LDL
• reduces risk of blood clots
• appears to have antioxidant effects on artery walls

are selling as a "wonder hormone" able to cure everything. One of my patients sent me just such a newsletter a few weeks ago, and I replied that if estrogen were lethal, why is it women feel better in the half of the menstrual cycle when estrogen is high and progesterone is low (and women certainly don't die routinely in that part of the cycle!), and why is it that women's worst health problems start occurring *after menopause* when estradiol is low? What's wrong with this picture??? I find it hard to fathom how such organizations get away with such blatantly wrong information and are seen as "right," and physicians trying to present new carefully done research results are routinely labeled as "pill pushers." I urge women to use some common sense in evaluating the various claims before throwing the baby out with the bath water. I also would like to see a better balance in the media articles, recognizing that neither "side" here has *all* the answers.

Progesterone and Progestin Effects in Cardiovascular Disease

The synthetic progestins have been added to postmenopausal hormone therapy regimens in order to reduce the risk of endometrial cancer of the uterus from taking estrogen alone. The drawback has been that the progestins have tended to offset the estrogen benefits on heart disease risks and to cause significant unwanted side effects such as breast tenderness, bloating, weight gain, and depression. These problems were particularly marked when higher doses of Provera (the standard progestin used in the U.S.) were common. The progestins *lower* the beneficial HDL cholesterol, and also alter insulin balance, which is another potential heart disease risk factor. The typical dose of Provera has been 10 mg daily for 10 to 15 days a month. Menopause specialists are now recommending that the progestin be decreased to 5 mg daily for a cyclic regimen, and 2.5 mg if given every day for a continuous regimen.

The adverse effects of progestins on the cholesterol profile are related to several factors:

- *duration of the dose:* Taking the progestin every day, even at a lower dose, has a more negative effect on HDL than does taking the progestin for only 10 to 14 days a month on a cyclic regimen.

- *degree of androgen-like properties:* Natural progesterone and the new non-androgenic synthetic progestins (e.g., desogestrel) so far seem not to have the unwanted effect of decreasing HDL, particularly if given transdermally, sublingually, or vaginally and if the doses used are in the therapeutic range for postmenopausal use. (This does not apply to the pharmacologic doses of progesterone often used in treating PMS).

- *route of administration:* Transdermal, sublingual, and vaginal types of progesterone bypass the liver and appear not to have the adverse effects on cholesterol levels that occur when the progestin is taken orally. Oral progestin therapy is standard in the U.S. The non-oral routes listed above are more the norm in Europe, and most of the European countries have a variety of forms of natural progesterone options as well.

Exciting results have just been released from the Postmenopause Estrogen Progestin Intervention (PEPI) studies, a three-year investigation into the benefits and risks of various hormone regimens. This was the first major study in the U.S. to use natural micronized progesterone as one of the therapy regimens and to compare its effectiveness with the standard progestin, Provera. Investigators found that the natural micronized progesterone protected the endometrium (not surprising, since that's what it did for women before menopause!) and did not have the drawback of decreasing HDL. The results of this study were hailed as a major breakthrough in this country by those of us who have long been advocating the use of natural progesterone for post-menopausal regimens. Hopefully we will now see this option made more widely available to women in the U.S., such as women in Europe have had for many years.

Testosterone and Heart Disease Concerns

I talked in Chapter 6 about the role of adding testosterone for some women after menopause, particularly if they have had an abrupt hormone drop from having a surgical menopause with the ovaries removed and are experiencing marked loss of libido. I do think this important hormone has a place in the options we offer women, but it is potentially a problem if a woman has a high risk of heart disease and has abnormal levels of total cholesterol with low HDL. In such a woman, testosterone may *worsen* the lipid profile by further increasing total cholesterol and *decreasing* the good HDL. For this reason, anyone on testosterone supplements must have regular monitoring of cholesterol levels. I have not found the doses I typically use for women to cause these unwanted changes in cholesterol, but *I am using lower doses than are often given* women. In controlled studies by Dr. Christopher Longcope, when testosterone was administered continuously in low doses (1.25 and 2.5 mg daily) with estrogen, there were no significant changes in cardiovascular or liver measures, including cholesterol profile. Testosterone may also increase blood pressure, but this is also related to dose and usually only happens at higher doses than I am suggesting. We now have a number of controlled studies showing that *low dose* testosterone therapy *does not cause increased blood pressure* in most women. As a general guideline, I do think that if you are taking testosterone with estrogen, it is a good health practice to have your cholesterol, HDL, LDL, and blood pressure checked at least annually as part of your usual checkup.

In the past, medical practitioners and women have been taught that heart disease does not strike women until after menopause. Recent research, and my own clinical experience with mid-life women, has shown that evaluation of ovary hormonal status may be more crucial in premenopausal women than we realized. Keep in mind that women *start* having increased risk for heart disease at whatever age they become *menopausal based on endocrine function, not just chronological age.* A woman who has either natural or surgical menopause at age forty, begins having the cholesterol and other changes that increase risk of heart disease. Those changes don't wait to start until she reaches fifty-five. Testing for the endocrine factor allows us to identify women at risk of cardiovascular disease *at a time when risk factors are reversible* and when lifestyle changes possibly along with hormone therapy can make the most difference.

I encourage all women, and their physicians, to take into account the *premenopausal* hormone changes, which can be readily assessed as part of an overall approach to optimal health care for women. If you think you are beginning menopause (regardless of how old you are) and you have a significant family history of heart disease, you may want to ask your physicians to do a simple blood test of FSH and estradiol on Day 1 or 2 of your menstrual bleeding, along with the usual multichemistry panel and cholesterol profile (make sure it includes HDL). This can help identify possible premenopausal changes adding to your cardiovascular disease risk. If you already have high cholesterol and/or high blood pressure, it is even more important to ask your physician to check your hormone levels so that this can be considered in your therapy. We have good screening and treatment techniques now available for reproductive cancers, so it is crucial that you *also* understand and address the greater risks of disability and premature death from osteoporosis, heart disease, and strokes, which increase as estrogen declines.

I have found it can be very rewarding as a physician to explain these mid-life endocrine changes and their effects on blood pressure, lipid profile, palpitations, and overall risk of heart disease. My women patients have been interested and even excited to learn about these connections and have been even more motivated, by the *knowledge*, to incorporate needed dietary and exercise approaches and to consider whatever hormonal therapy may be desired or appropriate. It also adds to your own sense of taking control of your health by exploring many options *after* having a medical assessment that focuses on what makes *your body different from male bodies.*

CHAPTER 14

Breast Cancer: Politics and Hidden Risks, What You Aren't Told!

The Hormone Controversy

Breast Cancer is the number one fear expressed by women when discussing hormone therapy, whether referring to birth control pill use or postmenopausal hormone use. A great deal of this fear was fueled by the publication of the "Swedish Study" in 1989 and the widespread headlines that hit the newspapers and magazines. I think women need to know the full story behind these headlines, because this is a classic example of the distortion of health information to sell products (TV ratings, magazine issues, newspapers, etc.) and to perpetuate the cycle of fear. It turns out that most of the brouhaha was *not* due to the actual study results, but rather to the *misinterpretation* of *preliminary partial results*, as I explain later in the chapter.

Let me say right off the bat: there are two *unchangeable* risks for breast cancer: being female and growing older.

I, for one, am happy being a woman, and I would like to keep growing older. So, no matter what else you do, all of us women have to keep up with our screening mammograms and breast self-exams as we age, whether you ever take hormones or not. I will talk more in this chapter about the various risk factors, how to put your individual risk in perspective, and some of the newest findings that give us all a more hopeful picture than what is portrayed in the press. At the outset, however, I really want to give you some important background on the Swedish study, and what happened with its publicity in this country.

The Swedish study by L. Bergkvist and team was intended to determine the number of cases of breast cancer in women on postmenopausal hormone therapy and compare this with breast cancer incidence in a control group of postmenopausal women who were *not* on hormone therapy. There were several major flaws in the design of the study itself:

- It was a *survey* study, not a double-blind, clinical *prospective study* which would be the type of study needed to address possible *causal* connections.

- The questionnaires were sent out to 23,244 women, but there was *only an 11 percent return* on the questionnaires sent out. Yet, this 11 percent response rate was *projected over the entire 23,244 women in the sample* to arrive at their conclusion about relative risk of breast cancer. I am astounded that such a small response rate would have been considered acceptable "science" for the study to be published in a major medical journal.

- The actual number of women in this sample who developed breast cancer was quite small: a total of 253 women, which is too small a study group to provide reliable comparisons.

- The type of estrogen used was a *synthetic estradiol*, estradiol valerate, not the native human estrogen, 17-beta estradiol, which is the natural estradiol typically used in this country for menopause hormone therapy. Estradiol valerate is also about *100 times more potent* than 17-beta estradiol, so one cannot make valid comparisons without adjusting for these differences. Estradiol valerate has a different chemical structure from 17-beta estradiol, and the two estrogens act somewhat differently in the body.

- Users of conjugated estrogens in this study (the most common estrogen used in the U.S.) had a relative risk of breast cancer of 1.7, which was not statistically significant different from the control group (another key point not reported in the media).

- The study's control population had a relative risk for breast cancer of 1.6, not 1.0 as is commonly used for comparison purposes.

- The authors' conclusions on the increased risk of breast cancer with *combined* estrogen and progestin use was based on *only ten patients!*

- In their paper, the authors stated: "whereas a number of the relative risks and associated trends in this investigation were statistically significant, *the number of observations on which they are based was relatively small. Some findings could be due to chance*"

(I italicized the previous material in order to illustrate what an important statement was left out of the media reports).

- In 1992, Bergkvist reported corrected relative risk data for breast cancer in estradiol and conjugated estrogen users. This time his group found a relative risk of 1.0, *exactly what the relative risk is without estrogen use.* Tragically for American women, this update was published in the British medical journal, *The Lancet,* and this important information, which could help reduce women's fears, did not make it into the American media.

- When the same Swedish group published the *results* of this initial study in 1989, in a more obscure medical journal this time, they reported that the relative breast cancer **survival rate** is **significantly higher in patients who had received estrogen therapy!**

  They found approximately a 40 percent *reduction* in excess mortality from breast cancer in the women *taking estrogen.* Why did we get such a distorted picture of the Swedish study in the U.S. press? Could it be that the scare tactics sold more magazines, newspapers, and news shows? Are you feeling angry as you read this? I was, both as a woman and as a physician sincerely trying to help women get accurate and up-to-date information.

Just as this book was in its final editing stage, another example of the fear tactics emerged with the release of an analysis of the Harvard Nurses Health Study showing a possible 30 percent increase in risk of breast cancer among the women taking ERT compared to those who did not. (To put this risk in perspective, instead of 7 cancers expected to occur over a 10 year period in 200 women over age 55, 10 such cancers would be found if *all* the postmenopausal women were taking hormones for longer than five years). Headlines again screamed the alarm and news magazines did sensationalized covers on the subject. Once again, the flaws in the study design were rarely brought out, and the balance of estrogen's benefits on other diseases was not portrayed accurately. Some of the other positive findings were not reported, and women were again left confused and scared. If you look at the summary graph (Diagram 14.1) on the following page, the picture isn't nearly as frightening as the newspapers and magazines presented.

In addition, I think a crucial point is being overlooked. When I read the NEJM article, I noticed that an overwhelming majority of the women in this study were taking the *conjugated equine estrogens* (Premarin and generic forms), *not the native human form* of estrogen (17-beta estradiol). I find it alarming that *no one* is

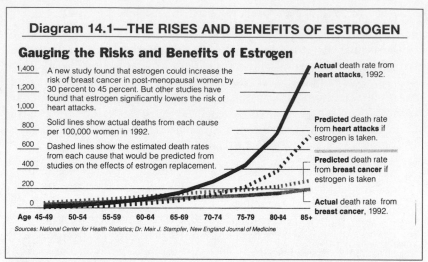

Diagram 14.1—THE RISES AND BENEFITS OF ESTROGEN

Gauging the Risks and Benefits of Estrogen

1,400   A new study found that estrogen could increase the risk of breast cancer in post-menopausal women by 30 percent to 45 percent. But other studies have found that estrogen significantly lowers the risk of heart attacks.

1,200

1,000

800   Solid lines show actual deaths from each cause per 100,000 women in 1992.

600   Dashed lines show the estimated death rates from each cause that would be predicted from studies on the effects of estrogen replacement.

400

200

0

Age 45-49   50-54   55-59   60-64   65-69   70-74   75-79   80-84   85+

Actual death rate from **heart attacks**, 1992.

Predicted death rate from **heart attacks** if estrogen is taken.

Predicted death rate from **breast cancer** if estrogen is taken

Actual death rate from **breast cancer**, 1992.

Sources: National Center for Health Statistics; Dr. Meir J. Stampfer, New England Journal of Medicine

addressing this issue, although I have been asking these questions in medical conferences for a number of years. I think it is imperative that we undertake research designed to address the potential for *different effects* on breast cancer which may occur using *different types of estrogen* therapy (see also Chapters 5 and 15).

The long-acting equine estrogens have unknown effects in the human breast, and are not cleared from the body quickly as is 17-beta estradiol. What effect does this long duration of estrogen effect, with a non-human type of estrogen, have on the potential for promoting growth of breast cancer? We *don't know* because leading researchers have simply failed to address these questions and have continued to assume that *all estrogens are alike.*

So where DO we stand with our knowledge about ERT/HRT and the risk of breast cancer? From analyzing all of the worldwide studies to date, menopause specialists and breast cancer researchers have found that the relative risk of breast cancer in estrogen users is hovering right around 1.0, which means that **estrogen is NOT acting as a carcinogen.** If estrogen were acting as a carcinogen, the relative risks would be ranging from 3 to 8 or greater, as is seen with endometrial cancer, in which estrogen does act to cause cancer when given alone (unopposed by progestin) to women who have a uterus. With endometrial cancer, taking estrogen alone gives a relative risk of 8.0, very different from what is seen in the breast cancer studies.

Estrogen appears to have the potential for *promoting growth* of existing cancers that are of estrogen-sensitive, rather than *causing* cancer. *Death rates* from breast cancer have *not increased* in women taking estrogen at the time of diagnosis, a point frequently not mentioned in the media. In 1979, Dr. Nachtigall published a double-blind, case-matched controlled study tracking any complications that emerged after ten years of hormone replacement therapy. Dr. Nachtigall's study did not show any increased risk of breast cancer in women on estrogen and progestin. All four of the breast cancer patients in this ten-year study were in *non-users* of hormones. There are a number of other studies that have shown similar results.

Another way to better understand the estrogen and breast cancer debate is to look at the pattern of breast cancer in women who *do not take any hormones after menopause*, and compare the pattern in breast cancer with the pattern seen in an estrogen-dependent cancer, endometrial (uterine) cancer. Dr. Don Gambrell, a leading menopause and cancer researcher, has summarized these cancer patterns in the following graph:

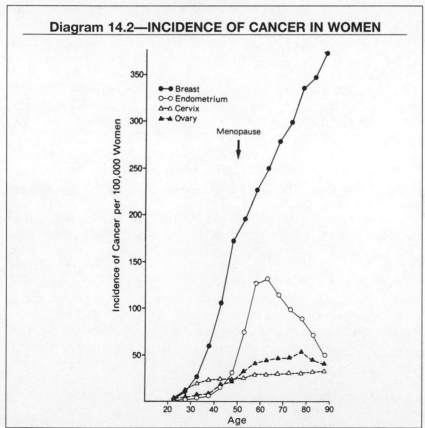

Diagram 14.2—INCIDENCE OF CANCER IN WOMEN

Since so many women are fearful that hormone therapy *causes* cancer, I want to emphasize that this graph shows data from women who are <u>not</u> taking hormones after menopause. This chart shows ages from twenty to ninety on the horizontal line, and on the vertical axis is the incidence of cancer per 100,000 women. Look first at the line for breast cancer. Breast cancer rates continue to increase as we get older, with 80 percent of all breast cancers occurring *after* menopause. A *crucial* point here is that, **even in women on <u>no</u> hormone therapy, postmenopausal women are the highest risk group for breast cancer.**

Next look at the line for endometrial (uterine) cancer, which is one where we know the risk is directly increased by high estrogen levels over prolonged periods of time. Uterine cancer rates rise through a woman's life until menopause, when estrogen levels drop. So, as expected, *in a woman who is not taking any estrogen after menopause, an estrogen-dependent cancer will decrease in frequency as estrogen levels diminish with years after menopause.* This is in fact what we see for endometrial cancer. If a woman with a uterus takes estrogen, she also takes a progestin or progesterone in order to protect the uterus from an increased risk of endometrial cancer.

Now compare the lines for breast cancer and uterine cancer. IF estrogen therapy after menopause *caused* breast cancer, we would see a pattern like the one for endometrial cancer in women *not* taking estrogen, but this is not the case. Clearly the two graph lines are different, and *breast cancer has a rising rate* when the body's *estrogen is decreasing*. This is one of the characteristics of breast cancer that helps us know that estrogen is not the dominant causative factor.

A comment about ovarian and cervical cancer. The major risks for these cancers is not hormonal. They are both diseases of aging. Ovarian cancer is now understood to have a significant genetic component. It is crucial that you know whether you have a family history of ovarian cancer so that you can be more closely monitored, since it is hard to diagnose and tends to spread early in its course. In addition to the increase seen with aging, cervical cancer is now rising in younger women due to the sexually transmitted viral diseases: human papilloma virus and herpes virus. Regular annual Pap smears help to detect cervical cancer early when it is easily treatable. Death rates from cervical cancer have dropped dramatically since annual Pap tests have become routine preventive care for women.

Data on women's survival with breast cancer continues to show that women **on estrogen** at the time of diagnosis have a better survival rate than women **not on estrogen** at diagnosis. There have been a number of studies, in different countries, that have shown this positive outcome, but information on these results doesn't appear often in the news. This pattern of longer survival is also true for women on hormone therapy who are diagnosed with endometrial cancer. It appears that the type of cancer that develops in women on estrogen therapy, as well as its aggressiveness, is different from the types that develop in women not taking hormones.

Even for women with atypical hyperplasia, a type of fibrocystic changes known to increase risk of breast cancer, some menopause and Oncology specialists feel that adding estrogen in the postmenopausal years does not increase their risk further. These women *need close scrutiny with or without estrogen therapy*. Women with fibrocystic breast changes (no longer called "disease" since it is now known to be a normal variation) take note: benign fibrocystic changes *do not give you a higher risk of breast cancer* if there are no atypical or proliferative changes associated with it.

What accounts for the differences in what we have found recently, compared to what has been presented in the past on this issue? One point is clear: the doses of hormones used now are lower than in the past, and we use new types and ratios of estrogen-progestin (or progesterone). Another key part of the answer lies in improved research methods and computer capability to analyze large volumes of data. Also, there is now better identification of other risk factors, better detection of early breast cancers, better understanding of the different types of breast cancer, and better treatment options.

The bottom line? As of this writing, the worldwide data *do not show* an increased risk of breast cancer in women who use birth control pills or women who take postmenopausal estrogen therapy in the currently recommended amounts. Studies as of this point **do not show that estrogen itself is acting as a carcinogen.** Estrogen may *enhance growth* of an existing estrogen-sensitive tumor. Some specialists feel that even this effect may have an indirect benefit: if an existing tumor grows more rapidly, it is likely to be discovered sooner when it can be effectively treated. A very few studies have found that postmenopausal estrogen therapy, used longer than twenty years, may *possibly* contribute to a *slight* increase in breast cancer risk, but this *slight* increase has to be weighed against the massive increase in heart disease and osteoporosis risk in elderly women (who would be those in the category of postmenopausal use greater than twenty years).

My recommendation? Each woman needs to (1) determine what her **individual disease risk** picture is; (2) weigh the potential benefits of hormone therapy against the risks, along with up-to-date information from her physician; (3) determine for herself what quality-of-life aspects may be helped by hormone therapy; and (4) decide what her health values are. And here, each woman will be different. One of my patients, who has severe bone loss, is absolutely terrified of taking estrogen, even though I know it would help prevent further bone loss. Given her fears and her beliefs, I will not push her to take estrogen. I will work with her in using a variety of other approaches she wants to use.

Another one of my patients, a woman in her fifties who seven years ago had breast cancer and now has severe osteoporosis and back pain, said to me: "I am terrified of growing older, having even worse osteoporosis, and living in such pain. It didn't do me any good to survive the breast cancer if I have to live like this, but my doctors don't listen to me. None of them will prescribe estrogen for me because I have had breast cancer. Will you prescribe it for me?" Her values and desires for her life are clearly different from the first woman, and I take this into account in helping her.

I tell my patients, "I can't tell you what to do. I can give you the best information I know, I can help you explore what is right for you, I can help you monitor your health, and I can be there to explore other options if you change your mind. The ultimate decision is what YOU *want* to do." And remember, you should reassess your benefit-risk profile regularly with your physician, perhaps at your annual checkup. You always have the option of changing your mind and taking a new approach, whatever your decision may be.

Media Influences

I have been alarmed at the degree of fear and terror I hear from women around the country concerning their risk of breast cancer. I think much of the fear is intensified and exaggerated by the images and headlines used to present the breast cancer story in our magazines and newspapers.

Am I against articles to educate the public? Absolutely not. But I am very much against the degree of sensationalism that is used to sell the product (i.e., magazines) by excessively dramatizing breast cancer and generating such overwhelming fear among women. I also oppose the portrayal of women as nothing but breasts. A woman is told she has to have a "perfect body." If the breast is "damaged," she's somehow less of a woman. Many women will say "I don't want to get a mammogram because I don't want to find anything wrong. I don't want a mastectomy. Because that disfigures me. That makes me less of a woman." This sequence of thought process is one many of us can relate to. Yet, today stage I breast cancer is more often treated with lumpectomy and radiation rather than mastectomy. Survival rates have been shown to be equally as good with lumpectomy plus radiation compared to mastectomy, *if breast cancer is detected early, before it has spread to the lymph nodes*. Unfortunately, I find that the majority of women at my seminars have not gotten that more hopeful message.

Going back to the Swedish study, what happened in the media is alarming as an illustration of how information is manipulated to grab headlines and attention. The first paper from the Swedish group was outlining the study design and preliminary results. This half of the material was published in *The New England Journal of Medicine (NEJM)*, one of the most prestigious, and widely read, medical journals in the world. This is also a medical journal that is closely monitored by health and science writers for the newest breakthroughs in medical research and advances of interest to consumers. So, when the Swedish study hit the pages of *NEJM*, the information was immediately picked up by writers on wire services for all the major newspapers. Many of these writers had the information about the latest issue of *NEJM* and the "Swedish breast cancer study" even before most physicians in this country had gotten their copies of *NEJM* in the mail!

Headlines around the country told *only a piece* of the story before most physicians had even the seen newly published medical article and could digest the information (or lack thereof!). Millions of women were alarmed, scared, and confused and stopped hormone therapy without being aware of their individual health risks and without being aware of the inaccuracies, distortions, and limitations in the headlines they had just read.

To compound the problem further, when the *outcome* study results from this *same* breast cancer study were published (in the same year, 1989), they did not appear in *NEJM*, but in *The American Journal of Epidemiology*. Now, you may say, "what's that? I've never heard of that journal." Well, neither have most physicians and certainly most health journalists! It is a medical journal with a narrower focus than *NEJM*, and a much smaller number of readers. So, why is this important to you? A very key finding emerged in this half of the Swedish study: the women in the Swedish study who were *on hormone therapy* at the time their breast cancer was diagnosed *had a better survival rate than those* women in the study *who were not on* hormone therapy when they were diagnosed with breast cancer!

This crucial information, buried in an obscure medical journal not seen by most practicing physicians and the press, provided an entirely different "slant" on the issue of hormone therapy and breast cancer risk. It is certainly a piece of information that women deserve to know and to be able to discuss with their physician. But in the world of academic gamesmanship on getting the most "pubs" (publications) from a given piece of research, *this highly significant result was buried* and never reached the headlines where women could see it and use it.

As much as I work hard to stay on top of such crucial information in order to responsibly inform patients, consumer groups, and other physicians of new research, it was *over a year* before I was able to find out the full story! The further follow-up came in 1992, when the corrected and more positive data was published, this time in the British medical journal, *The Lancet.* Of course, that didn't make it to the front pages of our newspapers. I was appalled by the blatant gamesmanship and commercialism that had been demonstrated by this manipulation of both the medical community and consumers. Women ended up being unduly alarmed about their individual risks based on faulty interpretation of statistics, inadequate numbers of patients in the study, and lack of full information on the outcomes.

The point here is not to devalue the role of media articles in providing education and more awareness about breast cancer for women. The point, I think, is to look at the total picture and be aware of imbalances in the information that often distort the true risk for women and frequently portray an overly negative view of progress and treatment options. Read articles with a critical eye on these issues; then talk over your fears and questions with a knowledgeable physician who will help you put your *individual risk* in perspective.

Dietary Fat and Other Factors

There have been a variety of studies over the last forty to fifty years that have demonstrated a significant connection between high levels of dietary fat, particularly saturated fat derived from animal products, and the subsequent development of breast cancer. More recent, detailed analytic epidemiological studies of the dietary links have failed to *unequivocally* establish quantitative associations between diet and breast cancer. You have seen these negative studies in recent headlines such as "Dietary Fat Not Linked to Breast Cancer." You may find yourself asking, "How can I make sense of apparently conflicting information? Has there been a 'cover-up' of important dietary factors? What should I do *now* to protect my health and reduce my risk of breast cancer?"

I have reviewed 104 articles in a Medline search of publications *since 1990* and found that the majority of these studies *did support the link between dietary fat intake and increased risk of breast cancer*. These studies have been done in a wide variety of geographic areas, from China and Japan, to Moscow, Italy, Australia, Europe, and the U.S. The link is stronger for saturated animal fat than for vegetable fat/oils. So, why can't we say definitively at this time that fat intake is a risk factor?

First of all, there are many reasons why *epidemiological studies*, even carefully done ones, may not show a clear, *unequivocal* link between diet and breast cancer:

- participants' recall of food intake may not be accurate
- study of dietary habits needs to be done earlier in women's lives
- weak associations are often obscured unless highly accurate dietary measures are used, and the number of participants in a study is quite large
- people may give answers about dietary practices that they think the questioner wants to hear, rather than what they actually eat
- dietary factors are more likely to act through *interaction* with other risk variables, rather than as direct (and easier to measure) cause-effect mechanisms
- dietary factors may play a more crucial role in cancer promotion at earlier stages in one's life (e.g., adolescence) and may be less important factors in later years (e.g., after menopause). *When* these factors are studied may be pivotal

What are some of the data that link dietary fat and breast cancer? The connection was first described in the 1940s, based on higher incidence of breast cancer in rats fed high-fat diets. In addition, observations for many years have confirmed lower incidences of breast cancer in countries where the fat intake is lower and where the diet is higher in vegetables, whole grains, and fruits. In countries such as the United States, Great Britain, and much of Europe where the fat intake is especially high, and there is more intake of animal fats, we have seen consistently much higher incidences of breast cancer. Following World War II, we have seen a significant rise in breast cancer in Japan, following along with the westernization of the typical Japanese diet toward much higher fat intake. Japanese women who emigrated to the U.S., and adopted the dietary habits of the American lifestyle, also began to have increasing rates of breast cancer equal to those of American women.

Even more striking has been the increased rates in the daughters of Japanese immigrant mothers, who have been exposed to higher levels of dietary fat in the U.S. from earlier ages than their mothers were. Another significant comparison is South African Bantu women, who consume about 15 percent of their calories from fat, have a breast cancer death rate of 5 per 100,000 women. Contrast that with black women in America, who average fat intake of about 40 percent, and have a breast cancer death rate of 23 per 100,000 women.

There appears to be from animal studies a *threshold level at about 20 percent* of total calories coming from fat in the diet which may be a key factor. Rats fed diets of 20 percent or less fat had a lower incidence of breast cancer. Rats fed diets *above* 20 percent had a greater incidence of breast cancer. Whether it was 30 percent or 40 percent fat didn't seem to make any additional difference in frequency of tumors. A recent evaluation of the dietary habits of nurses in the Harvard Nurses Health Study did not show a link between dietary fat and breast cancer.

The results of this study were headlined across the country, something like this: *Harvard study shows no link between breast cancer and dietary fat.* There was a crucial piece of information that *didn't make it into the headlines,* however, and that was that the *lowest dietary fat intake* recorded for the nurses in the Harvard study was somewhat above 30 percent fat! *All* of the women in that study had *too much fat* in their diets. It would be like looking at 89,000 women for reductions in lung cancer, but all the women are smokers. What the Harvard study had were high-fat eaters and very-high-fat eaters, so this study was not able to address the potential benefit from a *low-fat diet.* No wonder consumers are confused.

The studies we have now do show a very clear *trend* toward increased risk of breast cancer in women who consume high-fat diets, particularly if the fat is *saturated (animal) fat.* In fact, if you look at the data on identified breast cancer risks, and the percent of breast cancer cases *attributable to each risk factor, dietary fat has the highest attributable risk*: 27 percent of cases, compared to 12 percent attributable risk for obesity and 17 percent attributable risk if a woman is age 30 or older with first pregnancy. So it is important to pursue the "fat factor" as a breast cancer risk, especially in researching the degree of risk for young girls consuming high-fat diets.

In studies showing a positive link with dietary fat, *younger women* in particular appeared at high risk. Dietary fat has been shown to increase the secretion of prolactin and androgens, which can then be used by the body to make other types of biologically active estrogens different from estradiol. High prolactin levels are thought to be a potential risk factor for breast cancer. A 1990 Australian study of 424 women discovered that prolactin levels higher than the average in controls were associated with a more than two-fold increase in risk of breast cancer. Prolactin levels *decrease* with *first pregnancy, low-fat diets, and at menopause*, which fits with the observed decreased risk of breast cancer in women who have first pregnancy before age 30, and an earlier onset of menopause.

If you should develop breast cancer, it seems wise to clean up your diet by decreasing total fat to about 20 percent, decreasing animal fat and fried foods to the *least* possible, and reduce your intake of meats. Why do I suggest this after cancer has developed? It may have an important bearing on your risk of a *recurrence*. Dietary fat intake is thought to increase both the *growth* and the *spread* of breast tumors, with a greater effect on growth of estrogen-rich tumors. Studies have reported this connection over a number of years. In 1993, two new studies from Sweden and the U.S. came out showing that women with breast cancer had a lower risk of return of their disease if they changed to a low-fat diet, with about 20 percent calories from fat. So, being conscious of your fat intake is important both from a preventive standpoint and from a therapeutic standpoint.

Keep in mind there is a big difference between seeing a *trend* about a particular risk factor and finding a way to *prove* a cause-and-effect relationship. Are you someone who wants to perk up her ears and take notice at the *early* signs of a problem, or are you someone who waits until a problem hits you over the head before you take action? If you are in the first group of *proactive* types, you will probably want to reduce your dietary fat intake now, based on the last fifty years of *trends* in the clinical data, that show an increase in risk of breast cancer as dietary fat intake increases over time. If you are someone in the second group, who wants to wait until the facts are *proven* before you modify your food intake, stay tuned. We don't have the proof you seek on the breast cancer-fat connection. But since high-fat diets are *unequivocally known* to be a health risk for heart disease, hypertension, diabetes, stroke, and colon cancer, you may want to start reducing the fat in your diet while we wait for more information on fat's role in breast cancer!

Obesity is another risk factor for breast cancer. Obese women have a 2- to 4-fold increased risk of getting breast cancer. Excess body fat contributes to higher levels of estrogens (particularly estrone) and a male hormone dehydroandrosterone (DHA) circulating in the blood. It is *not* known which of these hormones is the culprit in the increased risk of breast cancer in obese women. Two factors imply that it is estrone: (1) 80 percent of breast cancers arise in women *after* menopause, when estrone is the primary estrogen present in the body (produced in the fat tissue and the adrenal glands), and (2) *the location of the fat on the body is important*: there is about a *six-fold increase in risk* of breast cancer in women who have *upper body* (truncal) fat compared to women whose fat is distributed more around the hips, buttocks, and thighs.

A 1991 summary of nutrition and breast cancer risk in Japan revealed that Japanese breast cancer patients were different from matched normal control patients by having *an increase in abdominal (truncal) body fat*. Upper body fat distribution is associated with *higher levels of estrone, androgens, and cortisol* than with high levels of estradiol.

Another issue, in addition to the *amount* of animal fat in our diet, is *what is in* the fat we eat. Most of the meat and poultry we consume come from animals that have been fed hormones to fatten them up and antibiotics to reduce infections. Pesticides and other toxic compounds become more concentrated in the fatty tissues of our meat sources the higher we go up the food chain. If you are eating more foods from the top of the food chain, meat, fish, chicken, dairy products, and organ meats, you are also getting more of these stored toxic chemicals, many of which have been clearly shown to be carcinogenic. Consider the issues in the next section on these environmental pollutants and their potential role in the breast cancer picture.

With most of the evidence pointing to strong links between dietary fat intake and increases in breast cancer, it is tragic that the Women's Health Trial (WHT) in this country was canceled in 1988. The WHT was a such a landmark project because it was a randomized, prospective ten-year study of the fat hypothesis. Its cancellation is a sad and complex story of political and economic interests put ahead of basic common sense approaches and needs in women's health. A telling point of the attitudes encountered by supporters of this study is found in one of the reasons opponents gave for the WHT cancellation: *women couldn't be trusted to change their diets and keep good records of their food intake.* Talk about negative stereotypes of women!

Alcohol and Tobacco

The case against alcohol is even stronger than the case against dietary fat. In 1977, the first study to link alcohol consumption with an increase in breast cancer risk was published. Since then, we have over a dozen studies giving similar results: even moderate alcohol consumption, *three or more drinks per week*, increased breast cancer risk anywhere from 20 to 70 percent. And drinking more than nine drinks a week increased risk even more. Alcohol intake is an independent risk factor for breast cancer. This means that the increased risk is *not* due to other confounding variables, such as total calories, fat, fiber, and vitamins.

Age at which you begin drinking is an important component of this risk factor. Mothers take heed and talk with your daughters! Drinking alcohol before age thirty increases breast cancer risk, regardless of alcohol consumption patterns later in life. As we are finding with fat in the diet, the main effect of alcohol on breast cancer risk seems to be in the vulnerable time of breast development during puberty. The mechanism for alcohol effect on cancer risk is not yet known. There is speculation that it may alter hormonal balance, by increasing estrone, some other estrogens, and the androgens in fat tissue. Alcohol also increases body fat deposited in the upper body areas, which further adds to cancer and heart disease risks. It may act through interference with normal immune function as well.

One more nail in the coffin for cigarette smoking: it increases your risk of breast cancer. **I cannot think of one single health habit that is more detrimental for women than smoking.** If all the other negatives about it haven't gotten your attention, does its role in breast cancer make an impact? The risk of smoking seems to be a stronger factor for premenopausal women than for postmenopausal women in adding to the risk of breast cancer. Tobacco smoke in the body contains many direct carcinogens, adversely effects immune system function, and alters the metabolism of estrogens and other important hormones. Two studies have shown that premenopausal women who have ever smoked daily may have approximately a two-fold increased risk of breast cancer, and women who are currently heavy smokers may have a four-fold increased risk. It's a "dose-dependent" relationship: the more you smoke, the higher the risk. While some studies have not borne out the relationship between smoking and breast cancer, the fact that some *have* is alarming to me in view of all the other terrible effects of smoking on women. Even if the connection with breast cancer is relatively small compared to other risk factors, doesn't it just make sense to eliminate this one factor over which you have some control?

Environmental Toxins

Radiation

A known risk factor for many cancers, radiation exposure also causes an increase in breast cancer. The younger a woman is at the time of excessive exposure, the greater her risk of later developing breast cancer. The danger from radiation occurs to the area of the body that received the radiation: for example, if you had radiation treatment to the cervix for cancer, it does not travel to the breast to increase risk of breast cancer. And the danger also comes from the total *accumulated dose* of radiation. The dose that causes increases in cancer is far greater than any you would get having screening mammograms or occasional diagnostic x-rays. For example, with modern mammography techniques, you would get about 1/4 rad of radiation. The studies that have shown an increased risk of breast cancer after radiation exposure have found that risk increases in a *dose-related manner* from ranges of 100 to 500 rads and up.

Terry Tempest Williams, a naturalist and writer from Utah, has written a powerful and poignant book about the human and environmental impact of the aboveground nuclear testing done in Utah and Nevada in the 1950s and 1960s. The "downwinders" (those living down wind from the radioactive fallout at the test sites) have a higher incidence of many types of cancers. The women have a marked increase in breast cancer, and this increase is found in a population dominated by Mormons, who do not drink alcohol or caffeine or smoke tobacco and tend to eat a lower fat diet. In addition, Mormon culture encourages large families, and women typically have their first pregnancy in late teens or early twenties, which normally seems to have a protective effect on later breast cancer development. Traditionally, statistics have shown that Mormon women have a lower than average incidence of breast cancer. Ms. Williams's mother was diagnosed with breast cancer at age thirty-eight, fourteen years after Diane Dixon Tempest, pregnant at the time, was driving with her husband across the desert not far from an area of atomic bomb testing and saw the fallout dust settling on their car. Listen to the voice of Terry Tempest Williams as she screams the pain of suffering seen in her family:

I belong to a Clan of One-Breasted Women. My mother, my grandmothers, and six aunts have all had mastectomies. Seven are dead. The two who survive have just completed rounds of chemotherapy and radiation. I've had my own problems: two biopsies for breast cancer and a small tumor between my ribs diagnosed as a "borderline malignancy." This is my family history. Most statistics tell us breast cancer is genetic, hereditary, with rising percentages attached to fatty diets, childlessness or becoming pregnant after thirty. What they don't say is that living in Utah may be the greatest hazard of all.

One by one I have watched the women in my family die common, heroic deaths. We sat in waiting rooms hoping for good news, but always receiving the bad. I cared for them, bathed their scarred bodies, and shot them with morphine when the pain became inhuman. In the end, I witnessed their last peaceful breaths, becoming a midwife to the rebirth of their souls.

When the Atomic Energy Commission described the country north of the Nevada Test Site as "virtually uninhabited desert terrain," my family and the birds at Great Salt Lake were some of the "virtual uninhabitants." I cannot prove that my mother, Diane Dixon Tempest, or my grandmothers along with my aunts developed cancer from nuclear fallout in Utah. But I can't prove they didn't.

—from *REFUGE: An Unnatural History of Family and Place* by Terry Tempest Williams, Vintage Books, 1991, pp. 281–87

Clearly, there will be more to learn from tragedies such as this, and I hope that all of us will benefit from those like Terry Williams who have had the courage to speak out and identify environmental sources of carcinogens. We are just beginning to understand the degree to which man has polluted and damaged our environment and the resulting long-term effects on human health.

Pesticides and Pollutants

Environmental Health Perspectives last year published a review article of forty-five different environmental contaminants or classes of chemicals that have been found to cause changes in animal and human reproductive hormone systems. Some of these chemical agents called xenoestrogens actually mimic estrogen effects in the body even though they are not the same chemical molecules as human estrogens. A number of studies already have revealed that women working in the petroleum and chemical industries have significantly increased rates of breast cancer compared to the general public.

I, like many others in the health field, have concerns about these *additional* sources of estrogenic compounds in our environment and what effects these substances have on a whole host of health problems, not just cancer development. These chemicals are everywhere in our environment: water supplies, food sources, body fat, breast tissue, and breast milk. Chemicals in these groups are toxic, tend to be long-lasting in the environment, and tend to be concentrated in fat tissue of fish, animals, and humans.

Dr. Mary S. Wolff of the Mt. Sinai School of Medicine in New York City heads a research team that has linked blood levels of DDT to a woman's risk of breast cancer. DDT is the highly toxic pesticide widely used prior to 1972, when its carcinogenic and damaging environmental effects were finally taken seriously. DDT has been banned in the U.S. since 1972, but due to its long-lasting effects, DDT still pollutes our environment from its use many years ago. It is still in use in Mexico and other countries today. All of us born prior to 1972 were exposed to DDT in our diet, because DDT was commonly found in dairy products and meats. Since it is stored in the environment and the body for decades, most Americans alive today carry some DDT residues.

In Dr. Wolff's study, women who had the highest levels of DDT is body tissues had *four times* the risk of breast cancer of women with the least amount of DDT residues. The rise in the rate of breast cancer in this country in recent decades followed the increase in use of DDT, suggesting to Dr. Wolff and others that DDT may be linked to breast cancer.

Similar observations and epidemiological date in Israel link breast cancer rates with the pesticides DDT, lindane, and BHC. After twenty-five years of *rising* breast cancer rates in Israel, two researchers noted that Israel was the only one of twenty-eight countries showing a *significant decrease in breast cancer rates* over the ten-year period which ended in 1986. Israel had allowed use of DDT, BHC, and lindane until the mid-1970s, when they were finally banned. Prior to the ban, all three of these pesticides were found in dramatically high concentrations in Israeli milk, dairy products, and human breast milk. Two years *after* the ban, in studies of human breast milk from residents of Jerusalem, lindane levels dropped 90 percent, BHC levels decreased 98 percent, and DDT levels showed a 43 percent decrease.

Within 10 years of the ban on use of DDT, BHC, and lindane, there was a marked drop of 30 percent in breast cancer mortality in women under age forty-four. Researchers could not identify any other significant lifestyle or environmental change to account for these differences except the prohibition against using the three pesticides. To date, the American Cancer Society and other U.S. cancer organizations have done little to explore the critically important evidence of the role of environmental pollutants in breast and other cancers.

Researchers are now looking at the effects on *male* reproductive function, such as lower sperm counts, from these estrogen-mimicking pollutants. The noncancer effects of these synthetic compounds may turn out to be far more wide-ranging than we have suspected. I bring this up to increase your awareness on these issues but also to help you put in better perspective your decisions about hormone therapy after menopause. After decades of tracking breast cancer patterns in women, therapeutic amounts of *native human estrogens* have *not* been shown to cause a significant increase in breast cancers. It appears clear, from what studies we do have on the environmental contaminants, that some of these chemicals, which *mimic* estrogen or have other types of adverse effects on the body's tissues and immune system, may be more dangerous than previously realized.

A Look at Your Real Risks

In addition to the problems I have already talked about in this chapter, we have to take a look at what the really mean. Statistics are often misleading and confusing. The one you hear repeatedly about breast cancer is "One in nine women will get breast cancer." How many of you think that one out of nine women right now, regardless of age, are at risk of getting breast cancer? Each time I conduct a women's health seminar, I find that the majority of the women in the audience raise their hands with a *yes* response to this question. This statistic has been used in ads and health headlines for a number of years with the goal of getting women's attention so they will get their mammograms for early detection of breast cancer. The problem is that most women, and quite a few physicians, don't understand what this statistic means and become terrified by it. This fear then keeps women from taking the appropriate preventive and early detection steps available. It's as if many women feel the weight of the statistic saying that there is an *inevitability* about getting breast cancer, so why bother? I constantly hear women saying "I don't want to get a mammogram, I'm afraid I'll be the one in nine."

What does this statistic really mean? It refers to the *cumulative lifetime risk* of getting breast cancer for Caucasian American women. It is *not* a number that can be applied to any one individual woman, since it represents an average risk, taking into account all causes of death over the life expectancy (in this case to age eighty-five). When you see the number change to "one in eight women will get breast cancer," it is actually a revised projection over the longer life expectancy to age ninety-five. It means that one in eight women *by age ninety-five* have a risk of getting breast cancer. It does not mean one in eight will die from breast cancer. And it does not mean that the incidence of breast cancer is increasing. It means we are expected to live longer and so our risk goes up slightly. These *lifetime risk estimates* will *overestimate* the actual risk for a woman who has no risk factors for breast cancer and will *underestimate* the risk for a woman who does have risk factors for the disease. I hope this helps put these numbers into a more balanced perspective.

You will see other terms used in articles reporting on breast cancer studies:

(1) *Attributable risk* refers to the amount of risk for an illness that can be traced directly to one risk factor. For example, with breast cancer, researchers have estimated that dietary fat has an *attributable risk* of 27 percent which means that 27 percent of breast cancers can be attributed to this risk factor. Obesity is estimated to have a 12 percent attributable risk. (2) *Relative risk* refers to the relationship between a person's exposure to a risk factor and the likelihood she will then develop the disease. It is determined by the following equation:

$$\text{Relative Risk (RR)} = \frac{\text{Incidence of Disease (exposed persons)}}{\text{Incidence of Disease (nonexposed persons)}}$$

A relative risk (RR) of 1.0 means that the group exposed to the risk has the same incidence of the disease as the nonexposed group. The **higher** the RR, the greater the risk. A relative risk of 1.6 means the exposed group has a 60 percent greater chance of the illness. If the RR is *less* than 1.0, it means that the exposed group has a *lower* chance of the disease. For example, an RR of 0.5 means the exposed group is 50 percent *less* likely to develop the disease. As I mentioned earlier, studies to date show a relative risk of 1.0 for postmenopausal estrogen therapy. For postmeno- pausal women on 0.625mg oral conjugated estrogens, the relative risk of ischemic heart disease is 0.5, based on most recent research. Keep in mind that relative risk will change as we age and other risk factors are added.

Cumulative Lifetime Risk of Getting Breast Cancer*

Age 25: one in 21,441
Age 30: one in 2,426
Age 40: one in 222
Age 45: one in 96
Age 50: one in 52
Age 60: one in 24
Age 75: one in 10
Age 85: one in 9
Age 95: one in 8

*Source: National Cancer Institute. All of the statistics are for white women in U.S.

One problem in applying these various risk statistics to you as an individual is that they don't take into account your specific health profile and the presence (or absence) of more than *one* risk factor (or variable). If you have several of the known risk factors for breast cancer, your individual risk will be higher than the num- bers above, and conversely, a woman with none of the risk factors will have a lower risk than the numbers suggest. Your physician will typically review your individual risk and benefit profile with you before recommending a particular therapy, and there are also lifestyle changes you can make to reduce your overall risk of a given disease. All of this has to be seen as a *total* picture in plan- ning your health care. Another problem with our perception of risk is the amount of publicity a given risk gets. All of us are familiar with the shock and fear that happens when we hear about a plane crash, and people rush to cancel flight reservations. Those people generally don't think twice about getting in a car and driving home. Yet, the chances of dying in a plane crash are estimated at 1 in 11 *million* in the U.S., and the chance of dying in a car accident are 1 in 5,000! Simply put, because the plane crash generates more publicity, it also creates more impact in the public mind than an automobile crash, and the *perception* of risk from flying appears greater. So the more media attention to breast cancer, and the less the emphasis on heart disease in women, the more you are likely to feel that you are at higher risk of getting breast cancer than heart disease even though the latter is far more common as women age.

We see a similar risk pattern for men with regard to prostate cancer: their two primary risks are being male and growing older. It used to be that most men typically did not live long enough to develop prostate cancer; they more often died at younger ages of heart disease and other causes. And, until recently, we did not have very effective early detection and screening tests for prostate cancer, so many more men had the disease even though they were not diagnosed and died of another cause.

A separate issue is the risk of *dying* of breast cancer. This number is much lower, at all age groups, than the risk of *getting* the disease. A woman's *lifetime* risk of dying from breast cancer is 2.8 percent—compared with a 38 percent lifetime risk of dying from heart disease. For a given *individual* woman, just how much lower the risk of dying is will depend largely on *how early* the cancer is diagnosed. That's why most physicians are so strongly in favor of regular screening mammograms. In spite of the current debate about whether annual mammograms in women under fifty will reduce total deaths, the mammogram is still the single most effective means of detecting early breast cancers when they are most treatable, are least likely to have spread beyond the breast, and the survival rates are the highest.

The majority of women who attend my seminars, even though they are generally knowledgeable and interested in health issues, simply do not know the high percentage of deaths in women over age fifty due to cardiovascular disease. Look at the dramatic differences in death rates on the graph (Diagram 14.3) on the next page: 4 percent of the deaths in women over fifty are due to breast cancer but 53 percent of the deaths in women over age fifty are due to cardiovascular disease! If you have a family history of heart disease, and a high cholesterol, then worrying about estrogen increasing risk of breast cancer (and *not* looking at estrogen's 50 percent decrease in heart disease risk) is a little like being worried about getting run over by a donkey cart coming down the road when you are standing on a track ignoring the freight train barreling toward you!

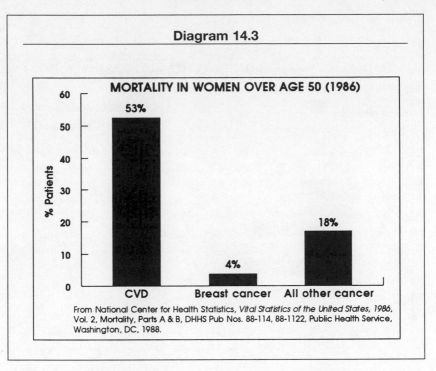

Diagram 14.3

MORTALITY IN WOMEN OVER AGE 50 (1986)

From National Center for Health Statistics, *Vital Statistics of the United States, 1986,* Vol. 2, Mortality, Parts A & B, DHHS Pub Nos. 88-114, 88-1122, Public Health Service, Washington, DC, 1988.

Research Advances: New Findings, Hopeful Outlooks

Talk with a hundred women and ask them what the outlook would likely be for a woman diagnosed with breast cancer, and I am confident that eighty to ninety of those women would list "death" as one of the three first responses. But is this accurate? Is the diagnosis of breast cancer the "kiss of death?"

Look at the graph (Diagram 14.4) on the following page, and notice that the picture for breast cancer is much more hopeful than for any other cancers that affect women. The **white** bars show the *new cases detected in one year,* while the **black** bars show *the death rates in that year* for each type of cancer common in women. It is striking that we are far better at detecting and treating breast cancer than we are at detecting and successfully treating any of the other cancers shown. I am concerned, that most women never get this hopeful message. Media articles on breast cancer, even today, still do not adequately describe this encouraging news about breast cancer.

Survival after breast cancer has improved consistently over the last thirty years: in 1960, the five-year survival was only sixty

Diagram 14.4

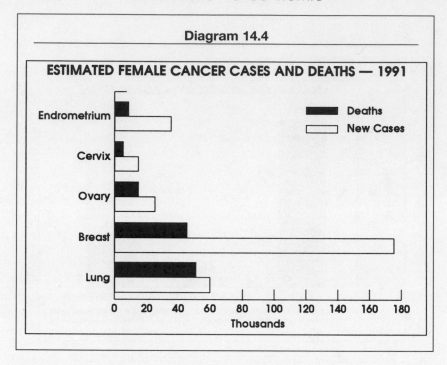

ESTIMATED FEMALE CANCER CASES AND DEATHS — 1991

Endrometrium

Cervix

Ovary

Breast

Lung

■ Deaths
□ New Cases

0   20   40   60   80   100   120   140   160   180
Thousands

percent overall; today the overall five-year survival is *better than eighty percent*, and the earlier the stage at diagnosis the better the survival. If diagnosed early on mammography before a lump can even be felt, the *cure rate* for breast cancer is now better than *ninety percent*. Notice I said *cure rate*. Breast cancer specialists now talk about **cures for Stage I cancers, not just remission.** But the most important thing for you to know is that **early detection** is crucial. It is our best hope at this time.

Mammography Updates

I want to state very clearly: mammography done in an accredited facility by experienced technicians remains our single most effective method of early detection of breast cancer. No matter what you read in the news about scientists debating whether annual mammograms in women under fifty will save lives, keep in mind that they are debating *statistical correlation*, not what relates to YOU as an individual woman. For you or me, the bottom-line issue is what gives you or me the best means of detecting a breast tumor early, because that's when we have the best opportunity to get it successfully treated and possibly cured. **Period.** Screening mammography has another benefit; based on a 1994 study from the University of Pennsylvania: detecting a tumor early with mammography *increases the likelihood* that a woman will be able to have a *lumpectomy* instead of a *mastectomy*.

As a woman's health advocate, I am incensed by what I see taking place on the mammogram issue and the way headlines screaming at us generate even more fear and confusion for women. Lurking not far behind the scenes on this subject is the issue of *cost*. Women are being given confusing information about the value of *annual* mammograms during their forties partly because if we move into a national health plan, it will be *more costly to screen all women in that age group every year*. So epidemiologists are looking for trends in death rates to see whether annual mammograms are "necessary."

What they leave out, however, is that we still know for *an individual* woman, her best chances of survival come from the earliest detection possible, which is greatly increased with mammography. Mammograms can detect tumors two years or more before they can be felt, and they only miss about ten percent of tumors overall. Correct, mammograms are not one hundred percent accurate, but then nothing is . . . except perhaps death. Missing just ten percent still means mammograms *pick up ninety percent of tumors*. In my book, those are good odds. If there were a device as safe and effective as mammography to screen men for testicular cancer, I doubt seriously that we would have any controversy at all about using the device annually for men.

Another dimension of the controversy is that the National Cancer Institute (NCI) analysis of the mammography data was flawed, according to leading cancer specialists. The American Cancer Society disagreed with the NCI policy change, and requested Dr. Daniel B. Kopans from Harvard to review the studies used by NCI in reaching its conclusions. Dr. Kopans, head of the breast-imaging division at Massachusetts General Hospital, reported that the NCI *used studies from 10 to 30 years ago, mostly done in countries outside the U.S.* Older mammography equipment frequently produced cloudy, difficult to read pictures, and x-rays from other countries were often read by technicians who were not as well trained as the radiologists (physicians) who read mammograms in the U.S.

The average American woman never knew about this crucial information. What you saw were the headlines questioning usefulness of mammography. The combined studies used by NCI had several other crucial flaws: they did not target women in their forties for study, and the sample numbers were too small and followed over too short a period of time. I find all this appalling.

Physicians and health activists from many fields have worked too long and hard to help women become aware of the potential life-saving benefits of mammography to have this kind of poor "science" cast doubt on the credibility of years of work and good research. This is one more example of women being manipulated through misinformation. Remember the key for you personally: if getting a mammogram regularly has the *potential* to save your life, is it important to YOU?

New and encouraging results just came from a ten year Swedish clinical study of 24,000 women ages 40 to 49. There was a *thirty-five percent decrease in deaths* in the 12,000 women who got regular mammograms compared to the half of the study group who did not have regular breast mammograms. A different type of study of 1000 women, done at Harvard, showed that in women under fifty the tumors detected on mammography were typically *smaller* and had *fewer metastases* at the time of diagnosis. These two tumor characteristics are associated with better survival rates.

I am also concerned about the significant number of older women who do not get annual mammograms. Only 17 to 20 percent of women over 65 in the U.S. get their screening mammograms done regularly. Since older, post-menopausal women are the highest risk group for breast cancer, that means that about 80 to 83 percent of the high risk population of women *do not get mammograms on a regularly scheduled basis*. I think one of the reasons for this disturbing trend is that breast cancer is often portrayed in the media as a young woman's disease, so consequently many women over sixty-five simply do not realize that *they are the high risk group*, not younger women. If I see that only a small percentage of well-informed, health-conscious women know their breast cancer risk increases with age, what are the implications for the rest of our society who may not be as well-informed? Add lack of knowledge to the confusion generated in the news, and it's not surprising that we have such a hard time getting more older women to have their mammograms done.

There's a recent ironic twist to all this: at a time when we clearly know that annual mammograms are very effective in reducing deaths in older women, Medicare has reduced coverage for mammograms to every *other* year in women over age fifty. It doesn't make much sense from a health standpoint, but it saves money. So

what can you do if you are on Medicare and want to get your mammogram annually? I would suggest checking local resources for free
or low-cost mammograms offered by hospitals and mobile units.

Promising Advances

There are a number of new approaches that have made mammography even more effective. Look into what facilities in your
area have these latest techniques: use of stereotactic X-ray-guided
needle biopsies, injection of radioactive tracers to enhance tumor
images, and equipment that can provide more comprehensive
views of each breast. University Medical Center and St. Joseph's
Hospital in Tucson have introduced an example of such innova-
tive approaches with a nonsurgical procedure for breast biopsies:
a woman lies face down on a special table with imaging equipment below it. The breast to be biopsied is exposed through an
opening in the table, images are taken and analyzed by computer
to give the precise location of a suspicious lump. The radiologist
uses a needle to remove a tissue sample from the area, leaving only
a quarter-inch scar instead of the usual one- or two-inch incision.
Only a local anesthetic is necessary, and typically this procedure
requires only cold compresses overnight to prevent swelling. This
new approach takes about an hour, results are available in twenty-
four hours, and the woman is able to return to usual activity the
next day, versus two or three days of rest after a surgical biopsy.
Women's satisfaction with this new procedure has been high. I
expect we will see even more improvements in the next decade.
Even with these advances, you are still in charge of taking the first
step: scheduling your appointment!

Vitamins and Minerals

A number of vitamins and antioxidants have been studied for
decades for their possible protective effects in cancer. **Antioxidants,**
described further in Chapter 9, include: **vitamin C** (ascorbic acid),
vitamin E (tocopherol), **beta-carotene** (provitamin A), **selenium,** and
glutathione. The 1994 study "Diet and Breast Cancer Risk: Results
from a Population-Based, Case Control Study in Sweden" had further good news about the role of beta-carotene. The authors found
that high dietary beta-carotene intake had a protective effect on the
risk of breast cancer development. Their results agreed with find-

ings from several other good studies of the role of diet in breast cancer risk and prevention. Beta-carotene, as most of us know, is an antioxidant compound, a fraction of which is converted in the body to vitamin A. Vitamin A and beta-carotene have both also been shown to have a protective effect on the development of lung cancer. In animal experiments, beta-carotene also inhibits tumor growth independent of its provitamin A activity, so beta-carotene has a significant overall role as a cancer-preventive agent.

There have been a few studies that have not shown the protective effect of beta-carotene, but since the negative studies were ones with small numbers of patients and limitations in the data collection on actual food intake, I think we are on pretty solid ground in suggesting that all of us would do well to increase our beta-carotene intake as part of a total healthy diet to help reduce cancer risk. Eat those sweet potatoes, carrots and dark green leafy veggies!

GUIDELINES FOR USING ANTIOXIDANTS

1. Take them in the recommended doses only—potential toxicity exist at higher doses, particularly with selenium.
2. Take antioxidants from a reputable source. Look for pure USP grade products, free of additives and contaminants. Make sure you know the complete ingredients in what you take.
3. Take the antioxidants as a combination regimen. They are more effective when functioning together to provide a positive synergy.

Antioxidant compounds have evidence of protective effects on several types of cancer development: lung, breast, colon, pancreas, and larynx, to name a few. There are several good studies which have shown a protective effect of ascorbic acid (vitamin C) on breast cancer, but so far, these studies have primarily shown this protective effect in *postmenopausal* women. Of course, this is the group of women at highest risk of getting breast cancer, but we also need more information about the role of vitamins in younger women. Maurice Black, at the New York Medical College Institute of Breast Diseases, found that women with Stage II breast cancer who had weakened immune systems *reduced* their five-year risk of *recurrence from 38 percent to 6 percent by taking vitamin E.* Since the supplement doses generally recommended (400 to 800 I.U.

daily) have no known harmful effects, it seems reasonable to add the antioxidants to your health plan. I typically recommend a good basic multivitamin, along with the combined antioxidants and a calcium-magnesium supplement as part of an overall "health maintenance" program for my patients. For women who have been diagnosed with breast cancer, or who are at high risk due to their family history or environmental exposures, I think it is even more important to add these nutrients to the daily meal plan.

Role of Exercise

Dr. Kenneth Cooper, the "father of aerobics" in this country, published in 1990 what I think is a landmark study of the role of physical fitness in reducing cancer deaths. I am very bothered by the fact that this study got so little media attention. It demonstrated such significant positive results and is using an intervention (exercise) which has few possible side effects, minimal cost, and a host of additional benefits. Maybe exercise benefits for cancer treatment just aren't "sexy" enough for our media appetite for the "high-tech" approaches.

At the Cooper Clinic in Dallas, they followed patients over more than ten years and tracked the correlation between level of physical fitness and cancer deaths. Dr. Cooper's research group found a marked *decrease* in cancer deaths as both men and women increased their level of fitness. Good news for women: his results showed a *greater decrease* in cancer death rates for women who were physically fit compared to males with a comparable level of fitness. There have been other studies that have supported this link between exercise and reduction of cancer, but none with such impressive numbers of participants and dramatic results. Another reason to put on those walkin' shoes and "JUST DO IT!"

Integrated Approaches for Healing Body, Mind, and Spirit

There's no question. Breast cancer is a disease that profoundly affects women physically, emotionally, sexually, spiritually and socially. The psychological impact is even greater because we live in a culture that directly and indirectly places value on women related to the perfection of the body, especially the breast. Anything that affects the breast has enormous meaning at all levels to our sense of self as a woman. Some women may be more traumatized by this diagnosis than are others, but at some level, we are all affected the moment the diagnosis is confirmed. There have been a number of deeply moving books written by women with breast cancer portraying their journey of healing. I encourage you to read one or more of these if you have breast cancer, because I think the encouragement and support will be meaningful and helpful.

At times of pain and struggle in our lives, we all need to know we aren't alone. I also encourage you to take time to reflect on what is important to you, what helps you feel more in control of the disease, what kinds of support you want or need, what gives meaning and purpose to your life, and where you want to put your priorities for time and energy. I find that taking a self-inventory such as this (and I am sure you will think of other aspects to include) provides focus and a sense of "owning" my life which helps keep me from feeling overwhelmed when I have been faced with a crisis.

Be sensitive to your spiritual needs, too. I think modern medicine too often overlook the importance of faith as a part of the healing process. Seeking support from one's spiritual community is just as important as seeking medical support from a physician or psychological support from a therapist or support group. In working with women who have been faced with breast cancer, I have been constantly impressed by how much better patients do overall when they address their spiritual needs and are also involved in taking an *integrated* approach with a variety of healing modalities they put together for themselves.

I like to help patients focus on improving what they eat and drink, taking vitamins and minerals, keeping up with exercise and physical activity, and incorporating visualization, imagery and meditation to aid the healing abilities of the body and reduce side effects of chemotherapy. I encourage them to find ways of *living more fully each moment*. There isn't space in this chapter to elaborate on all of these approaches; I simply want to express my philosophy that **all** of these dimensions are crucial to your emotional and physical health, especially when you are faced with a major illness. I encourage you to explore the many helpful resources—books, audio and videotapes, support groups, national organizations—that are available to bring knowledge, hope, and encouragement to you.

CHAPTER 15

Hormone Replacement Therapy: Facts and Fallacies

Taking a Look at the Big Picture:
Symptoms and Health Risks

So often, I hear women saying "I'm confused. There doesn't seem to be **an** answer. Every book I read says something different. Everybody I talk to is *doing something different*. Or, Everybody I talk to is on the same thing. Why? What about herbs for hot flashes? What about progesterone cream for osteoporosis?" Keep in mind these **two critical points** when reading *any* book on menopause or thinking about hormone therapy:

POINT 1. The *real* **issue is not an "either-or" approach:** "If I am having symptoms of menopause, do I take hormones *or not*?" I'm not having symptoms, so I don't need hormones, do I?" The key questions should not just be *symptom-focused*. You need to look at the big picture of your health and ask questions specific to YOU: "What are **my** health risks? Which of **my** health risks will be *helped* by hormones? Which of **my** health risks could be *made worse* by hormones? What **options** do I have?"

In my opinion, when women ask the question about taking hormones *just based on presence or absence of symptoms*, they are missing the most important points of all. Hormones are not the only way to manage symptoms. There are many other ways to minimize symptoms. The **crucial issue is whether you may be** *missing* **a silent health risk**, like bone loss or cholesterol changes. For example, both exercise and several Chinese herbs may reduce hot flashes, but may not be providing protection against bone loss that you might not know about for another ten years. How will you feel ten years from now when you have lost two inches in height from vertebral fractures and discover that you could have, should have been taking more aggressive steps than just herbs to prevent bone loss? When I do a bone density test and women discover the bone loss, I hear them say "Why didn't somebody tell me? I thought herbs were all I needed; I didn't have any more hot flashes."

POINT 2. Remember: **Every woman's body is different.** *Any* hormone options *must* be designed to provide what *you* need for your body. What you take *may* be, and probably *should* be, different from what your friends take. Women often say to me, "But my friend is taking Premarin and Provera every day, why are you suggesting something different for me?" The "cookbook" approach with everybody getting the same recipe (which has been the norm in this country) is *not* the way to do it! Your genes are different from your friends', your body chemistry is different, and your health issues are probably different as well. Not to mention that people have different *preferences*. Some women say they "hate" the patch on their skin; other women tell me they "hate" taking pills. Vive le difference! Today, there are many options. Keep in mind also that just because you enjoy trading kitchen recipes does not mean that it's a good idea to trade *hormone* recipes!

Each of us reaches a time when we need to make *our own* decision for our own health. How do you do this in an educated, informed way? I hope to give you suggestions and guidelines to help in this process. Let's examine some of the issues. First, do I think *all* postmenopausal women need estrogen? No. Many women are healthy and have no symptoms. How to determine who does and who doesn't? Is it just postmenopausal women with diagnosed disease who should take hormones? Yes, most women in this category probably should. But by the time a disease like osteoporosis is diagnosed, it may be too late to reverse it, and all you can hope for is to keep from *getting worse*. What about postmenopausal women with just symptoms? Some may really benefit from hormones, and some may still not need anything more than herbs, healthy diet and exercise. Some women have *marked symptoms* and *little* disease risk; others have *no* symptoms and *major* disease risk. You really need objective information to determine the best answer for you.

That's what CiCi did when she turned forty-four and came for a preventive medicine consult, saying she wanted to "take charge" of her health and do the "right things" before menopause. She was still menstruating regularly, she was five feet nine inches tall and had a heavy, sturdy body build. She had no symptoms of menopause, not even fragmented sleep! She had continued her walking program three to four times a week after an injury prevented her from running. She did not take calcium, but had been a milk drinker during childhood and continued to have skim milk daily as an adult. She did not smoke, but did drink one glass of wine with dinner on a regular basis. She had been in good health, and said "I want to stay that way as long as possible!" She asked about having a bone density evaluation done for a baseline, and we did this.

Amazingly, and quite unexpectedly, she was already *two standard deviations below the norm for her age.* She was shocked, and so was I. Neither of us had expected to find *existing bone loss*, since her health picture was so good, and she had not had any menstrual or other changes of menopause. This information changed the picture significantly. We determined what her options were. She said later, "I am so glad I looked at this whole picture *now*! What if I had just gone by the risk factors, and thought I was not at risk for osteoporosis? I'm so grateful to find out now when I can do something about it." As CiCi discovered, symptoms frequently do **not** correlate very well with risk of disease. We can only accurately identify about 30 percent of women with osteoporosis if we use risk factors alone.

I was an example of the other situation. I had no disease like bone loss and no heart disease risk but I was experiencing a great number of really disruptive symptoms: fragmented sleep, waking up many times at night and then feeling exhausted the next morning; and what must have been hot flashes but they didn't feel exactly like what I thought hot flashes were like. Because I was only thirty nine, neither my gynecologist nor I recognized these symptoms as the beginning of ovarian decline. Premenstrual mood changes that had not previously been a problem suddenly became noticeable and bothersome. I also started to have frequent ovarian cysts.

It turned out that these were all perimenopausal *symptoms.* My bone mineral density was above average, my cholesterol was 130, and I had an HDL of 70. My doctor said he had never seen a cholesterol/HDL ratio that good. I have been exercising most of my adult life, and I also have a heavier body build. Since I did have a lot of symptoms that were interfering with my quality of life, I elected to start a low dose of supplemental 17-beta estradiol, using the Estraderm patch. Within a week, it made a world of difference in my sleep and my energy level (from sleeping normally again, I decided). Even my clarity of thinking and word recall improved. I had not realized how much trouble I was having because of these subtle changes until I was given the estrogen patch. At the time, it definitely was not the standard practice to start premenopausal women on even a low dose of additive estrogen. My doctor and I were later vindicated in the validity of our decision as more data became available, and recommendations began changing around 1992 or so. Even before that, however, I felt validated by the rightness of my decision, *for me*, based on my significantly enhanced sense of *feeling well and feeling back to my normal self*.

Each of us must make our decision based upon knowledge of our whole health picture and our individual needs and desires. Gail Sheehy referred to osteoporosis, heart disease and dementia as the "silent thieves" of later life and health because they are ones that typically do *not* announce themselves with many *early* symptoms. As you consider your mid-life health management, and the possibility of taking hormones, look into the following:

1. Family history (especially heart disease, bone loss, diabetes, cancers)
2. Lifestyle habits (diet, exercise, calcium, smoking, alcohol use, etc.)
3. Your own health risks (illnesses, etc.)
4. Work with a physician who will do *objective* tests (in addition to physical exam):
   - measure your ovary hormones (if menstruating, cycle day one is best)
   - check your fasting lipid profile (cholesterol, HDL, LDL, triglycerides)
   - have your bone density done (DEXA of hip and spine is the most reliable)

If you and your physician decide that you may benefit from hormones, you need to know that the guidelines have changed in the last few years. It used to be that women were told to *wait a year after their last period*, but we now realize that waiting this long allows more bone loss to occur. Even if you are still menstruating it helps to know your objective measures, such as bone density, to enable you to make a decision that gives you the most benefit. It *may* mean starting hormone therapy *before* menopause for some who have low bone density. It may mean for other women that your health measures check out fine and you don't need hormones at all.

Current recommendations:

HORMONE THERAPY MAY BE STARTED WHEN:

1. symptoms appear,
2. when disease risks are identified,
3. actual disease, such as osteopenia or osteoporosis is present, or
4. a combination of these issues.

Synthetic Progestins versus Natural Progesterone

The primary reason any progestin (synthetic or natural) is added to a menopausal hormone regimen is to reduce the risk of endometrial cancer in women who have a uterus. Adding a progestogen (synthetic progestin or natural progesterone) causes the uterine lining to become *secretory* so it can then be shed when the progestogen is stopped. This protects against the buildup of endometrium that can later lead to cancer. *If you have had a hysterectomy*, the current consensus of the ACOG and menopause specialists is that *you do not need to take either synthetic progestin or natural progesterone* after menopause.

There are several terms that many women find confusing, so I will clarify these to help you understand various options.

Progestogen is the broad term used to describe *any substance* that has chemical effects to prepare the body for sustaining a pregnancy, called "progestational" activity.

Progesterone (found in humans and all vertebrate animals) is a biologically natural *progestogen*. *Human* progesterone is produced by the ovary primarily, and to a much lesser extent by the adrenal gland. Progesterone USP is the form of natural progesterone derived from wild yams and soybeans and purified to meet FDA standards for use as an injectable medication. It is also available as a powder that pharmacists may then use to compound individual prescriptions of tablets, suppositories and creams for patients. Progesterone USP is identical to the chemical molecule made by the ovary and has far fewer unpleasant side effects than the progestins (like Provera and others).

Disogenin (and others) is a plant precursor molecule found in wild yams, soybeans and a variety of other foods, that has some effects similar to progesterone and is used in many nonprescription creams. The plant precursors are technically **not** *proges-terone*, but can be made into progesterone by chemical processes.

Progestins are man-made chemical molecules with properties *similar to* progesterone but they have a *different* molecular structure and are many times *more potent* than natural progesterone. As a result, all of the progestins can produce very different effects in the body that are at times quite bothersome and undesirable. Progestins are technically a member of the larger group of *progestogens* because they do have progestational activity, but they are *not* compounds normally found in the human body. Synthetic progestins, whether in birth control pills or given in postmenopause, are the most common cause of unpleasant side effects associated with "hormone therapy." I will talk more about this issue in the next section.

Provera (generic name: medroxyprogesterone acetate, or MPA) is the most commonly used synthetic progestin in the U.S. for menopause therapy, although it has never been actually approved by the F.D.A. for use in menopausal women. Other brand names for MPA include Cyrin, and Amen. MPA was originally approved by the FDA in the 1960s for contraceptive use under the brand name Depo-Provera and has since been used to treat abnormal uterine bleeding and some types of amenorrhea. In more recent years, MPA and other progestins have been used for protection of the uterine lining in menopausal regimens. MPA is the *most progestational* and *least androgenic* of the synthetic progestins; other progestins have differing degrees of progestational and androgenic activity, which gives them varying therapeutic and side effect profiles.

Another group of progestins, such as norethindrone (brand names: Aygestin, Norlutate, Micronor) are derived from the male hormone 19-nor-testosterone, and as a result they have more *androgenic* effects similar to testosterone in addition to their progestational activity. This group of progestins is often used when women are experiencing a loss of libido since it has a better profile for this purpose than does Provera or other MPA progestins. My patients tell me that the androgenic progestins typically cause less bloating and breast tenderness than Provera and other brands of MPA. The more androgenic progestins, however, are not recommended for women with high cholesterol and low HDL, since the androgenic effects can worsen the risk of cardiovascular disease and decrease the benefits of estrogen.

I hope these examples begin to give you an idea how the different progestins ideally should be tailored to a woman's individual health risk profile. I will say it again: We should **not** be using a cookbook approach, giving 95 percent of women the same dose and type of hormones!

What about human progesterone? Why even use the synthetic progestins if they tend to cause so many side effects? Why isn't progesterone used as the progestogen for menopause regimens? It is . . . **in Europe,** where it has been widely available and used extensively for many years. Why isn't it available in the U.S.? Primarily for economic and political reasons: as a natural compound, readily derived from plant precursors found in wild yams and soybeans, progesterone cannot be patented as a unique product. As a result, there has not been a pharmaceutical company in this country willing to invest the millions of dollars needed to gain FDA approval if the company cannot patent the product and recoup their investment.

Progesterone has been available in the U.S. for many years in injectable form made by Upjohn, the company that also makes Provera and Depo-Provera. The injectable form of progesterone USP in oil has been widely used by gynecologists for years, but since most women understandably would not want to have to get an injection on a regular basis, this form has not been used for menopause therapy.

Oral progesterone hasn't been available until recently because the oral forms were inactivated in the digestive process. It wasn't effective to give progesterone *orally* until a new process, called "micronization" was developed and provided more reliable absorption and therapeutic effectiveness. More and more physicians are now using the oral micronized progesterone for menopause regimens because it can be obtained from independent pharmacists who compound the prescription individually for patients based on the physician's prescribed amount. I have used both the injectable progesterone and the oral micronized progesterone in individualized regimens for menopause, and the success has been dramatic. One of my patients, a woman judge, called me and practically shouted over the phone in a jubilant voice about my changing her to natural progesterone: **"It was 10 million times better than Provera, like night and day. I can live with this, I don't feel crazy and bloated like I did with the Provera. The Provera was really driving me crazy, I couldn't stand it."**

Two independent pharmacies with extensive experience compounding natural progesterone are *Madison Pharmacy Associates* (Marla Ahlgrimm, R.Ph., founder and long-time women's health advocate), and *Belmar Pharmacy* (Charles Hakala, R.Ph.). Phone numbers are listed in Appendix 2; you may call them for information on their products and services. Both pharmacies will work with your physician to provide doses right for you. I have found them to be reliable and reputable resources for my patients.

Listen to the voice of this fifty-three year old woman, who had been having very bothersome side effects of depression, weight gain, lethargy, and "all that PMS feeling again" with the Provera phase of her HRT, until I changed her to natural progesterone with the Estrace:

> I'm feeling great! I am so pleased with the changes and this combination. I'm floored by all of this. I can't believe the difference in how I feel taking the natural progesterone, it's nothing like what I felt on the Provera. I don't feel so depressed and slowed down like I did. I used to hate those 14 days on Provera, and sometimes I didn't even take it. I didn't want to tell my doctor, but I just didn't like how I felt on the Provera. I'm thrilled, the natural progesterone worked like clockwork, and my period started within 24 hours of stopping the progesterone. It was like a normal period, no pain or any problems.

Some women will find that they may actually be unable to tolerate the progestin completely because all synthetic progestins tend to cause depression and lethargy, as well as bloating, breast tenderness and weight gain. For these women, the American College of Obstetricians and Gynecologists (ACOG) published the ACOG Progestin Consensus Statement in 1988 which said if a woman is intolerant to the progestin, it is acceptable to use unopposed estrogen as long as she is willing to have an annual endometrial biopsy and report immediately any abnormal bleeding.

Many physicians are reluctant to use this approach because of the endometrial cancer issue, but it is an avenue you may explore with your doctor if you have not been able to find any progestin that you can use and natural progesterone doesn't work for you. The use of estrogen alone tends to be a greater concern in women who are not getting adequate health care and who have ongoing bleeding over a long period of time that is not being properly evaluated. For women who have a lot of side effects with the progesterone or progestin, and have severe cardiovascular risks or other problems precluding use of progestogens, the ACOG position does provide an option for you. You must take responsibility to see that you are appropriately monitored. There are really not any hard and fast rules in this situation, so it once again comes down to *an individualized approach.*

Progesterone and Wild Yam Creams: Analysis of Hormone Potency

The surge of interest in natural hormone options has resulted in a proliferation of over-the-counter products marketed as "natural progesterone" or "extract of wild yam." These products are not regulated by the FDA, and vary a great deal in the active hormone content and potency. I have found that most manufacturers will not release information about the contents of the products when I have sought this information so I could better advise my patients. I have also been concerned, as a women's health advocate, about yet another spate of misleading and, in many cases, blatantly incorrect advertising for these products.

Even though these products are touted as having no side effects, if a woman is sensitive to progesterone, there may still be enough hormone content to produce depression, loss of libido, increased appetite, acne, bloating, and other progesterone-induced body effects. I have had many patients who experienced these problems and had no idea it was the "safe" wild yam cream creating these unwanted effects. How do you as a consumer sort out the potential false claims and make an informed decision?

I met with researchers from Aeron Life Cycles Laboratories, who have been conducting pioneering work in hormone receptor assays for many years, particularly in regard to estrogen and progesterone receptors in breast tissue samples of cancer patients. This groups of concerned and dedicated scientists had similar questions to the ones I was asking about the over-the-counter creams. They decided to run *blinded* assays of a variety of the commercially available products. In the interest of providing sound information to women, so that women will be able to make informed choices for their health options, Aeron Life Cycles has given me permission to publish their results in the following tables. I am grateful to these men and their staff, and I think their work is providing a critically needed service to women who are being led astray by misleading advertising.

If you are using one of these products that has a higher progesterone content, you need to let your doctor know. If you have been having unusual symptoms since starting one of these products, you may want to stop it and observe what happens, or change to one from the list that has a lower progesterone activity. In any case, be aware that many of these products have *significant progesterone effects*, even though they are sold as "natural" and/or as "wild yam extract."

Myths and Misunderstandings About Side Effects

One of the common problems I encounter in talking with women about hormone therapy is *which* hormones typically cause *which* *side effects*. Most women, and the media, blame estrogen for all the various side effects attributed to the generic terms "estrogen therapy" or "hormone therapy." This is not the case. As I have described in other chapters, the *type and dose* of estrogen, progestin (or progesterone), and testosterone that you take makes a big difference in what side effects you experience. The *route* by which the hormone is given can also affect the degree of side effects. In addition, each hormone has a typical "profile" of possible side effects. An example I hear a lot is that the "estrogen" causes weight gain, bloating, depression and breast fullness. These are typical *progestin* side effects. These may be diminished by (1) decreasing the progestin dose and/or (2) changing to natural micronized prog-

---

RANGE OF PROGESTERONE CONTENT OF BODY CREAMS

I. Creams containing 400–700 mg Progesterone/oz Cream

A. Pro-Gest	Prof & Tech Serv, Inc	Portland, OR
B. Bio Balance	Elan Vitale	Scottsdale, AZ
C. Progonol	Bezwecken	Beaverton, OR
D. OstaDerm	Bezwecken	Beaverton, OR
E. Pro-Alo	HealthWatchers Sys	Scottsdale, AZ

II. Creams containing 2–15 mg Progesterone/oz Cream

A. PhytoGest	Karuna Corp	Novato, CA
B. Pro-Dermex	Gero Vita Int'l	Reno, NV
C. Endocreme	Wuliton Labs	Palmyra, MO
D. Life Changes	MW Labs	Atlanta, GA
E. Yamcon	Phillips Nutr	Laguna Hills, CA
F. Wild Yam Ext	Phytopharmica	Green Bay, WI
G. PMS Formula	PMS Relief, Inc	Auburn, CA
H. Menopause Form	PMS Relief, Inc	Auburn, CA
I. Femarone	Wise Essen. Inc	Minn, MN
J. Nutri-Gest	NutrSupplies, Inc	W.Palm Be, FL

III. Creams containing less than 2 mg Progesterone/oz Cream

A. Progerone	Nature's Nutr, Inc	Vero Beach, FL
B. Wild Yam Cream	Alvin Last, Inc	Yonkers, NY
C. Progestone-HP	Dixie Health, Inc	Atlanta, GA

Prepared by Aeron LifeCycles 5-9-95

esterone. In many of the newsletters from "alternative" practitioners (usually promoting progesterone skin creams), I have found a consistent pattern: editors mix up the side effects of estrogen and progestin and attribute progestin effects to estrogen, giving estrogen a further bum rap. Since many of these editors are male and don't live in a female body with our hormonal cycle, they don't realize the major differences between estrogen effects and progesterone effects. Think about how good you usually feel the *first* two weeks of your cycle then think about how you feel and what you typically experience a week or two before your period (the progesterone-dominant phase of the cycle). You'll know what I am talking about! **Just remember the PMS phase of the cycle, where *progesterone* is the main hormone (estrogen is lower at that time)** and you will have an easier time remembering *which hormone* is more often associated with **which side effects**.

In higher amounts than are usually needed for postmenopause therapy, estrogen may also contribute to breast tenderness and fullness. If this occurs, the most appropriate course of action is to decrease the dose, and/or change the type of estrogen. I find that the mixed estrogens (esterified, or conjugated equine types) generally cause more breast fullness than do the 17-beta estradiol products. My hypothesis on why this difference occurs is that the conjugated equine estrogens contain such a large amount of long-acting equine estrogens, which appear to be concentrated in the breast and contribute to overstimulation of the tissue.

The 17-beta estradiol products are much shorter in their duration of effect and don't accumulate in the body the way the esterified and equine estrogens do. For example, after stopping the conjugated equine estrogens, it may take eight to fourteen weeks for the equilin forms to be cleared from the body; when you stop one of the 17-beta estradiol forms of estrogen, it takes only a day, or perhaps two at most, for the levels to drop back to what they were before you started taking it. All of these differences have a huge impact on the degree of *positive response* as well as the type and severity of *side effects*.

Phillip Warner, M.D., gynecologist and founder of the Menopause Institute of Northern California, agrees from his years of observations of women on different hormone preparations. In a personal communication, he expressed concern about women on Premarin having *more* breast tenderness, *more* problems with an elevation in blood pressure, *greater* increases in triglycerides than did patients on other forms of estrogen (specifically 17-beta estradiol as tablets, patches, or pellets). In his letter to me, Dr. Warner

stated that "the effect of conjugated equine estrogen on liver parameters caused a *three-fold* increase in angiotensinogen compared
to estrone and estradiol. This has been well documented by Dan
Mishell and Rogerio Lobo [both well-respected menopause
researchers]." A rise in angiotensinogen is one factor which may
cause elevated blood pressure. Dr. Malcolm Whitehead, British
menopause researcher, reported this effect of the equine estrogens
in 1982, but it has been ignored as a potentially important issue
affecting menopausal women in this country.

The type of tablet formulation is another important issue to
consider if you have multiple medication sensitivities and/or allergies to dyes or binders in tablets. According to the advertisement
"Here is what makes Premarin different" (cited in the table
below), this brand of conjugated equine estrogens is prepared by
"a unique manufacturing process . . . with more than 63 *coatings*"
on the tablet (italics mine). Since so many of my patients have
experienced *complete resolution* of such symptoms as skin itching,
joint aches, muscle aches, and urinary (bladder and urethra) burning when I switched them from Premarin to Estraderm patches or

TYPES OF ESTROGEN (In order of amount present)		
Premarin* (conjugated equine estrogen	*Estraderm and Climara patches (17-beta estradiol)*	*Estrace tablets (17-beta-estradiol)*
* estrone sulfate * equilin sulfate * 17-α-dihydro equilin sulfate * 17-α-estradiol sulfate * d-8,9-dihydro-esrone sulfate * equilenin sulfate * 17-beta dihydro equilin sulfate * 17-beta-estradiol sulfate * 17-α-dihydro equilenin sulfate * 17-beta-dihydro equilenin sulfate	* 17-beta-estradiol * estrone sulfate	* 17-beta-estradiol * estrone sulfate
*Ref. Premarin advertisement, *Journal of the American Medical Assoc.,* Feb. 8, 1995.		

Estrace tablets, I have hypothesized that many of these symptoms may be triggered by the various dyes and coatings in the Premarin tablet (to which some women are sensitive, even if they do not have an actual allergy). I raise this issue for you to consider if you have been experiencing any of these symptoms, so that you can talk with your physician about trying another type of estrogen.

When you look at the chart on the previous page comparing what is actually in the leading estrogen products, I think it may be clearer to you *why* I find so many more side effects with the conjugated estrogens. Look at how many *more different types* of estrogens there are in this product and how many more "keys" there are to confuse the "locks" of our body's estradiol receptor sites. The three 17-beta estradiol products which are available in the United States provide *only the two types of human estrogen* our bodies are designed to use.

Dose Conversions: Human versus Conjugated Equine Estrogens, Progestins versus Natural Progesterone

As a general guideline, I am including the dose conversions here. Since Premarin (and the generic CEE) contain additional estrogen effect from the mixture of compounds, the dose used is smaller than the dose of tablets of oral micronized 17-beta estradiol (Estrace). Approximate comparable amounts are shown in the chart. Natural *progesterone* is much *less potent* than the synthetic progestins; the amount you needed to provide the protective effect on the uterine lining will be a larger number of milligrams to give the same effect as the usual dose of Provera.

PROGESTIN DOSE	PROGESTERONE DOSE	
Provera, Cyrin 10 mg	progesterone	300 mg
Provera, Cyrin 5 mg	progesterone	150 mg
Provera, Cyrin 2.5 mg	progesterone	75–100 mg

17-BETA ESTRADIOL (Estrace)	CONJUGATED EQUINE ESTROGEN (Premarin)
(Estrace)	(Premarin)
0.5 mg tablet (white)	0.3 mg tablet (red)
1.0 mg tablet (lavender)	0.625 mg tablet (burgundy)
2.0 mg tablet (aqua-blue)	1.25 mg tablet (yellow)

Cancer Risks: What's Real, What's Hype

I talked about the media emphasis on breast cancer giving women an exaggerated picture of their risk of this disease. What about the other cancer fears fueled by such articles? What is the real risk? How do you determine *your* personal risk? These are aspects to consider in deciding whether or not to take hormones, because the "payoff" in benefits is frequently seen in your later years. You are making decisions now that will have their full impact a number of years down the road. How do you make sense of the confusing, and sometimes contradictory, information? The cancer concern involves two types: breast cancer (I addressed this issue in Chapter 14), and endometrial cancer.

Endometrial Cancer

Endometrial cancer is a malignancy affecting the lining (endometrium) of the uterus or womb. It tends to be a slow-growing type of cancer, and most often, *erratic heavy bleeding* is an early symptom. Overall, it is a relatively uncommon cancer, particularly today when women are much quicker to seek medical attention for abnormal bleeding. Your risk of getting endometrial cancer is actually quite small: one in 1000 women (0.001 percent) per year. The following chart compares your lifetime risk of dying from cardiovascular disease, breast cancer, and endometrial cancer:

LIFETIME MORTALITY RISK FOR WOMEN

Disease	Lifetime Risk of Death
• Coronary Heart Disease	31%
• Breast Cancer	2.8%
• Endometrial Cancer	less than 1%

Cummings, et al. *Arch. Int. Med.* 1989; 149: 2445–2448

Today, it is even more rare for women to *die* from endometrial cancer for several reasons:

1. it is slow growing,
2. bleeding usually leads to early diagnosis,
3. metastasis, or spread to other organs, typically doesn't occur until

later stages in this cancer (unlike ovarian cancer which typically has already metastasized by the time it is diagnosed), and

4. it is very treatable, and women with a history of endometrial cancer generally live a normal life expectancy and die of something else. If you have *already had a hysterectomy* for other reasons, then you no longer have the endometrium present and therefore *cannot develop endometrial cancer.*

What are some of the risk factors for endometrial cancer? This is the *only* type of cancer in women that has been clearly demonstrated to be dependent on *sustained high levels* of estrogen for growth. The relationship of estrogen to endometrial cancer is a linear one: the higher the dose of estrogen and the longer the duration of sustained high levels of estrogen, the higher the risk of developing malignant changes in the lining of the uterus. No other cancer affecting women has been found to be estrogen-dependent in this direct way. This connection was discovered in the 1970s, after *estrogen alone* had been the recommendation for postmenopausal women. In women who had been on long-term estrogen *alone*, not taking a progestin, the incidence of endometrial cancer increased about three to eight times normal.

When this increased rate of uterine cancer was noticed, doctors studied the problem and found that *progestin* needed to be given *with estrogen* to convert the uterine lining to a *secretory* stage allowing it to be shed in a periodic bleeding. Progestin keeps the uterine lining from overgrowing into the thickened stage of *hyperplasia* which can then over a prolonged time become malignant. Now that standard practice is to prescribe a progestin along with estrogen in women who have a uterus, the incidence of endometrial cancer has dropped back to its usual *low frequency* in women.

If you are on a cyclical hormone regimen, you will have some degree of menstrual flow which is what you **want** to have happen in order to reduce the endometrial cancer risk. On the other hand, many women don't like having menstrual-type flow after menopause and may choose to take a progestin every day. This approach suppresses the lining and eventually stops all bleeding in about 80 percent of women. Whether the progestin is given cyclically or daily, we try to minimize the amount to the least possible dose that protects the endometrium.

Obesity is another key risk factor for endometrial cancer due to the high levels of estrone produced by the body fat tissue. Obese women *who do not take supplemental hormones* are still at higher risk of developing uterine cancer on the basis of sustained high levels of their own body estrogen even after menopause. Women who are significantly overweight and have never had children are at even higher risk, because these women have not had the high progesterone levels of pregnancy to help offset the many years of steady estrogen stimulation of the uterine lining. So endometrial cancer is not just related to *taking hormone supplements*; it may also be caused by estrogens in your own body. This is another reason we encourage women to reduce body fat and stay within a healthy body weight range.

Another interesting finding in recent studies is that the type of endometrial cancer that occurs in women on hormones after menopause has been found to be a *less aggressive* form of this cancer than the one that occurs in postmenopausal women *not* taking hormones. This parallels what has also been discovered with the differences in breast cancer in women on hormones compared to women not taking hormones. Examinations of the cellular patterns of endometrial cancer in women on hormone therapy showed a *well-differentiated* type, which has a *better prognosis* than poorly differentiated or undifferentiated cancer cells. Another positive difference that has emerged is that women *on ERT* who are diagnosed with endometrial cancer have a *95 percent survival rate*, which is significantly better than the survival rate for women who are found to have endometrial cancer and are *not* taking hormones.

Dr. Don Gambrell, Jr., a leading cancer and menopause researcher and clinician, has published findings from his nine-year study of cancer patterns in women on hormones and not on hormones. He found that the risk of endometrial cancer was significantly reduced in women using combined therapy with estrogen and progestin; in fact, his studies showed that the risk was *even less* in estrogen/progestin users than it was in untreated patients. Findings such as Dr. Gambrell's have been duplicated by other investigators as well. So I think the press reports have given most women an unfairly negative and alarmist view of both breast and uterine cancer risk from taking hormones.

Ovarian Cancer

This type of cancer is not common, but because it is difficult to treat successfully and it tends to spread to other organs early in the disease, ovarian cancer strikes a deep chord of fear for women. It occurs in about 4 percent of women in the U.S. and is primarily a disease of aging. It is also significantly influenced by heredity, which is the reason it is so crucial to know your family history. Many women have asked "Will hormone therapy increase my risk of ovarian cancer?" There is no direct hormonal association known, and certain types of hormonal options actually *decrease* the risk of ovarian cancer.

Women who have used birth control pills for five years or more have a 40 to 50 percent reduction in ovarian cancer risk, and the longer the pills have been used, the lower a woman's risk. The protective effect of the contraceptive pills is thought to be due to suppression of follicle growth and ovulation, since cells that are growing are more likely to undergo mutations into malignant forms as the person ages. The most recent research has found that women who have been on birth control pills continue to have a **lower risk of ovarian cancer for up to 10 years after stopping the OCs.** That's pretty impressive. With my family history of ovarian cancer, if I still had my ovaries, I would in all probability be taking the oral contraceptives to help reduce my risk. I know of a number of women physicians who have had tubal ligations, but are taking the OCs anyway because of this new information on the benefits. If you have a significant family history of endometrial or ovarian cancer, you may want to talk with your physician to see whether the oral contraceptives are an approach to consider.

CURRENTLY KNOWN RISK FACTORS FOR OVARIAN CANCER

- family history of ovarian and breast cancer
- disordered endocrine function (menstrual irregularities, difficulty conceiving)
- previous breast cancer
- frequent ovarian cysts
- obesity
- cigarette smoking
- residence in heavily industrialized area
- diets high in animal meat/protein/fat
- exposure to certain chemicals such as talc-asbestos (hydrous magnesium silicates).

Another controversial issue is the use of the CA 125 (ovarian cancer antigen) blood test. At this time, there is no definitive way to diagnose ovarian cancer early. The best available approaches for early detection lie in the combination of

1. careful pelvic examination by your physician,
2. pelvic and transvaginal ultrasound of the ovaries, and
3. the blood test for CA 125, a tumor marker.

The CA 125 is NOT a diagnostic test for ovarian cancer, but it is useful in women with a family history of the disease as *one part* of a complete screening program that also includes the other two tests listed above. The sensitivity of the CA 125 is about 60 percent, which means that about 60 percent of women with ovarian cancer will have significantly elevated levels of CA 125, while 40 percent of women *with cancer* will have a normal level of CA 125. Since there may be *false* positives AND *false* negatives with the CA 125, it is important that you discuss with your personal physician your particular risk profile and the need for any of these tests.

Women with a family history of ovarian cancer may want to have more frequent screening examinations, and should consider consulting with a geneticist specializing in oncology to more fully assess risk factors and appropriate testing. Several such programs are available. These are two I know well:

1. Hereditary Cancer Institute
   Creighton University School of Medicine
   Department of Preventive Medicine and Public Health
   P.O. Box 3266
   Omaha, Nebraska 68103-9990
   1-800-648-8133 or 1-402-280-2942

2. Joann Bodurtha, M.D., MPH; Director,
   Department of Human Genetics
   Medical College of Virginia-Virginia Commonwealth University
   Clinical Genetics Center
   P.O. Box 33, MCV Station
   Richmond, Virginia 23298-0033   1-804-786-9632

Hormone Therapy: Options and Choices to Individualize Your Program

For premenopausal women who are still menstruating but beginning to have either health risks like bone loss or menopausal symptoms such as hot flashes or fragmented sleep, one of the options to help provide hormonal stability is use of the newer low-dose oral contraceptives (OC), or birth control pills (BCP). "The pill," previously not recommended for women over thirty-five, has been found to not only be safe for perimenopausal women, but to actually provide a number of *health benefits*. Previous studies which linked birth control pills with increased risk of stroke and blood clots (1) did not take into account the independent risk of cigarette smoking on cardiovascular disease, including stroke, and (2) were based on the older very high dose pill formulations used in the 1960s. None of those high-dose pills are available today.

Today's OC formulas are a fraction of the hormone content used when the pills first came out. After reanalyzing the past data and evaluating current safety statistics from worldwide studies, the FDA approved the use of oral contraceptives in **non-smoking** women over age forty because they found that the potential **benefits** for many health problems in women at this age outweighed the slight degree of potential risk. Many women in this age group, even though they may not be ovulating regularly, still need and want contraception. I had one woman, age fifty-one, whose hormone profile confirmed that she had ovulated during her menstrual cycle, and she said (in a tone of shock and disbelief!) "You mean I could still get *pregnant*? I thought I stopped ovulating a long time ago. The last thing I need in my life right now is a baby!"

There is other good news about the **protective effects** of the oral contraceptives, and I have summarized this information in the chart below. The percentages given are the **degree of reduction** in that health problem when compared to nonusers of birth control pills. In addition to this list, studies from Italy published in 1994 showed a *significant protective effect on maintaining bone density* in women who used the OCs during the perimenopause.

BENEFICIAL EFFECTS OF ORAL CONTRACEPTIVES

Condition or Disease   Percent Decrease Compared to Non-Pill Users

Menstrual Disorders
• dysmenorrhea	63%
• menopausal symptoms	72%
• menorrhagia	48%
• irregular menstruation	35%
• intermenstrual bleeding	28%
• premenstrual tension (PMS)	29% (reduction in symptoms can be greater depending on which pill formulation is used)

Reproductive Organ Tumors
• breast: fibrocystic/fibroadenomas	60–75%
• breast biopsies	50%
• benign ovarian cysts	65% (using monophasic pills)
• uterine fibroids (fibroma)	59%
• ovarian cancer	40%
• endometrial cancer	50%

Other Reproductive Disorders
• endometriosis	50%
• pelvic inflammatory disease	10–70%
• toxic shock syndrome	60%
• uterine retroversion	24%

Other Health Problems
• Rheumatoid arthritis	50%
• iron deficiency anemia	45%
• duodenal ulcer	40%
• sebaceous cysts	24%
• acne	20% (higher reduction with low progestin pills)

Ref: Richard P. Dickey, MD, Ph.D. *Managing Contraceptive Pill Patients,* 8th edition, Essential Medical Information Systems, 1994.

If you use an oral contraceptive in the premenopausal years, you typically do not experience the hot flashes and other symptoms that mark the endocrine transition to actual menopause. How do you decide when to change over to the usual postmenopausal hormone options? Some women ask me why it is even necessary to make a change to another hormone regimen if the oral contraceptives are working well. The second question is simpler to address: it is important to make the change because even the *low-dose* oral contraceptives contain more estrogen and progestin than is needed for *postmenopausal* use. Conversely, keep in mind that **doses of hormones for menopause are *not enough* to provide contraception for the premenopausal women** who still ovulate and could become pregnant. After menopause, since contraception is no longer an issue, you can use the native human hormones which have even fewer side effects than the low-dose birth control pills.

Making a *smooth* transition to a postmenopausal hormone plan is best done with the assistance of a knowledgeable health professional, so you don't experience any unwanted effects from stopping oral contraceptives abruptly or from differences in potency of the birth control pills and the natural hormones. How is this best handled? I recommend that you have an annual blood test to measure FSH, beginning at age fifty-one or fifty-two. The FSH blood test should be done on days five to seven of the week you are *off the active birth control pills.* If your FSH is greater than 30 mIU/mL, you have reached the endocrine stage of menopause and can switch over to the usual postmenopause hormone options. If the FSH is still less than 30, you could *possibly* still become pregnant (although it is uncommon), and may want to stay on the oral contraceptives.

If the FSH is checked at the end of the week of placebo pills, you will have been off hormones long enough for FSH to rise into the menopausal range if you have reached menopause. You *do not* have to stop the oral contraceptives for several months in order to check the FSH, as many women have been told. If you have the FSH done while you are taking the *hormone-containing* pill, it will be suppressed and not give an accurate determination of your menopausal status. I want you to have this information because your physician may not yet be aware of how and when to check FSH, since it is still relatively new to use oral contraceptives for perimenopausal women.

Many patients ask about the difference between natural menopause and a surgical menopause: hysterectomy *with removal of the ovaries* is what is generally meant by "surgical menopause," although some people use the term to refer to removal of the uterus alone. If you have had a hysterectomy *without* removal of the ovaries, you will still have ovarian cycles and will be producing your own estrogen, progesterone, and testosterone. Correctly speaking, you are not in the endocrine state of menopause, although you will no longer have menstrual periods because the uterus is removed. If your ovaries are present, you may still have PMS because it is related to *ovarian hormone cycling*, not to the presence of the uterus. Women who have had a hysterectomy without removal of the ovaries do typically, however, have an *earlier* menopause. This is believed to be due to interruption of the blood flow to the ovaries during surgery. Dr. Sarrel from Yale Menopause Center recently published a study showing that 25 percent of women will have loss of ovarian function within three months of having a hysterectomy even though only the uterus is removed. He also found that *by three years after removal of the uterus*, about 50 percent of women will have *menopausal levels* of ovarian hormones.

It is crucial for YOU to know this, because *most doctors don't know it*. It is still a common belief that women who have their ovaries after hysterectomy *do not* become menopausal until about age fifty. If you begin to have symptoms of menopause following hysterectomy, no matter what your age, I think it is important to check your hormonal status, and other health risks, to see whether the ovaries have declined in hormone production. You may benefit from adding estrogen. Checking hormonal function becomes a little more difficult because you don't have the external marker of the menstrual cycle to know when to draw the blood tests. What I usually do is ask the person to let me know when she has any body changes like she had the week before her period (breast tenderness, mood swings, etc.). I draw hormone levels at that time, and again about a week or so later to get a picture of what's happening over time. I also encourage a woman in this situation to have a bone density test. Women who have had hysterectomies at a relatively early age, even if their ovaries are remaining, are still at higher risk of bone loss than women who have a gradual, natural decline in hormone production.

If you've had a hysterectomy with removal of the ovaries, then it is even more crucial that you have *adequate* hormone replacement. The younger you are when you have the uterus and ovaries removed, the more important it is to be sure you are on the proper replacement hormone amount. In this situation, it truly is *replacement* therapy, because your own ovaries were prematurely removed, and the body needs the ovarian hormones to function properly. The sudden loss of estrogen and testosterone can have a profound impact on all of the health concerns I have been describing throughout this book.

Many times a woman who may have a complete hysterectomy with removal of the ovaries at thirty-eight or forty may just be given the lowest dose of estrogen. That often is not enough for a younger woman. Her needs are different and the amount really has to be adjusted to what her body needs. Many women who have had a surgical menopause are also going to need the addition of testosterone. I listen to the patient, and I take my clues from what she describes. A patient may tell me "I've had a hysterectomy, my ovaries were removed and I'm on 0.625 mg of estrogen, but I don't have any energy. I don't have any libido. I'm still having hot flashes. I'm not sleeping well. And I just don't feel quite right." Her description tells me that she's probably not on the right type of estrogen or an adequate amount for her, and she may need testosterone also. And yet over and over women are told, "Well you couldn't possibly be having symptoms because you're on 0.625 milligrams of Premarin."

Remember: the *same dose doesn't fit for everybody*. Also, as you read in earlier chapters, not all estrogens are alike in the way they affect different women. When you are taking horse-derived estrogens or synthetic estrogens you may not get quite the same response at some of the body's estrogen receptors. Even though you may be taking estrogen, if you have not yet had an optimal response, I would encourage you to talk with your physician about other types of estrogen options available. Some of the newer ones may be much more effective.

The old way of prescribing hormones after menopause was 25 days of estrogen, generally Premarin. The progestin, usually Provera, was added for days 16 to 25 of the month. Then women were told to *stop both hormones* for 5 days a month. I often wondered how this was decided, because the interesting thing is that the ovaries don't **stop** making estrogen five days a month. They just produce *less* for those few days. If you listen to what women say about this schedule, they usually tell you they feel terrible for those five days: hot flashes come back, sleep is interrupted, aches and pains come back, memory isn't as sharp, palpitations hit again. It's miserable to experience both estrogen and progesterone withdrawal symptoms when the hormones are stopped abruptly! Obviously, it wasn't a woman who came up with that approach.

Today, the recommendations are finally more in keeping with what a woman's body normally does: take the estrogen *every day* and add the progestin or progesterone in a cyclic manner for 10 to 14 days a month. If one progestin bothers you and you don't feel well on it, try changing to natural progesterone or a different progestin at a lower dose.

As I listen to women, I find they know their bodies so well they tend to get smart after the first cycle or two of that regimen. They quickly realize that it's when they began taking the second pill (i.e., the progestin) that they started feeling *really bad*. I can't tell you how many women I have talked with around the country who tell me they just stopped the progestin, which made them feel miserable, and kept on taking the estrogen, which made them feel so much better. *But they were too embarrassed or afraid to tell their doctor they had made that change.* What we may have among menopausal women on hormone therapy, and not realize it, is a whole group of women who have taken themselves off the progestin and are taking estrogen alone unaware of the potential problems with doing this. **Physicians simply have to improve communication with patients** and work together to find hormone options that reduce side effects so that women feel well again!

I urge all of you readers to make sure that you do *communicate with your physician* about *any* medication changes that you may be making, or you think should be made in what you are taking. It's so important to your health and well-being for the long run for you to work in an active partnership with the physician you choose. She or he cannot do the best job for you if you don't speak up about your needs and communicate about things you may be doing on your own. If you stop taking a medication of any kind and you don't tell your physician, he or she may not know to see that you get monitored properly for possible consequences. Also keep in mind that there is a lot of fine tuning that can be done in order to come up with an optimal approach that works well for you.

The newest approach is to more naturally mimic the body cycle, and that is to prescribe the estrogen every day. For women who have a uterus, the progestin is given for ten to fourteen days of each month, in the lowest possible dose to provide appropriate shedding of the endometrial lining. In the past, the dose of Provera has typically been 10 mg. I find that is too much for most women, and produces an unacceptable degree of unpleasant bloating, breast tenderness, feelings of lethargy and depressed mood; or as some women tell me, "I feel like all that awful PMS has come back again." The more common recommendation today is 5 mg of Provera or equivalent amount of another progestin or natural progesterone. At the North American Menopause Society conferences for the past few years, more and more menopause specialists are recognizing the problems with the higher doses of the synthetic progestins and are urging physicians to use lower amounts.

Recent research has shown, whether the progestogen is given monthly or every two or three months, that it is the **duration** of the progestogen phase that is needed to protect the endometrium from hyperplasia. One study of 398 women found that in those who took the progestogen for only 7 days, 3.5 percent (14 women) developed cystic hyperplasia after several years. When the duration of progestogen was increased to 10 days or more, not a single woman developed cystic hyperplasia. If you are supposed to be taking a progestogen, make certain you take it for the full time your physician has recommended. There is some good news in all this: the longer you are on hormone therapy, what characteristically happens is that the uterine lining does not build up as much as it did earlier in your life so the actual flow is shorter and lighter.

For women who feel strongly that they do not want any more monthly bleeding, the newest combination or regimen being used is the continuous regimen of giving estrogen and progestin together every day, called continuous-combined therapy. After about six to eight months, this approach suppresses the buildup of the uterine lining, and about 80 percent of women on this regimen do not have any further bleeding. For a woman with no significant CVD risk and no history of depression, this option can work well.

There are some problems with it, however. It has not been studied long enough for us to have a clear idea of its safety and the relationship to later breast cancer. This is one of the reasons I don't recommend continuous estrogen-progestin regimens very frequently. Another reason I don't suggest this form of HRT is that it is not a physiologically normal approach. In our premenopausal years, our ovaries did not make progesterone every day of the month, so I don't feel very comfortable recommending that post-menopausal women take it every day either.

We still have a lot of other unanswered questions about the continuous-combined regimen, including potential negative effects on heart disease risk, more problems with weight gain, interference with optimal estrogen effects on the brain, and others. This last regimen still needs a lot of evaluation with regard to long term safety. It also tends to cause more side effects in women who are sensitive to the depression-causing effects of the progestin. For women with a family history of heart disease, the progestin every day *may* negate some of the benefits of the estrogen on the heart and the lipid profile. Daily use of the progestin may also contribute to difficulties regulating blood sugar in women with diabetes or insulin resistance. If you are considering this option you may want to review these pros and cons with your physician. Just keep in mind that this option is one for which we don't have as many studies on long term effects.

Another question that comes up frequently is "what about blood clots and the possibility of stroke?" The newest research from European centers, published since 1990 in the international menopause medical journals, has shown that the current doses and types of estrogen being used for menopause therapy *do not* cause adverse effects on clotting factors. The recently reported PEPI trials in the U.S. further supported the *lack* of adverse effects of estrogen on clotting factors, and also that women on ERT or HRT had *lower levels of fibrinogen* (one of the clotting factors) than women not taking hormones.

The issue of estrogen-related clotting disorders (thrombo-embolism, thrombophlebitis) has been more carefully evaluated with modern techniques and was found to be primarily due to use of the older *high-dose* oral contraceptives *in women who were also smokers*. Dr. Malcolm Whitehead in England published in 1982 his studies showing that the conjugated equine estrogens were more likely to adversely affect clotting factors than is the native human 17-beta estradiol. So the *type* of estrogen you are taking may be an important aspect to consider if you are worried about blood clots.

One of the things that has been very encouraging about the current research is that many diseases of the blood vessels, which can lead to stroke, hypertension, ischemia, and heart attacks, are *decreased by estrogen therapy*. With some of the newer forms of estrogen that are absorbed through the skin, such as the Estraderm skin patch and Estragel (only available in Europe), the estradiol doesn't pass through the liver so it has only the *physiologically* normal effects on clotting factors, an added plus. With our current knowledge of estrogen's protective effects on heart disease (see Chapter 13), a woman who is at high risk of stroke is someone who could likely benefit greatly and reduce her risk by using 17-beta estradiol to maintain premenopausal estrogen levels.

The following situation is one I commonly encounter, and it illustrates the kinds of side effects that can be reduced or even eliminated by making changes in the specific hormones used. Rya is 51, and was referred to me by her psychologist who had been concerned about her mood swings and headaches. He thought they might be related to her hormonal therapy, although she had been told by her gynecologist that this wasn't likely. Her gynecologist thought her mood swings and headaches were due to work stress. (An interesting switch: the psychologist thought the problems were hormonal, and the gynecologist thought they were psychological.) When I met with her, this was what she had to say: "I have terrible mood swings and constant headaches, and I have been so frustrated with this because I have always been so healthy.

I just want some answers with my hormones and what I can do to take something more natural and feel better. My psychologist heard you speak and feels you are the person I should see. I started out on Premarin and Provera and I just felt horrible on this. I tried it for three months, and I felt agitated, anxious, depressed, and had headaches almost constantly. Then I was switched to Ogen (a synthetic type of estrone) and Cyrin (a progestin) 5 mg for 10 days month. That's when I have the worst headaches. **I've ended up feeling like which do I deal with, my risk of heart attack or feeling lousy every day being on hormones?** That's why my psychologist suggested I see you."

Rya has a serious family history of heart disease in her mother, father, and her siblings. She expressed a lot of fear about going off the HRT because she's very worried about the heart disease risks, even thought she has made efforts to follow healthy lifestyle habits to minimize her CVD risk. I told her I thought we could find hormone options that didn't produce so many unwanted side effects, so that she would feel *well* on her hormones.

She was someone who had never had a problem with headaches before starting hormone therapy. She was also experiencing other menopausal symptoms when I saw her, in spite of being on estrogen: marked insomnia, with waking up about 2 or 3 A.M. and then having trouble going back to sleep. She took the Ogen (0.9 mg) in the morning, and I suspected that part of her waking up at night could be either that her estrogen was wearing off or that it wasn't the best type for her. Rya needed the cholesterol-lowering and cardiac protective effects of an oral estrogen, but she had not done well on either of the mixed estrogens she had tried.

I recommended a change to the oral 17-beta estradiol (Estrace), 0.5 mg in the morning and 1.0 mg in the evening (which is equivalent to the Ogen dose). Spreading out the estradiol provides better stability in blood level throughout the day, more like the estrogen production by the ovary. I find this works much better for most women than once a day and usually provides much better improvement in sleep. It also reduces headaches triggered by dropping estrogen levels between doses.

I also suggested that she try the natural progesterone, 100 mg twice a day for 10 days a month, which is equivalent to the 5 mg of Cyrin. At her follow-up appointment she described feeling "like a new person, it's wonderful not to have daily headaches, it's like a miracle. My husband has noticed a big change in my disposition, and said I'm not as irritable and short-tempered as I was. My mood feels more even, I feel a real difference in my ability to let things just run off and not get upset by them. I'm not as tired, and I'm sleeping better. This is a big change."

Where there's a will, there's (usually) a way!

Are Herbal Remedies Safe and Effective?

Don't be misled by the word "natural" when looking for remedies for PMS or menopausal changes. A variety of herbs have been well documented to have toxic effects on the liver, and may cause a variety of other symptoms as well. Just because compounds are *natural* to plants does not necessarily they are *natural* for humans (same reasoning I used in talking about the horse-derived estrogens, remember?). Two recent reports in *Archives of Internal Medicine* and the *Journal of the American Medical Association* reviewed cases of both severe liver and kidney toxicity from herbal products. The patient who had severe liver damage encountered the problem many of us have been worried about: the product had been *adulterated* with chemicals which were not shown on the label, so the woman had no idea what she was getting until she developed serious medical problems and ultimately *required a liver transplant.*

Since the FDA does not regulate the manufacture, safety, dosage recommendations and effectiveness of these substances, you are dealing with two major problems when you use them (1) the active ingredients simply are not known in many cases and (2) the bottles may not contain what the label says it does. Even though I am at times frustrated with the slow process of FDA approval for new medications, the advantage is that at least when I prescribe a *pharmaceutical grade* product, I know that its manufacture and labeling are closely scrutinized for safety, and there are standardized dosage forms and guidelines.

Another concern for menopausal women is that the *amount of hormone effect* obtained from skin creams and herbal products may not be enough to provide levels needed to maintain bone density and to avoid increased heart disease risk. So, deciding whether or not to use herbs depends upon your individual health needs and goals. If you *know* from testing that your bones and cholesterol levels are in desirable ranges, then you may decide to use an herbal remedy for reducing hot flashes. On the other hand, if your bone density is low, you really need to be sure that you are getting a reliable source of the right amount of estradiol to prevent further bone loss.

I hope this approach provides a rational, common-sense way of deciding what is right for you. The following is a brief list of some commonly available herbs with potential for severe adverse effects. This is not a complete list. I encourage you to contact a reputable source (several listed in Appendix 2) for additional information. Always let your doctor know if you are taking any herbal supplements, so that if you develop problems, he or she has more information to use to help you.

SOME POTENTIALLY DANGEROUS HERBS TO AVOID

- *Known to cause acute liver injury, chronic hepatitis, cirrhosis and/or liver failure:* chaparral, comfrey, coltsfoot, germander, margosa oil, mate tea, mistletoe and skullcap, Gordolobo yerba tea, pennyroyal (squawmint) oil, pyrrolizidine alkaloids, aflatoxins, *Amanita phalloides*, Jin Bu Huan (a Chinese herbal product), and others.

- *Known to increase heart rate, blood pressure (dangerous in people with CVD):* ephedra (Chinese name: mahuang), excessive amounts of caffeine (not generally shown on labels, but a common adulterant in "tonics"), and others.

- *Known to cause kidney damage (acute interstitial nephritis and/or renal failure): Tung Shueh* pills (the culprit for the woman who developed renal failure) found to be adulterated with an anti-inflammatory agent, **mefanamic acid**, not shown on the label; aristolochic acid; products adulterated with phenylbutazone; and others.

Decision Making: Thoughts to Guide You Through The Maze

There is such an explosion of information, some of it very helpful and reliable, some of it terribly out-of-date, and some of it blatantly wrong! I find that many articles and books still perpetuate old myths about menopause and incorrect myths about hormones. And some of the previous thoughts about contraindications to estrogen have changed dramatically just in the last three years. I think you have to be very selective about the resources you select in the way of books and articles, as well as the health professionals you choose. Not everyone is interested in, or knowledgeable about mid-life and menopause, as many of you reading this have probably already discovered!

You may not be able to get all of your questions answered in one place, because the specialists in different areas tend to know their own field well but may perpetuate inaccurate information about other areas. For example, I have an area of interest and expertise in the neuroendocrine issues and know a great deal about nuances of hormone therapy as well as how to incorporate a variety of other modalities to maintain good health. But I am not a surgeon and cannot take the place of a gynecologist when my patients need these services.

I know about herbal remedies and some basics about their use, but I am not a specialist in the use of herbs so I don't try to prescribe them. If a patient of mine wants herbal options, I would recommend a knowledgeable herbalist. Likewise, you can't expect a nonmedically trained herbalist to be as knowledgeable as I am about the current information on hormones. No one of us can know everything about other fields of specialty. If you are looking for resources, remember to *keep your expectations to the expertise expected for the person's area of specialty*. If you purchase a book on herbs for menopause, don't expect it to also provide current information on estrogen!

You will have to do your homework to select a variety of current, reputable books and other resources to help you develop your "health plan." I have included a list of selected books and information in the resources that I feel have a balanced, current view of the issues, and that I think will provide a good base for you.

We have different health needs at different stages of our lives. Women's health at mid-life and menopause is complex; it requires a great deal of integrated approaches and is not likely to fit exactly into any one specialty "box" based on our old models of health care. Just as when our financial goals and needs change, we change financial advisors; as women experiencing changes that have many ramifications on us physically, psychologically, socially, and spiritually, we may need to change our ways of thinking about who may be the best type of health provider to meet our needs and goals. Keep an open mind, and *be prepared to invest time, effort and money to find someone right for you*, someone who is really interested in mid-life and the integration of these important dimensions of your health.

CHAPTER 16

Still "Killing Us Softly" 1995 Update—Advertising Impacts on Women

Bombarded with Images: The Cumulative Impact of Cultural Messages

Commercials on television, advertisements in magazines and newspapers, jingles on the radio, billboards, bus and train signboards, advertisements on the back of public restroom stalls . . . images surround us constantly from our earliest childhood awareness throughout our entire lives. Most of the time, we are not conscious of the degree to which such images profoundly influence us, and over time, shape our very sense of self and self-worth. Dr. Jean Kilbourne has spent much of her career researching and teaching about the pervasive influence of advertising images in our lives. In 1979, Cambridge Documentary Films, Inc. produced a powerful and moving film called ***Killing Us Softly: Advertising's Image Of Women***, based on Dr. Kilbourne's work. I recall the first time I saw this film; I felt almost "shell-shocked" by the enormity of the problems she presented.

An updated version was produced in 1987 entitled ***STILL Killing Us Softly***, in which she illustrates further damaging portrayals of women, now with more emphasis on violent images and the erotic portrayals of young girls. Over the years, I have led many discussion groups using Dr. Kilbourne's films as a focal point. Even today, I find educated women have no comprehension of the degree to which the collective images we experience, through all forms of advertising, shape and alter our view of ourselves. I urge you to rent a copy of this film for discussion in your community organizations and schools.

If you look closely at most advertisements, a common theme emerges: in order to sell a product, the ad preys on our individual and collective fears and insecurities. A Nike ad from a short while ago summarizes this concept extremely well:

Fear of Failure
Fear of Success
Fear of Losing Your Health
Fear of Losing Your Mind
Fear of Being Taken Too Seriously
Fear of Not Being Taken Seriously Enough
Fear That You Worry Too Much
Fear That You Don't Worry Enough
Your Mother's Fear You'll Never Marry
Your Father's Fear That You Will
. . . it's not so surprising that there are a lot of conflicts and a lot of fears."

Nike has done a wonderful job with some of their recent ads (written by a team of women) which help to put things in perspective: fear of being taken too seriously, fear of not being taken seriously enough. This poignantly describes a double bind in which we as women often find ourselves. Throughout this book, I have talked about our unique physiological changes and cycles from puberty through menopause and how these hormonal shifts have many effects on our brain and body.

Another important dimension of understanding our unique needs as women is to consider how these *physiological* changes then interface with the external world and all of the *psychological* and *sociological* stressors that impinge upon us and require our physical self to constantly adapt. A great deal of this interplay occurs moment to moment without our conscious awareness. The cumulative effect on body, brain, mind-psyche, soul-spirit can lead to enormous consequences for our sense of *wellness* of being from day-to-day.

Why is this important to my concerns for women's health needs? I think it is crucial to be conscious of this dimension of our lives, and its impact, because it is in our *sociological* context that we as women *get our health information* and it is through these cultural filters that the information is distorted or biased. It is also through these filters and distortions of the sociological content that we end up feeling confused and uncertain about who to believe, who we are, who we should be, who we want to be, what we should do for our health, and a host of similar questions. We often find ourselves faced with conflicting information. In the next chapter, I will explore ways of becoming an "activated, involved, empowered patient" in the healthcare system. In order to help you understand *why* we are where we are today in our state of research about women's health, in our relationships with physicians, in the degree of confusion we feel about what choices to make I feel it is important to take a brief look at some of these underlying sociological and psychological filters, which collectively have an enormous impact on our ability to obtain the answers we seek to our health questions.

We also need to keep in mind that men and male physicians are not inherently *bad* or participants in some "evil plot" to overlook the needs of women. They too, are products of the culture in which they were raised and are steeped in cultural biases and stereotypes. Most men are probably not even aware of the largely unconscious influences that have shaped their attitudes about women. In this way, negative and destructive images of women in advertising *also* wound men in our culture, although advertising's adverse impact on men is usually more subtle than it is on women.

What is the image of "woman" we have been conditioned to believe is "normal" or desirable woman? Based on the pictures we see in all the magazines, billboards, TV shows, and movies, she is *thin; young; muscular; white; impeccably made up; beautifully groomed; has long legs; sexy feet; an incredibly vivacious smile; perfect white teeth; flawless skin; long thick hair*, I think you get the idea. Does that image describe you? It doesn't describe me or the majority of women I see around the country in my travels.

Collectively, we as women strive to reach this ideal because it is all we ever see around us. The bottom line is that these images are *designed* to sell us a product by playing on our insecurities about our appearance and fostering the idea that we, too, can *look just like that* if we would only buy the product. The cumulative effect of the daily immersion in the images of the "perfect" woman is that we have a lot of internal "tapes" about ourselves on continous play in our minds. These "tapes" produce a massive wound to our sense of self worth and value as a person when we don't measure up to what we are "supposed" to look like or be.

Many women tell me they feel selfish for taking time out to take care of themselves. Have you felt a slight pang of guilt or selfishness about taking time to read this book? The thoughts keep nagging: "There's a lot going on right now, and I have a lot of family responsibilities. How could I possibly take time out for me?" I think we struggle with this issue a great deal. In addition, women tell me how they experience in many settings being valued for how they look, rather than who they are as people and their contributions to the productivity and progress of the organization.

We also have been bombarded with many psychological messages that tell us there is going to be *someone else* to take care of us whether that "someone else" is a husband, a doctor, an attorney, or a business person. This also gives us the impression from the way we grow up that there will be other people to tell us what to do. The weight of the entire culture supports this message, so it is not surprising that health care became another *paternalistic* system, in which women are "told" what is best for them. I will elaborate on important aspects of this in the next chapter.

Body Image, the Media, and Self-Esteem

Today, more than ever, women are faced with the issues of the cultural emphasis on youth and ideal body size. We are bombarded again with images that thinness is the desired goal, regardless of its impact on our health, and we are bombarded with images of how to stay younger and how to fix ourselves so that we will look younger. There is not much emphasis on how you feel about yourself *as a person*. The focus is on making sure that at all costs, you *look younger and thinner*. Women are affected by these cultural images far more so than are men because our sense of identity is so tied up *culturally* with our appearance rather than our career. The desirability of extreme thinness for women to be sexy and attractive seems to have begun with Twiggy in the 1960s and has continued to this day. We have all been bombarded and barraged with messages that if we are not thin, we are undesirable, undisciplined, unattractive, unsexy, . . . and . . . , you fill in the rest!

The extreme emphasis on a thin body was effectively headlined on the cover of American Health in 1986 entitled "Thinness Mania." The lead article then addressed this distorted view of women's bodies as a major factor in the marked rise in eating disorders over the last twenty years (which, by the way, is another reason women in the U.S. appear to be entering the perimenopause at younger ages). Has there been any improvement so far? Look at the magazine, TV, and other media images and you tell me. It was in 1993 that the emaciated "waif" look was the hit feature for the fashion layouts surrounding us. In spite of a great deal of recent attention to these issues by women's health advocates, female bodies are still portrayed as lean, muscular, and above all, thin. The dramatic leanness and muscular development of the women in such ads has frequently meant dieting to the point of skipping or stopping menstruation, which then means that these young women are already losing bone, well before the usual age of menopause. For 90 percent of women, pushing our bodies to reach this unrealistic ideal is trying to overcome Mother Nature. Female hormones are designed to facilitate fat storage as part of our adaptation to being able to sustain pregnancies and nourish a growing baby. An important women's health issue for all age groups, beginning with young girls, is to overcome this pervasive message that thinness is beauty and acceptance. I recently came across this poem, which pretty well sums it up:

"Figure Problems"
by Allison Joseph

Our eyes are trained to search
for flaws, to see our bodies
as problems that must be solved—

thighs too heavy, ankles too weak,
hips too wide to suit an ideal
we did not create—trained to see

each body part as fundamentally
troubled, astray. We learn to
conceal, not reveal, not to show

the weakness each magazine cover
prompts us to hide, shrouding
or starving ourselves submissive.

What if we were to disregard
the slogans that keep us indoors,
to shun the shame that marks us

imperfect, using our bodies
as we please, pleasure more
important now, more necessary

than perfection, our senses
stirred as we walk outside,
moving thighs and hips however

we want, moving forward in
steady rhythmic motion,
feeling power deep in

calves, knees, arms,
pushing as if against
current, yet still mobile,

aware of the air we breathe,
the persistent throb of our
heart, pulse. What if our bodies

were ours to master,
not the province of pills
or diet shakes, our own machines

to use however we wanted,
with variations here and there,
room for the slim and the curved

the angular and the heavy,
each one of us pushing the other
on, not holding anyone back.

—from the book: *I Am Becoming the Woman I've Wanted*
Copyright 1994 by Papier-Mache Press

Each woman usually struggles with the burden of her perceived inadequacies alone, thinking that low self-esteem is somehow her fault. When you wonder why low self-esteem is so much more common in women than men, remember what I have said and keep in mind that these images affect *all* of us in our view of ourselves. You are not alone in these feelings. The solution lies not only in individual therapy to help you feel better about yourself, but in all of us working together to create a balanced view of women as valuable and important human beings in our society.

Cigarette Advertising and Women's Health

Beginning in 1986, **lung cancer** became the **leading cause** of cancer death in women, and every year since, lung cancer deaths in women **exceed** the deaths due to breast cancer.

Did YOU know that?

Most women don't.

The average woman in the United States still thinks that breast cancer is the primary cancer to worry about for women, and the leading cause of death for women. Based on health statistics, breast cancer is neither of the above. Lung cancer is more lethal and heart disease kills 10 times as many women as breast cancer. Why don't you and other women know what is happening with the rise in lung cancer? The main reason, in my opinion, is that **all but two** of the women's magazines in this country are heavily supported by advertising revenues from tobacco companies. The two exceptions are *Good Housekeeping* and the new *Ms.* Other magazines simply do not run articles on the health consequences of smoking due to the fear of offending significant advertisers.

If you survey the leading women's magazines for a year, you will find many articles on health topics. I doubt you will find even one on lung cancer and its relationship to smoking. Magazines just ignore that health issue altogether, even though it affects women now in greater numbers than men for the first time since World War II. Speaking of wars, I find that most people are terribly upset about the possibility of our country going to war and losing lives. Yet *in 1986 more people died of tobacco-related deaths than were killed in all of the wars in our lifetime*. That includes the combined deaths from World War I, World War II, the Korean War, and the Viet Nam war. That's right, you read it correctly: more people died in *one year alone* from tobacco-related causes than from all the wars since 1900.

One recent cigarette ad read: "Dare to be more." The implied rest of that sentence is *"you are not enough as you are."* The model is thin, she's glamorous, she's sexy, sassy, and provocative in her red sequined dress. These images are pervasive and are a major factor influencing young girls to *start* smoking. The emphasis on thinness is a primary reason girls and women continue to smoke, because nicotine helps suppress appetite. Women tell me every day "I don't want to stop smoking because I'll gain weight!" We have an epidemic of eating disorders in this country; we have an epidemic of early stage osteoporosis in young women who have been chronically dieting and/or smoking to stay thin. And yet we continue to see that the images convey the message: thinness is all that counts, don't worry about damaging effects on your health.

The ads don't talk about smokers' dramatically higher frequency of heart disease, lung cancer, osteoporosis, early menopause, emphysema, wrinkled skin, slower healing after surgery, and problems with poor circulation to hands and feet (and, as I noted earlier, poor circulation to the penis in men, causing problems having an erection!), among other health problems from smoking.

The bottom line is that tobacco companies sell glamour, glitz, thinness and the picture of good health in advertisement images that specifically target young women to buy a highly addictive product that will enslave and potentially kill them. When are we as women going to speak out and have our voices heard and heeded? Just as women have been outraged over the inadequate research and funding for breast cancer, we must raise our voices against this larger threat to the health of the next generation of women, our collective daughters. Tobacco-related costs and deaths affect all of us, whether we use tobacco products or not, whether we have daughters or not. We must all have the courage to work to end the glamorization of cigarette smoking and help our young people, especially vulnerable adolescent girls, make the choice to NOT start smoking.

Sexualized Selling and Violence Glorified: Devastating Impact on Women

There has been a more ominous trend in advertising themes in recent years. The rise in images of violence toward women as a sensationalized means of selling products has a frightening parallel in the societal statistics of increased rape, sexual assaults, battered women, and domestic violence. When we absorb images every day all around us showing women as targets of different forms of violence, it is a small step for society to develop the unconscious connection that *this is the way to treat all women.*

As we look at these images, keep in mind that over the next decade we can expect to see twenty-eight million children sexually abused. *Twenty-five million* of those abused will be little girls. The average victim of incest or sexual abuse is a *girl under the age of eleven.* As Dr. Jean Kilbourne said in the film *STILL Killing Us Softly* the advertising images do not themselves *cause* such violence to occur, but they create a climate in which such violent and assaultive acts are incorporated into our unconscious as *normal events*, and collectively we are desensitized to the suffering of victims of violent attacks.

These images surround us, affect all of us, whatever our age and whatever sex we are. As concerned as I am about these issues, I simply do not have the space in this book to go into the detail that this topic deserves. I urge you to read some of the excellent books on this subject, from scholarly research documenting the connection between media violence and the rising number of violent acts carried out every day in this country, to popular books voicing the same concerns and sharing the stories of women who have lived in the shadows of domestic violence. **Add your voice to those who are already speaking out to help create positive images for all of us.**

Violent images in ads may seem relatively innocuous, but they help to create a climate in which violence is accepted and tolerated. This in turn helps create an environment of fear for all of us when we have to stay on guard for possible danger when going about our daily activities: wondering if someone will assault us in the parking lot of a shopping center or try to car-jack us at a stoplight. These undercurrents of fear and having to be alert to possible danger add to the physiological stressors our body must deal with daily. The added surges of the "fight-or-flight" hormone adrenalin alters everything in our bodies, from mental fatigue to the immune system to ovary cycles. Living in a climate of constant fear of danger takes its toll on our physical, emotional, and relationship health over time and also wears down our spiritual well-being. I would be remiss as a women's health advocate if I did not address this topic and help you have a greater awareness for how crucial it is for all of us to begin to work for constructive change in our society.

Sorting Out Media Myths and Misinformation

Sometimes just reading women's health articles in the media may be hazardous to your health! Once ignored or relegated to the back pages, women's health has exploded in the amount of coverage given in newspapers, magazines, on TV and radio. But *more* coverage is not necessarily *better* coverage. All too often I see women being confused by contradictory information on health risks, sometimes even in the same issue of a magazine. Some health risks are over-emphasized, and others, which may actually be more common in certain age groups, are left out or underemphasized. What results is a significant gap between what health professionals know is a woman's real risk and what individual women perceive as their risks. I encounter daily in my medical practice the problem of women being unnecessarily frightened by the latest headline.

I don't think this problem is solely the fault of media editors and writers. Researchers are focused on one tiny piece of the health picture, and commonly do not look at the whole woman and her individual risks and needs. Practicing physicians are overwhelmed with acute illness and crisis management and don't have the time to devote to patient education, which could help correct misinformation from the media. Also remember that health writers are not physicians and they try to do the best job they can in making sense of medical articles to interpret them for nonmedical audiences. I think this is an important service and definitely needed.

The problem comes in when writers have to try to present nuances of medical data and studies, interpret the medical data correctly, see that consumers have the appropriate cautions, and at the same time try to sell the article and meet deadlines. What often ends up happening is that sweeping statements are made and then perpetuated by other writers over time. New information takes a long time to break in. I continue to read the same warnings about hormone therapy in all the magazine articles, even though some of these warnings are now at least four years out of date and incorrect as our knowledge, based on good research studies, has changed dramatically.

Bad press and dire warnings can be hard to erase as we gain new information. This is what has happened with birth control pills. Headline hysteria about risks in the 1970s is still with us, two decades later, in spite of dramatic worldwide confirmation of the safety and health benefits of the oral contraceptives. Recent polls have shown that American women still overestimate the risks of birth control pills and underestimate the benefits, even though studies from many countries have definitively demonstrated that birth control pills prevent more deaths and illnesses than they may cause. How many of you know that using the birth control pill for five years or more can reduce your risk of ovarian and endometrial cancers by about 40 to 60 percent? Physicians have had this information for about ten years and yet frequently run into the problem of women being too afraid of getting cancer to consider taking oral contraceptives.

Many times, TV, radio, magazine articles, and newspapers carry health information that's "hot" and helps to sell the show or magazine or paper. What's "hot" is not necessarily what is most important as a health issue for you to know. A recent example was an analysis of the frequency of various women's health topics in magazines targeted to different age groups of women. It turned out that breast cancer was the most frequent health topic addressed in women's magazines across all age groups, regardless of the risk of breast cancer for that particular age group. Accidents are the leading cause of death for adolescent women, not breast cancer, yet there were rarely articles addressing driving safety and other issues that contribute to such a high rate of accidental deaths among young women.

I think there is much we can do to improve the balance in women's health reporting, and this is one reason I do as much writing as I do to help educate women on various topics. Remember to read articles with a certain degree of skepticism and don't panic over each new tidbit of information that hits the headlines! The most important aspect for you as an individual is to be informed about your individual health risks and the ways of working to minimize them.

There is much more that could be said about such an important topic. I encourage you to read further with the resources I have included in the appendix. Constructive change comes from consumer demand for change. The answer does not lie in censorship. I encourage you to be a part of the process of creating positive images of men and women. Dr. Kilbourne described *why* this is important to *all of us*, men and women:

> I feel this is an issue which affects us all vitally. Advertising is a powerful force that keeps us trapped in very rigid roles based on rigid definitions of masculinity and femininity. I feel that one of the tragedies of our culture is the extent to which *human* qualities have been divided up and labeled masculine and feminine. Then the feminine is consistently devalued, which causes women to devalue ourselves and each other, and causes men to devalue women, as well as the qualities within themselves (men) which are labeled feminine. It seems obvious to me that we really need more than ever human beings who share *human* qualities: women and men who can be strong *and* gentle, logical *and* intuitive, powerful *and* nurturing, all of these... the full range of human qualities in each of us and the result will be positive for *all of us*. (italics mine)
> —from *Killing Us Softly* by Jean Kilbourne, Ed.D. and
> Cambridge Documentary Films, Inc.

CHAPTER 17

Patient and Physician: Imperative Agendas for The 21st Century

Stereotypes of Women: What Doctors Are Taught

I share this poem with you because it has triggered such over-whelming confirmation of our experiences as women whenever I read it to an audience. Niki Scott's words are unfortunately as true in 1995 as they were when she first wrote this piece in 1982 for the *Baltimore Sun*.

WHY ARE MEN ANGRY, BUT WOMEN HYSTERICAL?

"There is no need for hysteria," he said. Men get **angry**. Women get **hysterical**.

"Stop worrying," he said. Men **ask questions**. Women **worry**.

"Calm down," he said. Men are **adamant**. Women are **overwrought**.

Assumptions. Expectations. Labels. They diminish us when others apply them.

We sabotage ourselves when we buy them.

Furthermore:
Men get **annoyed**. Women get **bitchy**.
Men are **aggressive**. Women are **pushy**.
Men are **ambitious**. Women are **clawing**.
Men assess **their lives**. Women have **empty nest syndrome**.
If a man is **impotent**, it's the woman's **fault**.
 If a woman is **frigid**, she isn't trying.
Men are **assertive**. Women are **uppity**.
Men who are assaulted are **victims**. Women who are **raped caused it**.

Men are *versatile*. Women are *flighty*.
Men *change their minds*. Women are *unpredictable*.
Men are *virile*. Women are *nymphomaniacs*.
Men have *moods*. Women have *periods*.
Men are *concerned*. Women are *anxious*.
Men analyze *people*. Women *gossip*.
His doctor says it's *job-related stress*. *Her* doctor says it's *nerves*.
His doctor prescribes *tennis*. *Her* doctor prescribes *Valium*.
If a man is overworked, he is a *go-getter*.
    If a woman is overworked, she is *disorganized*.
Men pay attention to *detail*. Women *dither*.
Men *take charge*. Women *take over*.
Battering husbands need *help*. Battered wives *ask for it*.
Fathers *move* away. Mothers *desert* their children.
Older men are *experienced*. Older women are *over the hill*.
Men *react*. Women *over-react*.
A happily single man is *glamorous*.
    A happily single woman is *neurotic*.
Older men look *distinguished*. Older women look *dowdy*.
Men *communicate*. Women *talk too much*.
This list was fun. Labels are not."
      —by Niki Scott, *The Baltimore Sun*, 12/5/82

Niki Scott has really hit the nail on the head with this powerful piece illustrating what many of us have experienced: **the same behavior is viewed and labeled differently, depending upon whether the person exhibiting it is male or female.** Unfortunately, many of these same stereotypes are operational in medical education. When you look at this entire list and all that it implies about our typical experiences as women, I think it helps clarify some reactions women encounter in many medical settings. Physicians and nurses are also products of the culture in which these stereotypes are so prevalent, and all of us to some degree carry these cultural stereotypes of women ingrained in our unconscious minds.

In addition, qualities of women are always compared against the *societal norm based on males*: male bodies, male physiology, male behavioral patterns. If the male pattern is considered normal, then by definition women are considered "abnormal" in being *different* from males. For example, women have been labeled, in a negative sense, as "overutilizers" of health care services because we see doctors, have tests and undergo surgeries more often than do men. But this comparison assumes male bodies and male utilization patterns are "normal." It does not take into account the obvious source of some of the differences in healthcare utilization: women's bodies are physiologically more complex than men's, women have babies and therefore *should* be expected to have more medical visits than men.

It should be clear from reading this book that there is another factor why women average more doctor visits than men: women's questions, concerns, hormonal connections and health problems are frequently *not heard* or taken seriously, so women *continue* to seek help and try to find answers, often very *appropriately*, I might add. Many men may be *too stoic* for their own good and fail to seek medical help early in the course of an illness when consequences may not be as severe. Which gender behavioral pattern is then "normal" here: women who want to nip an illness in the bud at an early stage, or men who are stoic and wait until it's "crisis time?"

Women are more actively involved in all aspects of their lives and their health. I believe we are more closely attuned to our body, how it feels, what feels good for it. Through menses, pregnancy, and as ones often responsible for taking care of health problems in our immediate and extended families, we have a greater awareness and consciousness of the state of our bodies. Yet, women are still typically viewed as "neurotic" in their questions and focus on their health. The few studies that have been done on doctors' response to physical complaints from men and from women do indicate that physicians, especially male physicians, take those complaints from men more seriously and therefore do more extensive workups. The research indicates that in so doing, the doctors are responding to stereotypes that regard the male as typically stoic and the female as typically hypochondriacal. I have not seen any information that would indicate that female physicians are significantly *less* likely to show the same patterns, although studies have shown that women physicians are more likely to examine breasts and recommend mammograms than are male physicians.

Women not only have unique medical needs from a biological point of view, but from an emotional point of view as well. As a result of the dramatic social changes of last thirty years women have many more physical, emotional, and social expectations on them, and this has a significant physiological impact. Medical education and scientific research has also been based on the male norm, with the assumption that "what works for men works for women" (with the exception being reproductive function). As I have pointed out throughout this book, there simply has not been adequate recognition that the hormonal changes *normal for a women's body* have major effects on *all* organ systems in the body, not just reproductive organs. Doctors at all levels of training need to be taught how female hormones affect such functions as drug metabolism; the way alcohol is handled by female enzymes compared to males' enzymes; the effects of estrogen and progesterone on the motility of esophagus, stomach and bowel; how estrogen and progesterone alter insulin binding and glucose regulation and a host of other crucial dimensions affecting women's entire brain-body health.

I do not feel that this education emphasis should be limited to physicians specializing in Women's Health or just available to medical students and residents who are interested in Women's Health. I think female body physiology and hormonal influences should be taught to *all* physicians and health professionals who will provide services to women patients of any age. I think such an approach will further help to eliminate the negative stereotypes of women patients we see so much today.

Another stereotype *of women* perpetuated in medical education is that doctors have been taught to *beware* of a patient who arrives with a list of symptoms or questions because she is a neurotic, a hypochondriac. Men who arrive with a list of questions are typically *not* viewed as neurotic or anxious; they are seen as *helpful and organized*. The French name for psychoneurosis is "la maladie du petit papier" ("the illness of the little paper"), referring to the lists of symptoms brought in by the typically *female* patients. This concept about women has been around for hundreds of years, and is difficult to disspell.

It is also hard to speak up to an authority-figure physician in a white coat (male or female) if women have been socialized to be *passive* and are labeled "bitchy" or "difficult" when we are assertive. If we're not aware of this cultural background, our mental tapes may be telling us "it's all in my head," or "I'm making it up," or "I'm just weak," "I'm inadequate," "I'm somehow not coping." And there are certainly plenty of people around who are eager to attribute problems to mid-life stress. I think it's important that we are aware of these undercurrents of unconscious self-critical images so that we don't fall into the trap of *believing the stereotype instead of listening to our body wisdom*.

Even when we listen to our bodies, however, it may be hard to get heard when you are in a medical office. Current managed care systems do not encourage discussion because it decreases the volume of patients able to be seen on a given day, and administrators typically feel that spending more time with patients increases the cost of health care. I would like to propose that taking time to *listen well* may actually be more cost effective: if we take a few minutes to learn more information about what the problem may be, it may help refine options on what tests need to be done.

Studies have found that physicians on average interrupt patients within 20 seconds of asking the first question "What brings you in today?" That doesn't give you much time to respond. One thing I have found as a physician is that often the *first* symptoms mentioned may not be the ones that are most troublesome for the patient, and one brought up later in the interview may be more significant. In order for patients to feel free enough to talk about problems bothering them a great deal, they need to feel *listened to* in the early stages of the process. The physician and the patient must communicate; not just talk at each other, but *communicate*. By communicate, I mean YOU and the physician asking questions of each other, and each listening carefully to the answers so that you are each able to understand better what options will best suit your needs.

Restoring Trust in Physician-Patient Relationships

Traveling to different parts of the country giving seminars and workshops on women's health has been an eye-opening, rewarding, and frequently joyful experience. It has also been painful and sad for me, as a woman and a physician, to listen to the stories of women and the breakdown of trust in their physicians because many in my profession—male and female—have simply been unwilling to *really listen* to what their patients were telling them. As a result, there is so much anger and distrust of physicians in general right now, that we have a long way to go to rebuild that healing relationship.

Unfortunately this breakdown has potentially tragic consequences when women fail to seek a physician's help for what may become life-threatening problems, and/or turn solely to the myriad of "alternative practitioners" out there and miss out on the possible benefits of what modern Western medicine has to offer. I understand the undercurrent of frustration, dissatisfaction, and anger among women, and I certainly hear it all the time. Yet women want to like and trust their doctors and are generally very loyal to their physicians, sometimes undeservedly so in my observations. So where does the anger come from, and why do so many women, especially around menopause issues, now turn to nonphysician sources and therapists for help?

Fundamentally, what women tell me is that they are tired of not being listened to, of being discounted about their concerns, of being given pills for each symptom without time to discuss side effects, of being told they "have" to take hormones and then being given the same prescription as everyone else, of having their questions trivialized, or laughed off, of being told they were "neurotic," "stressed," or worse: "you just need some good sex, honey, and you'll be fine."

There is another aspect which may be underlying women's dissatisfaction with their physicians. For most women, their obstetrician-gynecologist is their primary care physician. This is the only physician many women see, and in the earlier stages of life, that may have been a good choice. As women move into mid-life, however, many of them tell me they feel that their Ob-Gyn physician "isn't interested," or "isn't listening to what I am experiencing," or "doesn't seem to know much about menopause." Perhaps "restoring trust" in the relationship with your physician will also involve *re-evaluating* just what type of physician is best for you *NOW*.

Ob-Gyn is a surgical specialty. There are some important differences in the education of physicians in surgical fields compared to medical fields. Surgeons are taught different skills and thinking processes from physicians in *medical* (not surgical) specialties such as Internal Medicine and Family Practice. Surgeons and Internal Medicine/Family Practice physicians *think differently* about clinical problems.

Surgery emphasizes the anatomy and *structure* of the body in health and disease, and how to *fix* body parts that are diseased, injured or abnormal. Medicine (Internal Medicine and its subspecialties, or Family Practice) emphasizes more of the physiological *function* of the body in health and disease. The *medicine* fields teach physicians to prescribe medications and use non-surgical approaches aimed at restoring balance and normal function for body organ systems. Both dimensions of the Medicine-Surgery spectrum are needed with today's complex body of medical knowledge and services; both areas of focus have their appropriate roles for optimum patient care.

As a mid-life woman, however, your needs are different from what they were when your focus was bearing children and having someone skilled in delivering them or ready to perform a surgery if needed. A physician from a *surgical* background may not be the optimal choice for your *primary care* physician if what you now need is someone to manage *interrelated* medical problems which do not necessarily need a surgical approach. If you think about it, this would be analogous to men having their *urologist* as their primary care physician (many women laugh when I point this out, and quickly see how such a scenario would be unlikely for most men). You may decide that a different type of physician with a medicine background would be appropriate at this stage in your life. If you have a good primary care physician (he/she may be a family practice or an internal medicine specialist) who also does pelvic exams, then you may not need to split your care with a gynecologist doing your pelvic exam and an internist checking the rest of you. Many women tell me they simply had not thought about this option. "I've always gone to my gynecologist for everything" is a phrase I hear frequently.

If your gynecologist is still doing a great deal of obstetrics, it may be difficult for this person to have the time to also keep up with the advances in the field of menopause health care. Your gynecologist may also not have a broad based adult women's *medicine* background to assimilate non*obstetrical* medical advances. So, this may not be the physician for the later phases of your life. It doesn't mean there's anything bad about that, it just means there's so much knowledge today that no one person can stay up to date on everything. I specialize in Preventive Medicine and Women's Health, with a neuroendocrine focus. I do not *also* do surgery, so I would not expect a surgeon to necessarily know all that I know about hormone effects on the brain.

You need to reflect on what your particular needs are and what type of health professional best suits those needs. You are not "locked in" to the physician you chose ten, or fifteen, or twenty years ago! You now have different needs. You may want to consider other options available to you now.

Another way to re-establish trust and build an effective working relationship with your physician is to look for someone who is willing to work with you in a partnership approach and who values your input and questions about your health. As we look at what's needed in women's health I clearly think that we must get back to the basics of the traditions and foundations from which medicine evolved. This means broadening the view of a physician's role from the post-World War II focus on medication and surgery, to the evolving role of a physician as a "teacher" and partner with you patient.

I use the word "patient"with a strong sense of the profound meaning of the physician/patient *helping relationship*. To me it means going back to the ancient traditions of Hippocratic medicine. The physician-patient relationship was seen as a *sacred* relationship; physicians still take the Hippocratic Oath when we receive our medical degrees, pledging to use our skills and abilities to the best of our ability to provide care to people who seek our help. The Hippocratic Oath includes a commitment to "do no harm." When I use the word patient, I am *not* using it as an indication of a subordinate relationship. I really see it as very much a partnership: you teach me about what you're experiencing, and I use my expertise to teach you how to improve your health.

For you to get optimal health care, particularly as a woman growing older, you are going to have to be more active, involved, and knowledgeable. You are the *patient* in the sense of someone seeking help; in my opinion, *patient* does not mean *passive* recipient of advice or medicine; your role is *active participation* in the process of becoming more well, the process of diminishing *disease* in your life, and the process of healing.

I also see *patient* as the name for the person to whom the physician has a responsibility to listen to, and take seriously. If this is not happening when you work with a physician, at some point you will need to be assertive enough to say "no more" if your needs aren't being met. Then look for other resources. I would encourage you to think of your health as one of the most important investments that you have; work with someone who is going to value you, listen to you, and value what you have to say about how you feel and what you are experiencing. You know that better than anyone else.

Listening to Women's Wisdom Again

I have been quite impressed over my years of medical practice with the body *"wise-ness"* of my female patients. I find that women are *far more* knowledgeable about their bodies, are more in tune with subtle as well as noticeable changes, and ask very well thought out questions about what is happening in their bodies. I find that typically women have reasoned out what might be a plausible explanation for their symptoms, and I am happily surprised to find that many of my patients are right on target with what they think is happening. Unfortunately, they have all too often been told by both male and female physicians that "this couldn't possibly be. Hormones (or dyes or whatever) don't cause that kind of problem." Or "No, that can't be, this medicine doesn't cause those kind of side effects."

When I had my first back problem I knew there was something terribly wrong, but I was afraid to question the pronouncement "There's nothing wrong with you" made by the attending neurosurgeon who was supposed to be the local expert. Besides, a medical student has even *less status* with a doctor than *you* would have as a private patient. If I had not listened to my body, and sought another opinion, I would have been ended up an incontinent handicapped woman on disability at *twenty-eight* years old. That was a crucial life lesson to learn at an early age, and I have been a better physician as a result.

A recent example from my practice is the forty-two year old woman who had migraines every two weeks, right before her period and again just after ovulation, like clockwork for several years. When she asked if it could have a hormonal connection, her doctor told her such a connection was not possible. I pulled out a copy of the menstrual cycle chart and showed her the drop in estradiol before the menstrual period starts and the drop in estradiol just after ovulation and told her I thought these hormone drops were the triggers for her "like clockwork" migraines. She later saw her other physician who told her that estrogen didn't drop twice in the cycle!

I can't figure it out. Every textbook on menstruation has a picture of this hormonal chart, which mothers and daughters often go over at puberty, doctors learn in medical school, and is a pretty well-documented hormonal pattern. I have years of medical practice filled with patient stories and quotes of exactly this type of experience, so I know hers is not an isolated case. I show patients the picture of the menstrual cycle chart and there it is! Exactly the pattern the woman (or her husband, mother, father or significant other) has been describing about the ebb and flow in her symptoms.

Is it that we have been dominated by the male model of body physiology and thinking for so long that people forget what is known about female physiology? Is it that we have collectively forgotten women's body wisdom, intuition, and insight? Is it that some physicians are so caught up in having to be right that they have forgotten to listen to their patients and have forgotten that one of the first tenets of medicine is that as physicians we should *never* say never? When you are dealing with the human body, there are all kinds of variations and almost *anything* is possible.

Is it that we are taught negative stereotypes about women patients who ask questions and who want to understand what they are experiencing? It has taken me a lot of years to undo those negative teachings about women and come to an appreciation of just how wonderful it is to have a "partnership" with a patient who is observant about her body, shares with me her insights and thoughts about possible connections causing or aggravating her symptoms, and writes down her symptoms and questions. An involved, interested patient makes my job easier, not harder!

I encourage my patients to keep records of their physical and emotional sensations, not only when they are feeling ill, but also when they are feeling *well* so they have a baseline. I also encourage women to keep a list of health questions they want answered. That way their thoughts are focused, and things don't get overlooked in the discussion and not answered. I *like* to see lists. It shows that the patient cares and is doing her part in our partnership. It makes the office visit more efficient in the first place, much more effective for the patient getting her needs met, and also easier for the physician in determining what is expected of him/her. As I explain in the next section, it is also crucial for you to gather your family health information.

Finding the Right Doctor for You: Questions to Ask

I do think that it's important to ask a potential physician or nurse practitioner what her/his interest is in preventive medicine as well as "wellness" or "complementary" approaches. What is this person's interest in women's health and has he/she been attending update medical education programs in mid-life and menopause health issues? If the answers to those questions are negative, then I would encourage you to interview someone else. It may be worth an extra consult fee to find someone whom you really feel comfortable talking with and whose medical philosophy, empathy, and competence you feel confident about. If you want to be involved in making decisions, find a health professional who is willing to work with you in a collaborative way.

The type or specialty of the physician is not as important as finding the right individual physician. My suggestion for mid-life women is to locate a broad-based adult medicine generalist as the physician to oversee and coordinate your care. In such a situation the majority of your ongoing care can be managed by one doctor with referral to specialists arranged when needed. Feel free to ask questions about to training, interests, and payment policies. Of course price is important, but it is a little different from muffler repair! You can always get another muffler, but it is tough getting a new body.

Unfortunately your choice of health benefits for you and your family may well be determined to a great extent by your employer, their insurance company, and/or your legislators. If you get a chance to choose from several plans, be sure you do the time consuming but important task of reading all of the descriptive material. Make comparative charts, noting things like fitness and disease prevention programs, mental health services, physical therapy, and long-term care. The plan that has the lowest premium and co-payment may be the most expensive in the long haul if you have to cover such expenses from your own pocket. Obviously you need to read the directory of doctors and hospitals and ask questions about them. If the physician you have been assigned on your health plan doesn't seem to communicate adequately with you, speak out and request a change.

One of the first requirements of most current health insurance plans is to designate a primary care physician who will become the focal point of your health care. Not only will that doctor be responsible for evaluating your general state of health and treating most of your aches and pains, he/she will also be the keeper of your health information. That person will be approving prescriptions, authorizing mammograms and other screening tests, and very importantly, making referrals to specialists. You need someone you trust, respect and feel comfortable with. *Select Your Physician Carefully.* Don't be afraid to speak up. If you don't understand something, *say so.* Treat your physician with respect for her/his time and intelligence and expect the same response in return. Do not be afraid to change doctors if you are not satisfied. Surveys have indicated that over 90 percent of patients consider it very important for a physician to: (In order of importance)

1. Be knowledgeable and competent
2. Answer questions honestly and completely
3. Explain medical problems in clear language
4. Spend enough time with patients
5. Really care about patients' health
6. Make an effort to get patients to explain problems and symptoms completely.

It is equally important for physicians to realize that they too have a communication responsibility, as the above list indicates. Good communication, caring, clear communication, particularly in drawing out patients' concerns and responding to their questions to their satisfaction goes a long way toward establishing patient loyalty and compliance. Patients are more concerned with the *perceived* value of the care they pay to receive than with the dollars per se. Fees are not of primary importance with most patients, providing they are satisfied with the amount of time and attention they receive from the physician. A significant number of malpractice suits are triggered by poor communication, not bad results.

Ferreting out Family History: Connections Between Your Ancestors and Your Health

I was in my early forties, preparing for a hysterectomy due to major problems with fibroids, and deciding about whether to have my ovaries out. My gynecologist told me that at my age, removal of the ovaries wasn't usually done, but he would be open to my preference. We talked at length about my overall health at the time, my reasons for wanting the ovaries removed, and his medical opinions about the potential advantages and drawbacks of either option. I was aware that my grandmother had ovarian cancer, which I knew has a significant hereditary dimension. My grandmother had developed ovarian cancer in her mid forties.

After giving this a great deal of thought, I wrote a letter to my gynecologist outlining her family history, my concerns about my own tendency to have recurring ovarian cysts which increases risk of ovarian cancer. I just didn't want to have the continued worry in the back of my mind about developing ovarian cancer, since I knew my risk was quite a bit higher than normal. My doctor was reluctant to remove my ovaries, but he agreed it made sense after he listened to my concerns. I did well after surgery with a hormone regimen of 17-beta-estradiol and natural micronized testosterone.

Two years later, my mother was able to locate additional key family history: there were two other women on my grandmother's side of the family—a sister, and a niece—who had also developed ovarian cancer, with all of them having it in the *early to mid forties*. With a shiver, I realized I was right smack in the "window of risk" based on my family pattern of ovarian cancer! I am glad I made the decision I did. The genetic counselor who reviewed my family data confirmed that it was fortunate I had already undergone removal of my ovaries (oophorectomy) due to my high risk of developing the disease. If I had not been proactive about my health, I may very well have been in an entirely different situation today. I did what I am suggesting you do: I made it a point to find out her family history, and I used this information in making the decision which felt right for me. **Become empowered with infor-**

mation, explore your options, find out what you need to know to make the decision that fits you!

As science advances, as we understand diseases better, and as we have better ways of tracking family patterns, it turns out that an astonishing number of health problems, both common and rare, have some type of hereditary, or genetic, link. Many very common disorders are now known to have a strong hereditary component: alcoholism, Alzheimer's dementia, allergies, asthma, many cancers (breast, lung, colon, ovarian, prostate, skin), depression, diabetes, heart disease, glaucoma, osteoporosis, rheumatoid arthritis. If you find that you are more susceptible to a disease because it runs in your family, you have several ways of reducing your own risk of having more serious illness:

- having earlier, or more frequent, screening tests
- regular check-ups
- eliminating nongenetic lifestyle risk factors: such as smoking, alcohol, high-fat diet
- being alert to early symptoms

It really isn't all that difficult to get the information and draw a *genogram*, or family tree. Patients tell me they don't think they can find the information about people who have died. Often there is a family "historian" who knows the family traditions and problems, and it usually isn't necessary to go back many generations since the most important links are your parents, brothers, sisters, grand parents, aunts and uncles. A second cousin would only share about 3 percent of the same genes you do, so going this far out on the branches of the family really is not relevant in most situations unless you are trying to track down an inherited cancer pattern. The types of health history information you should gather include the following:

	RELATIVE	YR BORN YR DIED
ILLNESSES (especially cancers, diabetes, stroke, heart attacks, osteoporosis, thyroid disorders, dementia, depression, alcohol abuse, autoimmune disorders,etc.)		
SURGERIES/INJURIES		
ALCOHOL/TOBACCO OR DRUG USE		
OCCUPATION		
TOXIC EXPOSURE?		
AGE OF MENOPAUSE		
PROBLEMS W/MENSES OR PREGNANCIES		

You simply MUST take the time to find out and write down your family medical history, before it is too late and records are lost. You need to know it, and your children and family members need to know it. *Your Lifetime Health Planner* is a handy loose-leaf notebook created by two women in Tucson as a convenient way of keeping all of this information in an organized and concise fashion (ordering information for this is in the Appendix). Sue Giles, the primary creator of this project, said she realized how needed it was when her son got ready to have his precollege physical exam, and she had trouble finding all of his health information and their family history. Having the family medical information can be an important gift to yourself, to your children, and for generations still to come. You are connected to your ancestors; knowing more about *them* is a link which may have a profound effect on *your future* health.

Becoming an "Activated Patient": Getting Involved to Protect Your Health

I cannot say it strongly enough: you must become an "activated" patient in your health care. What does "activated" patient mean? This is my list:

- Become proactive about getting information, exploring options and taking action
- Find out your family health history
- Know your health risks
- Know your past and present "health data" (physicians call this database your "medical records")
- Pay attention to your "numbers" (medical results); ask for copies of your lab reports and key medical test results and keep these at home for your records and to show other physicians you may consult
- Do your homework investigating resources for physicians and other health professionals who will best suit your needs for your health "team"
- Speak up and ask questions
- Keep track of your symptoms (charted with your menstrual cycle)
- Keep records of your over-the-counter medications, vitamin, mineral and herbal supplements

I know this kind of involvement takes time, and many of you may be saying to yourself "I don't have time to do all of that." You are like most women, juggling multiple roles, meeting many demands and expectations in your life. "Isn't my doctor supposed to take care of all that?" Yes and No. Just like the way you would work with your financial planner, your tax advisor, your hairdresser, or any other person helping you, your input and your desires are crucial to a result that meets your needs. Your physician is no exception. Ideally, she or he should welcome and value your input and your questions, as well as your desire to be actively involved in the decisions about your health care options. And you have to do your homework about yourself and your health needs in order to give your physician the input needed to make suitable, intelligent recommendations for you.

There is a lot of information out there. Most libraries have good publications on health issues. I have provided a list of resources I think are helpful and worthwhile. I do find that a lot of magazine articles either contain information that is old news or are written with more sensationalism than substance and are slanted to promote a particular bias. Talk with your friends about health concerns, but always remember: their cure won't necessarily be yours, their symptoms are not exactly the same as yours, and their body chemistry is not exactly the same as yours. If you are *reading a research report*, don't forget to check *if women were included* in the study population!

What are some resources to help you locate a good physician for you? Typical sources of information about doctors include friends' experiences and state and local medical societies. A doctor or nurse you know personally may have recommendations. Yellow Pages can give you a start, and most have a section that lists those who are board certified in their specialty. An excellent resource for women in mid-life is the North American Menopause Society, based in Cleveland, Ohio. Members are physicians who are interested in women's health and are attending the update conferences to learn about advances in the field. If you live in a city with a hospital-based referral resource center, these people may be able to tell you who the local health professionals interested in prevention, wellness, and mid-life women's health are. You may also contact the state board of medical examiners if you have questions about whether or not a physician has ever been sanctioned for inappropriate medical practices or has had a number of malpractice suits. Don't be afraid to ask questions.

Another resource I hope to have available soon is a network of health professionals in different fields who have an integrated approach to women's health concerns. When women have consults with us, I would like to be able to help them locate health resources in their own area to follow through on my suggestions. Since one of my major interests is teaching physicians from many different specialties who see patients such as you, I often meet receptive and appreciative male and female doctors who want the latest information and are genuinely concerned about being more effective in women's health issues. I make an effort to keep their names in my resource file, and I also record patient recommendations of health professionals who are caring, knowledgeable, and compassionate.

And another important point: you may have in your life all the money, friends, family, relationships, and anything else you desire, but if you don't have your health you cannot fully enjoy all the rest. As someone who has *been there* in the experience of having a major health crisis and watching my good health slide rapidly into a deep, dark hole, I can emphatically say that without one's health, all the other assets seem to lose a lot of value too. I came to appreciate a quote I came across a few years ago: *"your health is your greatest wealth."*

Healthcare Reform, Women's Issues, and Women's Centers: Marketing Ploy or Genuine "New Approach"?

With all of the recent publicity about health care reform in the United States, and the need to improve access and control spiraling costs, I think an even more *pressing* need has been *grossly* overlooked: how do we pay better attention to the specific need of female patients? With an emphasis on cost containment (yet at the same time still providing bottom line profits for health systems and insurance carriers), are we missing the boat in taking care of crucial health problems in female patients which have been ignored, overlooked, undertreated and mistreated?

I find increasing evidence that the frightening answer to this question is *yes*. Women are often denied important diagnostic tests, which may be critical, and are told "you're just over-worried, there's nothing wrong," "you're just under a lot of stress," "you're not at risk for anything serious," "you look healthy." I have seen this happen with everything from blood tests to treadmill stress tests (for heart disease), to bone density evaluation, and even to mammograms. There is now a significant amount of research that confirms the gender preference: when similar types of health problems affect men, men are far more likely than women to have rapid access to and insurance reimbursement for the diagnostic tests deemed important.

Mammogram coverage is a case in point. Women's health advocates finally succeeded in getting insurance reimbursement for screening mammography, and we now find that reimbursement for mammograms by Medicare has been *reduced* to coverage for a mammogram every *other* year over age fifty. This change comes at a time when the national guidelines for adequate cancer screening are for women to have a mammogram *every* year after age fifty.

Bone density testing gives another illustration of these problems and concerns. We have more data emerging to show that women actually start losing bone long *before* menopause. I continue to hear physicians say bone density testing isn't needed, and yet we have no better way to identify women with early bone loss. Bone loss in this stage of life is silent—it doesn't cause any symptoms to warn a women that it is happening until much later, when she may notice a decrease in height. The only way women can know whether or not they have beginning bone loss is to have a specific test, usually Dual-energy X-Ray absorptiometry (DEXA), which measures the bone mineral content of the hip and spine. I find that not many of my patients and women in my seminar audiences *even know that simple, reliable bone density testing is available*, and yet I first started doing bone density testing for peri-menopause patients back in 1985, a full decade ago! In a strange twist of logic, some insurance plans will pay for the *more expensive (and in my opinion, less useful)* computerized tomography (CT) bone density test but not the DEXA.

We also know that osteoporosis and its consequences and complications are one of the most devastating robbers of quality of life, independence, and longevity for older women. Why are we not using the information and technology that is available to help women avoid these problems? Many physicians and insurance carriers often reply that "it's too expensive" to do bone density testing in broader groups of women.

The sad fact is that we could dramatically *reduce* the existing and projected health costs associated with osteoporosis if we just evaluated women sooner, when bone loss is typically minimal and can be prevented or reversed. And this statement is based on reducing actual dollars—it doesn't even include the potential reduction in human suffering from the pain, hospitalizations, surgeries, and other "costs" of osteoporosis. Women understand this logic once they know that such tests are available, and many women are willing to pay for the test, if need be, in order to have the information they need. But for the most part, bone density testing remains largely unknown to women consumers and unused as a tool to improve women's knowledge of their health data. Are women once again getting the short end of the stick on health care? In my opinion, yes.

We address the issue of health care reform to benefit the people in this country who do not have insurance, and that is a worthwhile goal. But are we addressing the major overhaul that must be undertaken to better provide better health care and treatment options for fully *half* the population in this country who are female? I have not yet seen much evidence that many of our leaders are even aware of this aspect of the problem, much less focusing on ways to address and correct the deficiencies in our knowledge and care of women patients.

Many of the health problems that affect women do *not* fit neatly into our fragmented, specialty "boxes" based on organ systems and body parts. Women need more of an *integrated, or multidisciplinary* approach, which can help identify such things as endocrine changes that cause diverse symptoms and also provide

more effective treatment. So, will health care reform actually benefit women? Not unless we women speak up, make our voices
heard as to the issues important to us and vote with our economic
clout to insure that our health needs are included in health care
reform proposals and plans. AIDS activists have achieved remarkable results in getting their research, education and clinical services agenda met. Women must be equally as devoted to moving
forward all phases of the women's health agenda as well.

There are lots of newspaper ads promoting a new concept at
many hospitals and medical practices, called women's centers.
Read these very closely. I have seen so many that are nothing but
dressed-up birthing centers with drapes, a rocking chair and a
beauty salon. Is this really any different from what we have
always had? In my view, *a good women's center must provide a
new model* of health services aimed at meeting women's unique
needs, not just aimed at new paint colors and a beauty shop on the
floor. Does that approach make you feel valued? Is "women's
health" only addressing services based on the body from breasts
down and thighs up? It shouldn't be.

As an experiment, I produced a flier showing a woman's body
from the neck down and had the headline question at the top:
"What's wrong with this picture?" At a women's health confer-
ence for both professional and lay population, no one gave
responses other than "she's overweight." I was surprised. No one
noticed that the women's *head* was missing! We often don't consider the brain-mind and its functions when it comes to women's
health. I mean not only emotions, but hormones. We have many
health needs for all parts of our body, which are monitored by our
brain. If you are looking for a women's center where you can have
many dimensions of your health care *integrated*, read the fine
print, and find out what programs they offer and what physicians
and alternative practioners they have on staff. Just as you need to
ask questions about your physicians, so you need to ask questions
about a women's program. Is it fluff or substance? Don't settle for
window dressing or a program that is just another product of a
marketing effort. You may find it helpful to use the questionnaire
in Chapter 18 to evaluate a potential women's center.

Where Do We Go from Here?

Sorting fact from fiction, myth, misinformation becomes a difficult challenge for the average consumer. I encourage you to keep

in mind that all of the consumer "short pieces:" you read in the news have to give you just that: a "piece" of the whole picture. You are going to have to *know yourself, your health history, health risks, and your values for yourself* in order to make some informed, intelligent choices among the many options available to you today. One article said about hormone therapy said"it's one of the most important and difficult decisions a woman ever has to make." Women are faced with hundreds of difficult and important decisions throughout our lives. **How do you make *other* decisions in your life about matters that are important to you?**

In my opinion, *most* of the decisions we make have some degree of benefit to us and some degree of downside or drawback or even risk. If I take a position in Tucson, I can't live in Norfolk. If I leave Virginia, I will miss my family close friends and patients I have worked with for many years. I want to try the new challenges available to me in Tucson, but I can't have both. How do I decide? Think about it for you. Each choice means a road taken and a road not taken. You weigh what is meaningful, important, and beneficial against what "downsides" you are willing to face. There are ways to get information regarding important decisions of all kinds in our lives: **the problem is, few of the really important decisions are going to be easy, and each of us has to do our homework to make them.**

We re-evaluate other decisions and choices we have made as new information comes in or as our needs change. Media articles may have good, accurate, and helpful information but they also may have incorrect and out-of-date information. You will have to do your homework to find out more complete answers to questions that are important to YOU to have addressed. You will also have to be assertive and diligent in seeking out a knowledgeable health professional to keep you up on new developments and to work with you in a partnership have *your individual* health concerns addressed optimally.

The other side of that coin is to remember this admonition from Ecclesiastes: **"If you wait for perfect conditions, you will never get anything done."** This observation is true for us today as we look at some of the issues in women's health. Women ask me, "Well, what about the studies and the fact that there's conflicting information? We don't have a definite answer and we don't have information about that." This is true. There are still many answers to be determined. The problem is that many of us early "baby boomers" are at a point *now* when we have to make important decisions about our course of action for our health. We can't wait another ten years for "definitive" answers to come in from research. If I had waited for the confirming research to answer all my questions before I decided to address my immediate needs with the Estraderm patch, I would likely have had reduced quality of life now, as well as progressive bone loss before I even reached menopause, even though I exercised and had good calcium intake.

Each of us needs to make a personal decision as to whether we can afford to take more time in making a health decision or whether we need to *act now*. We will each have to make the best choice we can in light of the information available to us and our own individual values, and then stay informed as new information becomes available. I foresee that with the current interest in and demand for more information tailored to women, we will have an explosion of new information over the next decade. Hang on, we will *all* have to keep learning and discerning, and not just be blown like leaves in the wind with each new fad. As a foundation for this process, each of us must continue to seek the relationship with a health professional that is right for us as individuals.

Being *proactive* also means, at another level, getting involved with health advocacy organizations around the country, which are working to improve services, access, education, and research into the specific health needs of women. These organizations, some of which are listed under the resources at the end of this chapter, are actively getting the message out to health professionals, insurance companies, legislators, researchers, and others that the specific and different health questions for women must be taken seriously and addressed.

Your voice, your wisdom, your insight, and your energy are all needed in these endeavors. Tell your story, talk about your experiences, share your ideas about how you would like to see things done differently. Get involved and speak out. Help to make sure that women's needs will be adequately addressed in the coming insurance plan changes.

It does make a difference when women take charge in this way. All you have to do is look at what has been accomplished in this country by *one* mother got who became outraged about the problem of drunk drivers when her daughter was killed by one, and you begin to see what the power of women can accomplish when working together on common goals that in some way will affect us all. "Mothers Against Drunk Driving (MADD)" as a grassroots organization did more in a short time to address the serious and potentially lethal consequences of intoxicated drivers than any other single agency or legislative group in this country.

No matter what direction this organization now takes, it remains a prime example of the effect *one concerned woman*, and those working with her, can have for the broader needs in the U.S.

Vicki Ratner, M.D., who founded the Interstitial Cystitis Association, is another example of a woman who, after a long personal ordeal to have IC diagnosed, became an advocate for other women suffering from this unrecognized problem. Our increased breast cancer awareness and advocacy has come from small groups of concerned women and concerned breast cancer survivors all over the country, who have worked together to make their voices heard.

Screaming to Be Heard has evolved from my own experiences as a physician advocate for women and as a patient in a health system that has not listened well to the voices of women. I think a major focus of change in medical education for the 21st century needs to be on integrating women's health into all aspects of the medical education curriculum. This process has just begun in one or two medical schools in the country, so we have a long way to go.

I have been, and plan to continue to be, a voice for change in how we educate health professionals and how we can better serve the needs of all patients, but especially women, who have been so overlooked and unheard for so long. I hope you will join me in these efforts, in whatever way fits into your life and community. You have taken a crucial first step in that change process by coming with me on the journey through the pages of this book, so don't stop now! Margaret Mead said **"Never doubt that a small group of concerned, committed people can make a difference; indeed, it is the only thing that ever has."** Women make a difference. YOU make a difference.

CHAPTER 18

What's Wrong? Quiz Yourself Before You See the Doctor

Self Test: Do You Have PMS?

PMS, premenstrual syndrome, is characterized by a wide variety of emotional and physical symptoms that appear regularly before a woman's period (sometimes as long as two weeks before menstruation), end with the onset of menses, and are followed by a *symptom free phase* EACH cycle. The following questions are aimed at helping you identify whether or not you suffer from a cluster of PMS symptoms. Please answer each question as accurately as possible. **At about the same time each month, prior to the beginning of your menstrual period:**

1. Do you experience any of the following mood changes?

    a. anxiety   ___YES ___NO
    b. irritability   ___YES ___NO
    c. feeling nervous and tense   ___YES ___NO
    d. mood swings   ___YES ___NO
    e. crying spells   ___YES ___NO
    f. depressed mood   ___YES ___NO

2. Do you experience any of the following changes in your behavior?

    a. impulsivity   ___YES ___NO
    b. anger outbursts   ___YES ___NO
    c. becoming withdrawn   ___YES ___NO
    d. lethargy   ___YES ___NO
    e. fatigue   ___YES ___NO
    f. craving for sweets, chocolate   ___YES ___NO
    g. craving for carbohydrates, alcohol   ___YES ___NO
    h. craving for salty foods   ___YES ___NO

3. Do you experience any of the following symptoms related to the central nervous system?

a. forgetfulness	___YES	___NO
b. indecision	___YES	___NO
c. difficulty concentrating	___YES	___NO
d. memory problem	___YES	___NO
e. lack of coordination	___YES	___NO
f. restless sleep	___YES	___NO
g. altered sex drive	___YES	___NO
h. marked appetite changes	___YES	___NO

4. Do you experience any of the following physical symptoms?

a. weight gain	___YES	___NO
b. breast tenderness	___YES	___NO
c. bloating	___YES	___NO
d. swelling of hands and feet	___YES	___NO
e. constipation	___YES	___NO
f. headaches	___YES	___NO
g. heart palpitations	___YES	___NO
h. dizziness	___YES	___NO
I. low back pain or joint pain	___YES	___NO

Discussion of Results

If you answered YES to more than *five* of the above questions, and you feel that the symptoms regularly affect your daily functioning, you may have PMS and I suggest you consider the following steps:

- Read one of the recommended self-help books listed in the Resources (Appendix 2)
- Seek a comprehensive medical/psychological evaluation from physicians who are knowledgeable about PMS and who will do appropriate lab tests also.
- Seek the guidance of trained professionals to help you make lifestyle and dietary changes that will help reduce PMS symptoms.

PMS affects women of all backgrounds, races, ages, and nationalities. About four out of every ten women have moderately severe premenstrual symptoms. Five to ten percent of women with PMS have symptoms severe enough to disrupt their personal and professional lives. PMS symptoms are not caused by psychological or mental problems, but stress may make the PMS symptoms worse. There is no one established theory as to what causes PMS; it is generally considered to be a biochemical disorder involving the interacation of many hormonal systems.

PMS is a problem that has *many* approaches to help reduce your discomfort. Ideally these approaches should be combined in an integrated program suited to your individual needs. Options to help you feel better include diet changes, stress management, vitamins, herbs, acupuncture, a variety of medications for severe symptoms, and for some, hormonal therapies may be beneficial. Don't just sit there and feel terrible, seek the help that is available!

PMS Self-Check by Elizabeth Lee Vliet, M.D., 1984 and revised 1990

Self Test: Are You Beginning or in Menopause?

Current Medications/Hormones_____

Hysterectomy: ___No   ___Yes   (Date:_____)
Ovaries Removed: ___No   ___Yes

Directions: Circle number that best describes *degree* of symptom intensity you have experienced over the past month(s):

No	Mild	Moderate	Severe
0	1	2	3

1. Hot flushes, perspiration and/or chilly sensations?

0	1	2	3

2. Sensations of numbness and/or tingling of the skin?

0	1	2	3

3. Insomnia or restless, fragmented sleep?

0	1	2	3

4. Irritability, feeling anxious or apprehensive?

0	1	2	3

5. Feeling of depression and unhappiness and/or being miserable without any obvious reason?

0	1	2	3

6. Sensations of dizziness or swimming in the head?

0	1	2	3

7. Feeling of weariness of mind and body associated with desire for rest; disinclination to make further efforts?

0	1	2	3

8. Pain of any kind affecting joints or muscles?

        0   1   2   3

9. Headaches of any kind (tension, migraine, etc.)

        0   1   2   3

10. Quickening or acceleration of heartbeat or a fluttering/pounding heartbeat in a sitting or resting position?

        0   1   2   3

11. Sensation of ants or other insects creeping over the skin ("crawly skin")?

        0   1   2   3

Directions: Circle number that best describes *degree* of symptoms' intensity you have experienced over the past month(s):

Never	Infrequently	Sometimes	Most of Time	Always
0	1	2	3	4

12. Vaginal burning or itching?

      0   1   2   3   4

13. Painful urination or increased frequency of urination?

      0   1   2   3   4

14. Leaking of urine when coughing, laughing, sneezing, or on hard work?

      0   1   2   3   4

15. Leaking of urine when walking, running, climbing steps, or on light work?

    0   1   2   3   4

16. Leaking of urine, regardless of activity, even when in a lying position?

    0   1   2   3   4

Reference: Kupperman Menopausal Index; modifications by Elizabeth Lee Vliet, M.D., 1992

Scoring and Discussion

To calculate your total score:

Question 1: **Multiply** the number corresponding to your response **by 4** and write the resulting number on the line   _____

Questions 2–4: **Multiply** the number corresponding to each answer **by 2** and then **total the points**, write the total points on the line   _____

Questions 5–16: **Add** together all of the numbers corresponding to your response for each question, and write the total points on the line   _____

Total from Above: _____

If your total score is **between 7 and 15**, you *may* be in the early phases of the menopause transition, or (if taking hormones) your HRT regimen may not yet be optimal for you.

If your score is **between 16 and 30**, you clearly have menopausal symptoms, and I think you would benefit from having hormone levels checked (ovary and thyroid) along with your usual medical checkup. There are many lifestyle changes, herbs, vitamins and/or hormones that may be helpful to you and should be discussed with your primary physician or an experienced and knowledgeable menopause specialist.

If your score is **greater than 30**, you have marked to severe menopausal *symptoms, which also suggest the presence of other risk factors such as bone loss and cholesterol changes.* You would be wise to have a *comprehensive midlife women's health evaluation* to determine the best options to improve your immediate well-being as well as to reduce the risks of later diseases such as osteoporosis and heart disease. You may want to have this done by your present physician, or consider one of the centers around the country where the comprehensive evaluations, tailored to midlife women, are provided.

Self Test: Cancer Risk Questionnaire for Women

Name_____ Date of Birth_____ Age:_____

YES NO GENERAL HEALTH

___ ___ I have had cancer
___ ___ There is a history of cancer in my immediate family
___ ___ I am 15 or more pounds overweight
___ ___ I eat a diet high in meats/dairy products and fat content
___ ___ I eat fewer than 5 servings of fruit and vegetables per day
___ ___ I use chewing tobacco or snuff, or smoke cigarettes
___ ___ I have not had a complete physical in at least five years
___ ___ I drink alcohol regularly
___ ___ I have not been to a dentist in over three years

YES NO BREAST CANCER

___ ___ I have had breast cancer
___ ___ Someone in my family has had breast cancer
         Who? _____ **Risk increases if person with cancer is
         mother or sister**
___ ___ I am over 50 years of age
___ ___ I have had surgery for "lumps" in the breast
___ ___ I have had a female cancer (ovary or womb/uterus)
___ ___ I gave birth to my first child after age 35
___ ___ I am 35 or older and have not been pregnant to full term
         (9 months)

YES NO ENDOMETRIAL CANCER

___ ___ My mother and/or sister(s) have had endometrial or
         breast cancer
___ ___ I have had breast or ovarian cancer
___ ___ I am over 50 years of age
___ ___ I am more than 20 percent over the recommended body
         weight for height
___ ___ I have never had a full-term (9 months) pregnancy
___ ___ I have high blood pressure
___ ___ I have a uterus and have taken estrogen **alone** (without
         progestin or progesterone) for a long period of time
         (more than two years)

YES NO OVARIAN CANCER
___ ___ I have a family history of ovarian cancer
___ ___ I am over age 50
___ ___ I have had either breast or endometrial cancer
___ ___ I have never had a full-term pregnancy
___ ___ I have a history of infertility and/or menstrual irregularities,
            cycles with no ovulation
___ ___ I have a history of recurring ovarian cysts
___ ___ I am or have been a cigarette smoker
___ ___ I have taken fertility drugs such as Clomid and/or Pergonal
___ ___ I regularly used talcum powder in underwear and/or on
            sanitary pads

YES NO COLON CANCER
___ ___ I have had colon cancer
___ ___ A family member has had colon cancer
            Who? _____
___ ___ I have had polyp(s) in the colon
___ ___ I have had Crohn's disease or ulcerative colitis
___ ___ I have had a recent change from my usual bowel movements
___ ___ I have noticed blood in my bowel movements
___ ___ I am over 50 years of age
___ ___ I eat a diet high in meat, fat and/or grilled foods
___ ___ I eat very few fruits, vegetables and whole grains

YES NO LUNG CANCER
___ ___ I smoke cigarettes
___ ___ I have smoked cigarettes How long?_____ When quit?_____
            (If you stopped smoking more than 15 years ago,
            risk decreases almost to the normal expected risk
            based on your present age.)
___ ___ I am over 40 years of age
___ ___ I am exposed regularly to other people's cigarette smoking
___ ___ At work, I am exposed to arsenic, asbestos, chromates,
            nickel, organic solvents, uranium, or petroleum products
___ ___ Someone in my family has had lung cancer. (**Risk is higher if
            parent or sibling has lung cancer, especially if person is a
            non-smoker**)

YES NO SKIN CANCER

___ ___ I have light colored hair, eyes, or complexion

___ ___ I have a large number of "moles" or moles that are large or irregular in shape or color

___ ___ I frequently work or play in the sun

___ ___ I rarely use sun screen or sun block when I am out in the sun

___ ___ I was sunburned (blistered) several times before age 20

___ ___ My skin is frequently exposed to chemicals or radioactive materials (arsenic, coal, petroleum, uranium, radioisotopes)

___ ___ I have a family history of skin cancer

___ ___ I have been to tanning salons

Discussion of Results

The more YES answers you have, the higher your cancer risk. If the YES answers are clustered in a particular type of cancer, you should take this self-test information to your physician and discuss what preventive screening is desirable for you to have and how frequently such screening evaluations should be done. Even if you do not appear to have a high risk of a particular cancer, I would encourage you to copy this information for your physician to have as part of your medical record. Then you and your physician should reassess your risks whenever you have your annual checkup.

Adapted from "SPOT: Cancer Risk Questionnaire": A joint program developed and funded by the University of Texas, M.D. Anderson Cancer Center, and the Texas Academy of Family Physicians. Copyright UTMDACC 1993. Material added by Elizabeth Lee Vliet, M.D., 1994.

Self Test: Are You at Risk for Serious Bone Loss?

Osteoporosis is called a "silent enemy" because you may not find out you have it until significant irreversible damage has occurred. Even if you do not have any clear symptoms, use this test to evaluate your risk level according to factors that have been scientifically identified through extensive medical research.

Directions: Answer each question, then write down the number of risk points shown for each answer, and total your score.

I. Risk Factors that Can't Be Controlled

_____ Do you have a family history of osteoporosis?   **No** (0 points) **Yes** (4 points)

_____ Are you White, northern European, or Asian?   **No** (0 points) **Yes** (3 points)

_____ Do you have a fair complexion?   **No** (0 points) **Yes** (2 points)

_____ Do you have a small-boned frame?   **No** (0 points) **Yes** (4 points)

_____ Are you over 40 years of age?   **No** (0 points) **Yes** (2 points)

_____ Are you over 70 years of age?   **No** (0 points) **Yes** (4 points)

_____ Have you had both your ovaries removed? (and NOT taking replacement hormones)   **No** (0 points) **Yes** (4 points)

_____ Have you breast fed at least one child?   **No** (0 points) **Yes** (1 point)

_____ Are you allergic to milk or other dairy products?   **No** (0 points) **Yes** (3 points)

_____ Have you not had children?   **No** (0 points) **Yes** (2 points)

_____ Did you menopause occur around age 45?   **No** (0 points) **Yes** (3 points)

_____ Have you lost more than 1/2 inch in height?   **No** (0 points) **Yes** (4 points)

_____ **Subtotal for risk factors that can't be controlled**

II. Risk Factors that Can Be Controlled

_____ Do you smoke cigarettes? **No** (0 points) **Yes** (4 points)

_____ Do you drink alcoholic beverages? **No** (0 points)
        1–2 ounces a day (2 points)
    3 or more ounces per day (4 points)

_____ Do you avoid milk and other **No** (0 points) **Yes** (3 points)
    dairy products?

_____ Do you exercise? Little or none (3 points)
    Regular exercise (0 points)

_____ Are you a person who exercises **No** (0 points) **Yes** (4 points)
    a great deal, with irregular or
    no menstruation?

_____ Is your diet high in animal **No** (0 points) **Yes** (2 points)
    protein, such meats?

_____ Do you add salt to foods at **No** (0 points) **Yes** (3 points)
    the table?

_____ Are you a vegetarian, or have a **No** (0 points) **Yes** (2 points)
    diet heavily weighted toward
    vegetables?

_____ Do you have an eating disorder, **No** (0 points) **Yes** (4 points)
    or consume too little
    nutritious food?

_____ Do you have high amounts of **No** (0 points) **Yes** (4 points)
    fiber in your diet?

_____ Do you have 3 or more cups of **No** (0 points) **Yes** (2 points)
    coffee a day—or an equivalent
    amount of caffeine from other
    sources, such as cola-type beverages?

_____ **Subtotal for risk factors that can be controlled**

III. Risk Factors that You Might Be Able to Control

_____ Do you have a low percentage of   **No** (0 points)   **Yes** (4 points)
body fat (less than 18% of total
body weight)

_____ Have you ever used anticonvulsants   **No** (0 points)   **Yes** (2 points)
(medications designed to prevent
convulsions or fits)?

_____ Have you had hyperparathyroidism   **No** (0 points)   **Yes** (3 points)
(an excessive secretion of the
parathyroid glands which causes
loss of calcium from the bones,
formation of cysts in the bones,
and kidney stones)?

_____ Have you ever used steroid   **No** (0 points)   **Yes** (4 points)
(cortisone) drugs?

_____ Have you had biliary cirrhosis   **No** (0 points)   **Yes** (3 points)
(an inflammatory disease of
the bile system connecting the
liver and the intestines)?

_____ Have you had an overactive thyroid   **No** (0 points)   **Yes** (4 points)
gland with symptoms such as fast
pulse and heart rate, loss of weight,
"hyped up" bodily metabolism?

_____ Have you had stomach or small-   **No** (0 points)   **Yes** (4 points)
bowel disease?

_____ **Subtotal for risk factors that you might be able to control**

_____ **To Evaluate Your Level of Risk, Add ALL Subtotals.**

Your **total point level (from I, II, and III subtotals)** determines your risk
category:

0–8 Low-Risk Category: As you grow older, your risk will increase. So
take steps now to minimize threats to your bones by paying close attention to good nutrition, exercise, and the other controllable risk factors.

9–16 Moderate-Risk Category: Pay close attention to changeable risk factors. Ask your doctor about drugs that may be causing bone loss. If you're past menopause, discuss estrogen replacement therapy if you aren't already on it.

17–25 and Above: High and Very High Risk Categories: Take steps immediately to counteract bone loss. With your doctor, formulate a personal bone-protection program. You may want your doctor to measure the density of your bones to evaluate their present condition and to serve as baseline to be sure the bone loss is not getting worse.

From: *Preventing Osteoporosis*, by Kenneth Cooper, M.D., M.P.H., 1989, Bantam Books

Self Test: Do You Have a Sleep Disorder?

1. Do you have an irregular or abnormal sleep-wake schedule? ___YES ___NO

2. Do you have a problem falling asleep at night ___YES ___NO

3. Do you regularly wake up several times during the night? ___ YES ___NO

4. Do you regularly wake up too early, unable to go back to sleep? ___YES ___NO

5. Do you have difficulty getting up and functioning effectively the first thing in the morning? ____YES ___NO

6. Do you frequently feel overly sleepy or drowsy in the daytime? ___YES ___NO

7. Do you regularly have discomfort or pain disturbing your sleep? ___YES ___NO

8. Do you snore loudly on a fairly regular basis? ___YES ___NO

9. Do you have any abnormal breathing during sleep? ___YES ___NO

10. Do you have abnormal movements, jerkiness of the legs, or excessive restlessness during your sleep? ____YES ___NO

11. Do you need medication to help you sleep at night? ___YES ___NO

12. Do you need stimulants or medication for daytime alertness? ___YES ___NO

13. Does your bed partner or anybody else who has observed your sleep say that you snore too much, are too restless, have jerky movements, or ever stop breathing briefly during sleep? ___YES ___NO

Sleep Disorders Questionnaire by Elizabeth Lee Vliet, M.D., 1988

Scoring and Discussion

If you have *two* or more YES answers, you should discuss these problems with your physician. Ask the question "Could I have a sleep disorder which needs to be checked further?" I encourage you to *avoid just taking sleeping pills* thinking that is treating the problem. Sleeping pills lose their effectiveness after about two weeks, and most are addictive when taken for longer than seven to ten days. These medications can actually be dangerous if you have sleep apnea, since these medications may further depress breathing.

For women in midlife, restless sleep with several awakenings may be one of the earliest indicators of declining estrogen. This is even more likely if the waking episodes are also accompanied by "fluttering" or racing heartbeat, sweating, feeling too hot and/or suddenly chilled. If the cause of the sleep disturbance is an endocrine change, it won't help to just take sleeping pills.

If you answered yes to *any* of the questions 8 through 12, you should be evaluated for sleep apnea, myoclonus, "restless legs syndrome," and narcolepsy. Sleep apnea, if unrecognized and untreated, can cause sexual dysfunction, major depression, high blood pressure, chronic fatigue, problems with memory and concentration during the day, and potentially a heart attack.

It is important to have sleep problems such as these checked properly by a physician knowledgeable about sleep disorders. If your physician dismisses your concerns, seek a consultation with a sleep specialist.

Self Test: What's Your Stress Index?

How do you cope with the stress in your life? There are numerous ways, and some are more effective than others. In addition, some coping approaches you might turn to can actually be as *harmful* as the stress they were intended to alleviate. This scale is a self-assessment *educational* tool, not a *diagnostic* one. Its purpose is to inform you of ways in which you can effectively cope in healthy ways with the stress in your life. Using a point system, this self-test is designed to give you some indication of how important or desirable specific coping strategies are.

Directions: Simply answer the questions, score each one as directed. Then total your points and see how you did! Do you see some ways to improve your score?

_____ 1. Give yourself 10 if you feel that you have a supportive family member near you.

_____ 2. Give yourself 10 points if you actively pursue a hobby.

_____ 3. Give yourself 10 if you belong to some social or activity group that meets once a month (other than your family).

_____ 4. Give yourself 15 points if you are within five pounds of your "ideal" body weight for your height and bone structure.

_____ 5. Give yourself 15 points if you practice some form of "deep relaxation" at least three times a week (such exercises include meditation, imagery, Yoga, etc.)

_____ 6. Give yourself 15 points *for each time* you exercise thirty minutes or longer during the course of an average week.

_____ 7. Give yourself 5 points for each nutritionally balanced and wholesome meal you consume during the course of an average day.

_____ 8. Give yourself 5 points if you do something that you enjoy and that is "just for you" during the course of an average week.

_____ 9. Give yourself 10 points if you have some place in your home that you can go to relax and/or be by yourself.

_____ 10. Give yourself 10 points if you practice time management techniques in your daily life.

_____ 11. Subtract 10 points for each pack of cigarettes you smoke during the course of an average day.

____ 12. Subtract 5 points for each evening during the course of an average week that take any form of medication or chemical substance (including alcohol) to help you sleep.

____ 13. Subtract 10 points for each day during the course of an average week that you consume any form of medication or chemical substance (including alcohol) to reduce your anxiety or just calm you down.

____ 14. Subtract five points for each evening during the course of an average week that you bring work home (work that was meant to be done at your workplace).

____ 15. Subtract five points for each day during the course of an average week that you overeat or "binge" to cope with feelings (anxiety, anger, depression, etc.)

_____ NOW CALCULATE YOUR TOTAL SCORE

A Maximum Score Would Be 115 Points.

This stress assessment test was created by Dr. George S. Everly, Jr., University of Maryland. Available from U.S. Gov. Department of Health Education.

Discussion and Reflection

If your score was *less than 30,* I encourage you to seek a professional in stress management, counseling, or psychotherapy to help you improve your stress-coping skills, behaviors and attitudes, which will lead to improved"psychological hardiness" and a better sense of wellness in your life.

If your score was *between 30 and 50,* it's time to take a serious look at your lifestyle and think about the choices you are making that cause stress to mount up and have a negative effect on your health. Time to wake up and practice some new (or unused!) stress-coping skills!

If your score was *over 50,* you probably have adequate coping strategies for the common sources of stress. Keep in mind, the higher your score the greater your ability to cope with stress in an effective and healthy manner. The higher your score, the better your "resilience" when major stresses hit!

You may have been surprised with your results. Maybe you thought you cope pretty well with stress but got a lower score than you expected. Maybe you found you were doing pretty well but would like to improve more. Whatever the case, each of us can find ways to bring more joy, playfulness, and spontaneity into our lives to reduce tension and over-load. Create fun rewards for yourself as you carry out adding new coping skills.

Self-Reflection and Exploration

Another important dimension of "stress management" is to feel good about the way you live your life, that your life has meaning and purpose, and that you are reaching those goals that are important to you. You may find it helpful now to jot down your thoughts, feelings, and reactions to these "reflection" questions.

1. Describe an experience in which you had the feeling of being totally alive. How long ago was this? When are you going to schedule time for such an experience again?

2. What makes you feel life is really worth living?

3. Make a list of at least five things you like about yourself and another five things you feel you do very well. Put these lists in a place where you will see them daily.

4. List at least five things in your life that you are happy with and do not want to change. Put this list where you will see it daily, and *add* at least one item a month!

5. What ways have you found to maintain these positives in your life?

6. What are the five most pressing things in your life that you are *not* happy with and would like to change?

7. Which of these are within *your control* to change and which are *not* within your control? Begin a list of ways to change the things within your control.

8. What are some ways to help you accept the things that are not within your control? Do you need an objective outside person (e.g., therapist) to help you with this accepting?

9. List at least five ways you contribute positively to the lives of others?

10. List at least five things you can do for your own well-being without the assistance of anyone else. Pick one of these when you are tempted to overeat or drink alcohol.

11. Make a list of your five to ten most important aspirations. What do you have yet to learn to do? Is it time to take a class or tackle learning something toward an aspiration?

12. What are some self-destructive or self-defeating behaviors you want to stop? List several ways to "neutralize" or eliminate obstacles to your success that are created by your old behaviors.

13. What are several things that you tell yourself you "should/ought" to do that you really *do not want to do*? List several ways you may **begin now** to eliminate these "shoulds" and "ought tos" and be gentler on yourself.

Reflection Self Inventory: by Elizabeth Lee Vliet, 1989

Self Test: Do You Have a Problem with Alcohol ?

The AUDIT, or "Alcohol Use Disorders Identification Test" was designed to help physicians and patients better identify people who have problem drinking patterns and encourage treatment interventions *before* the addictive illness of alcoholism develops. I have included the self-assessment part of the AUDIT here so that you can answer these questions in a private setting. In our culture, women who are problem drinkers or alcoholics are more adversely stigmatized than are men; as a result, women are usually too ashamed to bring this up to their physicians. Even when they do talk with their physicians about drinking problems, women are commonly *not* referred for appropriate substance abuse treatment as early in the disease as are men. Consequently, women are more seriously ill and have experienced more destructive onsequences of alcohol abuse before they get help.

Be honest with yourself when you answer these questions. If you are not, you hurt primarily yourself and those who love you. **I *urge you to get professional help* if you have a score of 4 or more on this self test.**

AUDIT Self-Assessment: The following questions are about the past year.

1. How often do you have a drink containing alcohol?   <u>POINTS</u>

    _____Never   (0)
    _____Monthly or less   (1)
    _____2 to 4 times a month   (2)
    _____2 to 3 times a week   (3)
    _____4 or more times a week   (4)

2. How many drinks containing alcohol do you
    have on a typical day when you are drinking?

    _____None   (0)
    _____1 or 2   (1)
    _____3 or 4   (2)
    _____5 or 6   (3)
    _____7 or 9   (4)
    _____10 or more   (5)

3. How often do you have six or more drinks on one occasion?

    _____Never   (0)
    _____Less than monthly   (1)
    _____Monthly   (1)
    _____Weekly   (3)
    _____Daily or almost daily   (4)

4. How often during the past year have you found that you were unable to stop drinking once you had started?

    _____Never   (0)
    _____Less than monthly   (1)
    _____Monthly   (2)
    _____Weekly   (3)
    _____Daily or almost daily   (4)

5. How often during the past year have you failed to do what was normally expected from you because of drinking?

    _____Never   (0)
    _____Less than monthly   (1)
    _____Monthly   (2)
    _____Weekly   (3)
    _____Daily or almost daily   (4)

6. How often during the past year have you needed a first drink in the morning to get yourself going after a heavy drinking session?

    _____Never   (0)
    _____Less than monthly   (1)
    _____Monthly   (2)
    _____Weekly   (3)
    _____Daily or almost daily   (4)

7. How often during the past year have you had a feeling of guilt or remorse after drinking?

    _____Never   (0)
    _____Less than monthly   (1)
    _____Monthly   (2)
    _____Weekly   (3)
    _____Daily or almost daily   (4)

8. How often during the past year have you been unable to remember what happened the night before because you had been drinking?

   _____Never   (0)
   _____Less than monthly   (1)
   _____Monthly   (2)
   _____Weekly   (3)
   _____Daily or almost daily   (4)

9. Have you or someone else been injured as the result of your drinking?

   _____No   (0)
   _____Yes, but not in the last year   (2)
   _____Yes, during the last year   (4)

10. Has a relative, friend, a doctor, or other health worker expressed concern about your drinking or suggested you cut down?

   _____No   (0)
   _____Yes, but not in the last year   (2)
   _____Yes, during the last year   (4)

11. Have you ever experienced blackouts, "D.T.s," or loss of consciousness from drinking too much?

   _____No   (0)
   _____Yes, but not in the last year   (2)
   _____Yes, once during the last year   (4)
   _____Yes, more than once in the last year   (8)

Reference: Schmidt, et.al.

Self Test: Do You Have Fibromyalgia?

Fibromyalgia is such an elusive medical problem that it is difficult to design a questionnaire that would be specific for this pain syndrome. I have provided these questions as a guide for you to evaluate what you are experiencing. If you answer YES to **more than 3 questions,** I suggest you review the chapter on fibromyalgia, write the resource organizations in the appendix for more information, and consult with your physician or a pain management specialist in your area. The more you know about this pain syndrome, the better you will be able to put together effective approaches to reduce pain and feel better overall.

1. I have trouble sleeping on a regular basis due to pain. ____YES ___NO

2. I notice the pain on a constant, almost daily basis. ____YES ___NO

3. I experience pain in multiple areas of my body: neck, shoulders, back, hips, joints, head, etc. ____YES ___NO

4. My pain is not usually relieved by aspirin, Tylenol, or over-the-counter anti-inflammatory (pain) medications. ____YES ___NO

5. I have reduced or eliminated activities that I used to enjoy due to limitations caused by my pain. ____YES ___NO

6. I no longer enjoy sexual activity due to constant pain. ____YES ___NO

7. I experience a worsening of my pain in cold, damp weather. ____YES ___NO

8. I have experienced a decrease in my ability to work at home or in my outside-the-home job due to pain. ____YES ___NO

9. I have been depressed or irritable and tense to a degree that is unlike my usual self because of the pain. ____YES ___NO

10. I experience numbness, burning or cold sensations in my muscles and/or my arms and legs. ____YES ___NO

11. I have generalized stiffness and soreness,   ____YES ___NO
    often worse in the mornings.

12. I have a lot of tender places where muscles   ____YES ___NO
    come together around my joints, shoulders,
    back, and neck.

13. My memory and concentration are getting   ____YES ___NO
    worse due to the pain.

14. My pain is so difficult for me to live with,   ____YES ___NO
    I have had thoughts of taking my life.
    (If this answer is YES, **you must get
    professional help NOW.**)

Self Test: Do You Have a Major Depression

Directions: Answer each question below according to the following key:

	None of the time	Some of the time	Good part of the time	Almost always
1. I feel downhearted, blue and sad				
2. Morning is when I feel the best.				
3. I have crying spells or feel like it.				
4. I have trouble sleeping through the night.				
5. I eat as much as I used to.				
6. I enjoy looking at, talking to, and being with interesting women and men.				
7. I notice that I am losing weight.				
8. I have trouble with constipation.				
9. My heart beats faster than usual.				
10. I get tired for no reason.				
11. My mind is as clear as it used to be.				
12. I find it easy to do the things I used to do.				
13. I am restless and can't keep still.				
14. I feel hopeful about the future.				

	None of the time	Some of the time	Good part of the time	Almost always
15. I am more irritable than usual.				
16. I find it more difficult to make decisions.				
17. I feel that I am useful and needed.				
18. My life is pretty full.				
19. I feel that others would be better off if I were dead.				
20. I still enjoy the things I used to.				

Make sure you answer every question. You cannot accurately score this quiz according to the formula below unless there is a response to each question!

Scoring and Discussion

Questions **2, 5, 6, 11, 12, 14, 16, 17, 18, 20**: Score according to the following key:

    None or a little of the time = 4 points
    Some of the time   = 3 points
    Good part of the time   = 2 points
    Almost always   = 1 point

Questions **1, 3, 4, 7, 8, 9, 10, 13, 15, 19**: Score according to the following key:

    None or a little of the time = 1 point
    Some of the time   = 2 points
    Good part of the time   = 3 points
    Almost always   = 4 points

After you have given the proper points to each of your responses, add all of these numbers to get your total raw score. To convert your raw score to the "Depression Index" score, use the following formula:

$$\text{INDEX} \quad = \quad \frac{\text{Raw Score Total points}}{\text{Max Score of 80 points}} \quad \times \quad 100$$

Once you have calculated your index score, you can then interpret it based on the following ranges:

Index Score Less than 50:   normal range
Index Score of 50 to 59:   presence of minimal to mild depression
Index Score of 60 to 69:   presence of moderate to marked depression
Index Score of 70 and above: presence of severe to extreme depression

Depression is a very treatable problem! If your score is over 55, I encourage you to consult with your personal physician or a psychiatrist to see that you have a more indepth evaluation for possible medical factors affecting your mood and well-being and to also evalutate the possibility of a major depression, which could respond well to medications and supportive therapy.

W.W.K. Zung, "A Self-Rating Depression Scale" *Arch.Gen.Psychiatry*, 1965; 12:63–70. Zung Depression Scale also copyrighted 1974, 1989.

Self Test: Do You Have An Anxiety Disorder?

Directions: Answer the following questions according to the following key:

a. **None or a little of the time**
b. **Some of the time**
c. **A good part of the time**
d. **Almost always**

1. I feel more nervous and anxious than usual. _____
2. I feel afraid for no reason at all. _____
3. I get upset easily or feel panicky. _____
4. I feel like I'm falling apart and going to pieces. _____
5. I feel that everything is all right and nothing bad will happen. _____
6. My arms and legs shake and tremble. _____
7. I am bothered by headaches, neck and back pains. _____
8. I feel weak and get tired easily. _____
9. I feel calm and can sit still easily. _____
10. I can feel my heart beating fast. _____
11. I am bothered by dizzy spells. _____
12. I have fainting spells or feel faint. _____
13. I can breath in and out easily. _____
14. I get feelings of numbness and tingling in my fingers and toes. _____
15. I am bothered by stomachaches or indigestion. _____
16. I have to empty my bladder often. _____
17. My hands are usually dry and warm. _____
18. My face gets hot and blushes. _____
19. I fall asleep easily and get a good night's rest. _____
20. I have nightmares. _____

Make sure you answer every question. You cannot accurately score this quiz according to the formula below unless there is a response to each question!

Scoring and Discussion

Questions **5, 9, 13, 17, 19**: Score according to the following key:

a. None or a little of the time = 4 points
b. Some of the time = 3 points
c. Good part of the time = 2 points
d. Almost always = 1 point

Questions **1, 2, 3, 4, 6, 7, 8, 10, 11, 12, 14, 15, 16, 18, 20**: Score according to the following key:

a. None or a little of the time = 1 point
b. Some of the time   = 2 points
c. Good part of the time   = 3 points
d. Almost always   = 4 points

After you have given the proper points to each of your responses, add all of these numbers to get your total raw score. To convert your raw score to the "Depression Index" score, use the following formula:

$$\text{INDEX} \;=\; \frac{\text{Raw Score Total points}}{\text{Max Score of 80 points}} \;\times\; 100$$

Once you have calculated your index score, you can then interpret it based on the following ranges:

Index Score Less than 45:   normal range
Index Score of 46–59:   presence of minimal to moderate anxiety
Index Score of 60–74:   presence of marked to severe anxiety
Index Score of 74 and above: presence of extreme anxiety

Anxiety Disorders are very treatable problems. If your score is over 55, I encourage you to consult with your personal physician or a psychiatrist to have a more in-depth evaluation for possible medical factors causing your anxiety symptoms and negatively affecting your well-being. It is also important to evaluate the possibility of Panic Disorder or a significant generalized anxiety disorder, which could respond well to medications and supportive therapy.

Many types of alternative or complementary therapies are very useful in alleviating anxiety disorders. Among the ones I have recommended for my patients are those in the list that follows. You may find others to be helpful as well. I do think it is crucial to your health to have a good medical checkup, before assuming that your problems are "just" due to anxiety. There are over a **hundred different medical disorders** that can cause identical symptoms and may need specific and different treatments. Make sure your physician and your alternative therapists are working together to help you with the anxiety problems!

Complementary Therapies Helpful For Anxiety

- acupuncture
- biofeedback
- hypnotherapy
- visualization and guided imagery exercises
- therapeutic massage for deep muscle relaxation
- jacuzzi herbal baths (using calming herbs)
- dietary changes and proper vitamin balance
- brisk walking
- aerobic exercise (to relieve build-up of excess adrenalin)
- eliminating alcohol, caffeine, and over-the-counter decongestants and sinus medications

Reference: WWK Zung: Self-Rating Anxiety Scale, 1974.

Self Test: Do You Have an Eating Disorder?

This quiz is not diagnostic for the presence of an eating disorder. It can serve to alert you to problem areas that need to be changed or improved, and it will also alert you to the possibility that you may have an eating disorder. Both anorexia and bulimia may have serious medical complications, so it is important to have a professional evaluation if you suspect you may have an eating disorder. Anorexia nervosa is often called the "starvation disease" and it is far more common in women than men, particularly adolescents and college-age women. It is potentially fatal if not treated in a comprehensive approach by experienced medical and psychiatric professionals. Bulimia is often called the "binge-purge disease" and is also seen in the same age group as anorexia, with a similar prevalence in women. It may be cyclically aggravated by the menstrual cycle hormonal effects on appetite regulation mechanisms.

Directions: Answer each question YES or NO, then total the number of YES answers and the number of NO responses.

Are you presently at the optimal body weight for your height? ____YES ___NO

Do you feel overcome with fear of becoming fat? ____YES ___NO

Do you feel totally preoccupied with weight and thinness? ____YES ___NO

Do you feel fat most of the time? ____YES ___NO

Do you avoid letting people close to you see you without any clothes? ____YES ___NO

Do family and friends tell you that you are too thin or underweight, even though *you* feel *fat*? ____YES ___NO

Have you regularly restricted the amount of food you eat daily? ____YES ___NO

Do you tend to fuss around the kitchen, fixing food for others and not eating it? ____YES ___NO

Do you take laxatives or diuretics on a regular basis? ____YES ___NO

Have you ever taken laxatives and diuretics to lose weight? ____YES ___NO

Have your menstrual periods gotten *lighter, less frequent, or stopped completely?* (not due to hysterectomy or birth control pill use)   ____YES ___NO

Has your body and scalp hair become thin and fine, or are you losing a lot of hair?   ____YES ___NO

Do you exercise frantically trying to burn off calories and keep your weight down?   ____YES ___NO

Have family and friends told you that you appear to eat a large quantity of food, but you don't gain weight?   ____YES ___NO

Do you fast (not eat) for long periods of time?   ____YES ___NO

Have you become *secretive* about eating, the food you buy, and other food-related activities?   ____YES ___NO

Have you made yourself vomit after large meals to keep from gaining weight?   ____YES ___NO

Have you frequently had weight fluctuations greater than 10 pounds due to alternating binges and fasts?   ____YES ___NO

Do you frequently binge on high calorie, easily consumed food like ice cream, cookies, fast food, snacks, etc.?   ____YES ___NO

Do you frequently end such eating episodes due to falling asleep, to abdominal pain, or self-induced vomiting?   ____YES ___NO

Scoring and Discussion

The more YES answers you have, the more serious the eating disturbance. A score of 2 to 3 YES answers suggests that you have abnormal eating behaviors, may lead to a serious eating disorder. You would benefit from seeking professional help to make healthy changes in your eating habits.

A score of 4 or more YES answers suggests that you have an existing eating disorder, which may already have created significant hazards to your health, such as bone loss and menstrual disruption. It is very important that you seek professional help **now** from an experienced eating disorders specialist. You should also talk honestly with your physician about your eating problems and ask to have a complete medical evaluation to determine what medical problems may be present or likely to happen. Eating disorders can be lethal. They are treatable, and help is available. Choose to *use* it!

Eating Disorders Questionnaire by Elizabeth Lee Vliet, M.D., 1988

Self Test: Do You Have OCD?

Obsessive Compulsive Disorder is another type of biological illness, thought to be due to dysfunction in the serotonin-regulating mechanisms in the brain, that is manifested by intrusive unwanted thoughts (obsessions) and actions (compulsions). In its milder forms, it may not be noticed or may be seen as simply "odd" behavior. In its severe forms, it can be debilitating and may interfere with one's ability to live a normal life because the sufferer is so preoccupied with carrying out the actions that he or she is unable to carry on normal activities. It is much more common than previously thought, and is no longer considered to be due primarily to unconscious *psychological conflicts*. This illness is now treated, usually very successfully, with the new serotonin-augmenting medications such as Prozac, Paxil, Luvox, or Anafranil. In some cases, behavior therapy is also used as a component of treatment.

If you have checked several of the items on this list and are troubled by OCD symptoms, I encourage you to consult with a psychiatrist knowledgeable with the newer treatment options, or you may want to call the national OCD Foundation for a list of specialists in your area.

Obsessions and Compulsions Checklist

Answer each question with one of the following choices (points in parentheses): **rarely or never (0) occasionally (1) frequently (2) almost always or daily (3)**

I. Obsessions
  1. I have fears I might harm others   _____
  2. I have fears I might harm myself   _____
  3. I experience violent and/or terrifying mental images   _____
  4. I have fears of doing something embarrassing   _____
  5. I am afraid I will act on undesirable impulses   _____
  6. I am afraid I will be responsible for things going wrong   _____
  7. I have fears something terrible might happen to
     someone   _____
  8. I am disgusted by bodily waste or secretions
     (e.g., urine, feces, semen, saliva)   _____
  9. I am preoccupied with concerns about contamination
     with dirt, germs, household chemicals, and/or
     environmental contaminants   _____
 10. I am preoccupied with concerns I will get ill   _____
 11. I am preoccupied with forbidden or perverse sexual
     thoughts, images, or impulses   _____

12. I am preoccupied with hoarding or collecting nonvaluable items _____
13. I am preoccupied with religious thoughts, images, experiences _____
14. I am preoccupied with thoughts of exactness, symmetry, order _____
15. I have fears of not saying things just right _____
16. I experience intrusive nonsense sounds, words, or music _____
17. I am preoccupied with thoughts of lucky/unlucky numbers, colors with special significance, and/or my body sensations and experiences _____

II. Compulsions
1. I engage in excessive or ritualized handwashing _____
2. I engage in excessive or ritualized showering, bathing, toothbrushing, or grooming _____
3. I engage in cleaning household items or other inanimate objects to avoid contact with contaminants _____
4. I engage in counting and recounting of objects _____
5. I engage in excessive checking of doors, locks, stove, appliances, emergency brake on car, etc. even though I may know I have just checked these _____
6. I engage in checking to see that I have not harmed others or myself _____
7. I engage in checking that nothing terrible has happened _____
8. I frequently check for contaminants _____
9. I engage in ordering, arranging, and rearranging items _____
10. I hoard or collect nonessential or nonvaluable items _____
11. I have urges to touch, rub, or stroke other people and/or objects _____
12. I take extra precautions or steps to prevent me from harming myself or others _____

SCORING: Many people experience some of these thoughts and actions occasionally. A score of **15 or more**, however, indicates the *possibility* of OCD, particularly if the your thoughts and actions are interfering with your normal day-to-day activities and performance. If you score higher than 25, I urge you to have a consultation with a psychiatrist knowledgeable about OCD who can determine whether medication may improve your quality of life.

Checklist by Elizabeth Lee Vliet, M.D., 1995. Modified from Yale OCD Checklist

Self Test: Are You at Risk for Heart Disease?

These questions address some of the common genetic, lifestyle, and medical factors that increase risk of *atherosclerosis*, or disease of the heart and blood vessels. If you are a *postmenopausal* woman, you will want to know what your estradiol level is in addition to cholesterol and other measures of risk. The items shown here do not all have the same degree of importance in determining your heart disease risk. They are ones that you should be taking into account as you make healthy lifestyle changes. Your physician can discuss the relative importance, or weighting, given to each of these risk factors, based on your individual health profile as a whole.

The items shown in bold are ones that should be checked by your physician. If you do not know the answers to the statements shown in bold, I urge you to *find out*. This is information you should keep in your personal health file to help you keep track of how you measure up on heart disease risk.

Directions: Answer YES or NO to the following questions:

No one in my family has heart problems, high blood ____YES ___NO pressure, strokes, diabetes, or is overweight.

My body weight is in the normal range for my age, ____YES ___NO height and sex.

My waist-to-hip ratio is <u>less</u> than 0.85 (divide ____YES ___NO waist measurement by hip measurement, with hips measured 7 inches below the waist).

I walk briskly or do other aerobic exercise three or ____YES ___NO more times a week.

I never used or have stopped using cigarettes and ____YES ___NO tobacco products.

I drink alcohol occasionally or only one drink a day. ____YES ___NO

I manage stress in my life effectively. ____YES ___NO

I have eliminated or reduced my intake of meat, ____YES ___NO butter, cheeses, lunch meats, and salty and fatty snack foods.

I take regular vacations and weekend breaks. ____YES ___NO

I feel pretty calm most of the time, able to relax after work. ___YES ___NO

I take a low dose of aspirin every other day (low dose is one-quarter to one full tablet of regular strength aspirin, 325 mg per tablet) ___YES ___NO

My total cholesterol is 200 or less. ___YES ___NO

My HDL-cholesterol is 50 or higher. ___YES ___NO

My blood triglycerides are in the normal range. ___YES ___NO

My blood pressure is in the normal range for my age. ___YES ___NO

My fasting blood glucose is in the normal range. ___YES ___NO

My estradiol levels are in the normal premenopausal range. ___YES ___NO

(If you are postmenopausal) I take estrogen therapy daily. ___YES ___NO

Scoring and Discussion

The more **NO responses** you have, the *higher* your risk of heart disease. You will notice that *all* of the risk factors above, *except* for your family history, are ones that YOU CONTROL by CHOICES you make each day and by how effectively you work with your physician as an active partner in your healthcare. Think about this: If YOU don't take care of your heart, who will? Review chapters 13, 15, 19, and 20 for more help on heart disease and how to decrease your risks.

Women's Heart Disease Risk Checklist by Elizabeth Lee Vliet, M.D., 1987

Self-Test: How's My Sexuality?

Most women I talk with say they are embarrassed to initiate discussion of their questions about sexuality. I think it will help if you take time by yourself to consider these questions, write down your responses, and then make a list of the specific questions you would like to ask your doctor or a therapist. There are no right and wrong answers to these questions. I have written them in hopes it will help you reflect honestly about areas you may wish to improve, or possible health issues that should be addressed with a professional you trust.

1. *Am I satisfied with the frequency of my sexual activity?* Has it declined in recent months or years? If so, what ideas do I have about causes? (Suggestions for reflection: think about your body (are you satisfied with how you look and feel?), your partner, your lifestyle (do you drink too much alcohol, use drugs or medications, smoke tobacco?), your stresses (are you overworked and too tired to relax and enjoy sex?), and others.

2. *Am I as interested in sexual activity as I have been in the past? Is my partner healthy and interested in sex? Do either my partner or I have any difficulty performing sexually?*

3. *Have I noticed a change or decline in my level of sexual desire?*

4. *Am I experiencing any pain or discomfort (burning, itching, etc.) with sexual intercourse?*

5. *Have I been having decreased vaginal lubrication and feeling too "dry" to enjoy sexual activity?*

6. *Does it take longer or is it harder to achieve an orgasm, making me feel like it's just too much effort to try?*

7. *Am I experiencing any painful muscle (e.g., uterus) contractions with intercourse or with orgasm, inhibiting my interest or desire?*

8. *Am I angry or upset with my partner and not communicating these feelings?*

9. *Are there other relationship problems (including my relationship with MYSELF) affecting my sexual activity and enjoyment?*

10. *What would I like to see changed or improved in my sexual activity and relationship with myself and others?*

"How's My Sexuality?" by Elizabeth Lee Vliet, M.D., 1982, revised 1992.

*Take Charge of Your Health! Personal Prevention
Guidelines for Periodic Screening*

There are many different resources and recommended frequencies for health risk screenings. These are the recommendations that I feel are important for women and that will provide the best possibilty of identifying disease in early and more treatable stages.

1. Keep an up-to-date list of diseases present in your family.

2. Self-exams:
   Breast—monthly, just after menses
   Skin—a nurse practitioner colleague calls this "Your Mole Patrol," giving yourself a good look to see if any moles or skin "bumps" exhibit changes in size, shape, or color over time. **Frequency:** every six months from adolescence through age 35, monthly along with your breast exam after age 35. Report any suspicious changes to your physician, or nurse practitioner.

3. Physical Examination by your physician:

   Blood Pressure: Every year ages 14 to 40.
   Two or more times per year after age 40
   Two or more times a year **before age 40 if you have**
   • elevated or borderline blood pressure
   • take oral contraceptives
   • have had a hysterectomy (with or without ovaries removed)
   • have a history of heart disease
   • smoke cigarettes or use other tobacco products
   • are more than 10 percent overweight
   • have chronic diseases that require periodic blood pressure screening
   • take corticosteroids
   • have kidney disease.

   Breast: Every 1 to 3 years, ages 16 to 39; *annually after age 40.*

   Pelvic Exam: Every 1 to 2 years beginning when you become sexually active. *Every year after age 40.*

   Pap smear: Begin when you become sexually active. Ages 18 to 39, every 1 to 3 years after two negative results. *Every year after age 40.*

Endometrial (uterine) tissue biopsy: American College of Obstetrics and Gynecology recommends an *annual* biopsy in women who are intolerant to progestin or progesterone and are taking estrogen alone. American Cancer Society recommends *one screening test* for the following situations (frequency of additional tests based on physician recommendations):
- a woman is anovulatory
- has a history of infertility
- has abnormal uterine bleeding
- if the woman is postmenopausal and is considering estrogen replacement therapy (ERT)
- is taking Tamoxifen.

Rectal exam for occult blood (digital): Once a year after age 40.

Proctosigmoidoscopy: for polyps, tumors, bleeding, etc.
Every 3 to 4 years after age 50; annually if at high risk for cancer.

4. Laboratory/Screening Tests

Bone Density measurement: I recommend this be done for a baseline by age 45, or earlier if multiple risk factors for bone loss are present. Waiting until after menopause is too late in my opinion. I recommend Dual Energy X-Ray Absorptiometry (DEXA) as the safest and most useful procedure. DEXA uses far less radiation and is much less expensive than CT scans.

Electrocardiogram: Baseline at age 40, then every 3 to 5 years. There is controversy about the value of screening exercise (treadmill) "stress" EKG in women. I recommend that this be done if you are beginning a new exercise program and are overweight or have existing medical problems. Such testing may also be recommended by your physician if you develop chest pain or shortness of breath with mild exertion.

Mammogram: Baseline exam at age 35 if no family history of breast cancer.
If there is a **positive family history** of breast cancer in mother or sister(s), the baseline should be done **before age 35**.
Normal risk: every 1 to 2 years from age 40 to 50.
High risk (positive family history): annually from age 40 onward.
Normal risk: Every year after age 50.

Cholesterol testing (must include HDL cholesterol to be useful): Every 5 years, beginning in early teen years. Twice or more per year if the following situations exist:
- extreme changes in weight
- marked changes in level of activity have occurred
- if you have been ill or begin new medications that may affect cholesterol
- if you become menopausal (after surgery or naturally) and do not take estrogen; once a year if taking estrogen
- if you had previously been found to have high cholesterol or triglycerides
- if you smoke cigarettes or use other tobacco products
- if you drink more than 2 glasses of wine (or equivalent) daily
- with any other life changes or chronic diseases that require cholesterol testing.

Hemoglobin and hematocrit: Every 5 years, unless anemic (then annually until stabilized).

Fasting blood glucose (sugar): Every 3 to 5 years after age 20, if within normal limits. **Annually after age 35 if you are at high risk of diabetes based on:**
- family history of diabetes
- overweight
- have gained more than 20 pounds in the last year
- experience new onset sweet cravings, increased thirst, increased urination

Thyroid: Baseline test at age 35, unless indicated earlier. Then every 2 years. **Should include TSH for women, since this is a more sensitive indicator.**

Sexually Transmitted diseases: Annually or more often if high risk.

Tuberculosis: Annually if in health care profession. If high risk, as indicated.

Check List: Questions to Ask Your Women's Health Center

Many facilities are now calling themselves "women's health centers," but the resources and types of staff available vary considerably. Some are just traditional medical practices repackaged under a new name designed to attract women. Evaluate *your* center by asking the following questions. Is the women's health center you are visiting the real thing? It probably is if the answer to most of these questions is YES.

1. Is the first step a careful and thorough assessment of you as a total person, rather than just treating the presenting symptom? Are hormonal factors checked?

2. Is the initial visit at least 45 minutes, with subsequent visits at least 20 minutes?

3. Are the physicians interested and do they listen to YOUR ideas about your health.

4. Are the physicians willing to take time to talk with you about your concerns and to answer your questions about your health?

5. Does the care you receive emphasize **prevention** of health problems in addition to the treatment of acute problems?

6. Does the center utilize a range of health care providers including such professionals as nutritionists, exercise physiologists, massage therapists, chiropractors, and others?

7. Is there an emphasis on noninvasive treatments (such as lifestyle changes) first, rather than just giving medications for symptoms?

8. Do the physicians offer a choice of treatment options and explain the pros and cons (or the benefits and risks) of each, rather than using only the medication approach?

9. Does the center offer evaluation of your emotional well-being as well as your physical problems?

10. Does the center offer counseling and psychotherapy with psychiatric physicians who are able to treat the mind *and* the body together?

11. Does the center have or urge patients to use a medical library that includes non-technical resources for the layperson? Does your physician give you references to read further about your health concerns?

12. Are there free or low-cost educational programs and self-help support groups available on site?

13. Does the staff make you feel comfortable, secure, and confident that they care about you as a woman and treat you as an individual?

14. Does the staff take your concerns seriously, and do you feel they listen?

15. Does the center make an effort to solicit your feedback and ideas about how to improve services?

The more YES answers you have, the more likely you will find that this women's center is able to meet your individual health needs and provide you with additional resources beyond those provided on site at the center.

CHAPTER 19

Fat to Fit: Making Healthy Lifestyle Changes for Mid-Life and Beyond

> Women are not frail. By widespread consumer educa-
> tion early lifestyle behavior modification and the pro-
> ductive use of modern technology the image of the
> shrunken little old lady we hope will be condemned to
> history and replaced by women imbued with vitality
> and a zest for an active and productive old age.
>
> —Unknown

VR's Story

"I'm the third girl in a family of four girls. My sisters and my
mother had serious medical problems (mostly cardiovascular)
while they were alive and they've died too soon. I enjoy life, I want
to be physically and mentally active. I don't want to be sickly or
to die young. This is the reason for my story.

"In 1984 I was fifty-four years old, a widow for a year, and the
mother of four adult children. I was enjoying my work with young
people, my family and friends, and life in general; however, I sensed
something was wrong with my physical condition. I had been diagnosed as having essential hypertension when I was *twenty-nine*
years old. Over the years, physicians had prescribed a variety of
medications which usually kept my blood pressure below the
150/90 threshold. I was taking four different medicines for five or
six years and my blood pressure was staying within normal limits.
But I knew something was wrong.

"My body just didn't feel like me. Everything was taking more
effort than it usually did. I felt like I had to push myself to swim and
play golf, my two favorite sports. I would go to aerobic class and
really be working out well and never could get my heart rate into
the target range. Very frustrating for someone who likes to follow
directions and achieve my goals!

"When I mentioned this to friends, they made the usual comments, 'Remember you're older now, VR!' I knew too many active people much older than I was, so I didn't buy into my friends' excuses. I went to my doctor whom I'd been going to for seven years. I told him how I felt and suggested that I needed a reevaluation with an up-to-date cardiac stress test (remembering my sisters and their heart problems, it seemed like a reasonable request to me) and then a review of my medications. He looked over my record and said "No, there is no sign that you need a cardiac stress test. Your blood pressure is well-controlled and you seem fine to me." I believe he thought this was true, but I think he was also influenced by the fact that I was on an HMO insurance plan and this would add to his medical expenses. He had indicated there would be problems justifying the cardiac stress test.

"At this point I did some serious soul searching. *I felt something was wrong with me physically*. I knew I couldn't prove it, but I wasn't going to let a doctor keep me from getting a correct diagnosis! I thought about my mother and sisters: Mother started having heart attacks in her fifties, had two operations on her carotid arteries in her sixties, had strokes in her seventies and eighties, and died in a nursing home at eighty-five out-of-touch with reality. My sister Rae, who was seven years older than I, started having heart attacks in her forties. At forty-eight she had a severely damaged heart, was bedridden, and died at fifty-one. My older sister Anne, who is ten years older than I, started having heart attacks in her fifties, and at sixty-four had a quadruple bypass. She is now very limited in her activities because of her poor health. My younger sister Mary died at age thirty-two of leukemia, so I don't know what her cardiovascular condition might have been. With this kind of family history, I knew I needed help immediately.

"At the library I picked up a brochure on *Preventive Medicine* by Dr. Lee Vliet. Could this be the doctor I needed to see? Just walking into her office was a healthy experience: relaxing music was playing, the colors of everything were soothing, the art work was thought-provoking and creative; Dr. Vliet and her staff were obviously interested, caring people. I shared my story with Dr. Vliet. She asked many questions and then ordered a cardiopulmonary exercise test plus some labwork. I had never had such a comprehensive stress test. It was stopped suddenly because my condition rapidly declined. The test report stated I was heavily overmedicated, my heart was blocked so much by the beta-blocker that it couldn't get to a higher heart rate even though I had already passed the aerobic threshold! The cardiologist's report said I was in danger of sudden death if I participated in physical activities. And here I had been pushing myself in aerobic classes three times a week. I was flabbergasted with this news. I knew my body had been trying to tell me something, I just didn't realize how serious it was. Needless to say, Dr. Vliet urged me not to go on my planned wilderness hiking trip, but to take time to get my medication changed and my body in better shape. After the abnormal results, my primary care physician then said, 'Oh, well, I guess this did need to be done. I'll send the prescription to the insurance company.'

"I believe Dr. Vliet saved my life. She *listened* to my concerns and accepted the possible validity of them. She ordered the tests that would give her the factual information she needed to confirm or deny my subjective feelings about my body. Dr. Vliet did a complete reevaluation, and with her colleague, provided me with a new regimen of preventive medicine and appropriate medications.

"Now, eleven years later, I follow the basic tenets of preventive medicine: low-fat foods, regular physical activity, relaxation techniques, caring relationships, and periodic medical checkups with required medications. I have lost weight, yes, but more importantly I have *gained* good health. My blood pressure is controlled; exercise four times a week. I take only two medications now, instead of *five*, and I am off the beta-blocker. I work full-time in a high-pressure job I love, I go jet-skiing and swimming with my grandchildren, and have just taken up scuba diving. Good living for a sixty-five-year-old woman! And my younger friends now say, 'Gosh, VR, I hope I can be like you when I'm your age.' And *my doctor keeps thinking I'm fifty-five instead of sixty-five*!"

VR wrote her story herself when she learned I was writing a book, because she wanted her voice to be heard by other women who may be listened to, and wanted to encourage other women to *listen to their own body wisdom*. I feel gratified by her words and inspired by all that she has done to take charge of her life in spite of the "bad genes" she's inherited! She has truly made the efforts that are within her control to change her lifestyle, move from FAT to FIT, and do her best *not* to end up like her sister who was for years a respiratory cripple due to emphysema from cigarette smoking and a cardiac cripple from her severe vascular disease. Two women from the same family, living in the same town, one active and fit at sixty-five heading off to scuba dive and the other housebound for years, dead at sixty-eight. Which will you be? You choose. There is a great deal that is indeed within your control.

Why else is VR's story so important here? To me, she illustrates the many integrated issues I have raised throughout this book and encapsulates what has been wrong in women's health care. She is an articulate, educated, health-conscious professional woman; she knew her body and trusted her instincts; she very appropriately consulted her physician with her concerns; *she was not listened to, not taken seriously, not evaluated properly for her health history and risks, and she was overly medicated **and then told she was fine!***

Given her ability to speak up for herself, if she was dismissed and discounted, it makes it even more alarming to think about all the women out there who do not have VR's knowledge and asssertiveness, who quietly become more debilitated or die from not being listened to and taken seriously.

Her story is critical in illustrating another problem for women. Weight loss is key to reducing hypertension and heart disease risk. Doctors know that, but all too often don't refer patients for nutritional consultations to help with healthy weight loss plans and tend to prescribe pills to control blood pressure instead. It's faster, it's what they are taught, and many patients expect and want the "magic bullet." But VR was different. She had been actively involved in a regular exercise program for a number of years, and she had worked hard to decrease her body fat, cut out added salt, reduced alcohol, and stopped smoking. What she did not know, and what was potentially lethal, was that the very medications given to decrease her blood pressure were also directly interfering with her ability to lose weight and her ability to accomplish the benefits of her aerobic exercise.

And she had never been checked for hormonal changes, nor had any physician talked to her about the potential cardioprotective benefits of estrogen therapy so she could consider that option. She was on *five* different antihypertensive medications and cholesterol-lowering drugs when she came to see me, but no one had ever looked at the estrogen factor, which is so crucial to preventing heart disease in women! For the "bottom-line" folks out there, *if* you ignore all the quality of life issues for VR, and *if* you ignore the risk of premature death she was facing, and *just* look at the dollar cost of her care (over $500 per month on mendications alone) it is far more cost effective to provide a woman-oriented evaluation, decrease her expensive medications, help her with lifestyle changes, prescribe hormone therapy if appropriate than to continue multiple medications and treat the complications, and heart attack, when these occur. Put in this context, a hormone blood test doesn't seem so expensive, does it?

The specific type of medication VR was taking added an additional impediment to her own efforts to lose weight. Beta-blockers (like Inderal, Corgard, Atenolol, and others) have several *unwanted* effects: (1) they slow down metabolism, (2) decrease insulin release from the pancreas, which then impairs glucose regulation and increases the tendency to gain weight, (3) they block the normal heart rate response to exercise, which impaired VR's ability to safely exercise and monitor her heart rate, and (4) they decrease one's energy level and tolerance for physical activity. Here was a well-motivated and disciplined patient who was being thwarted in her efforts to achieve her health goals *by unaddressed side effects of the medication she was taking.*

Doing the right type of evaluation in situations like this allows both the physician and patient to design a therapeutic plan that *enhances*, not *blocks*, the individual's health goals. I am increasingly concerned, as I conduct seminars around the country and do individual medical consults for women, that the beta-blocker antihypertensive medications are prescribed too quickly in mid-life and menopausal women without appropriate consideration of endocrine factors in high blood pressure, weight gain, and high cholesterol. There are better options with medications, and we need to emphasize healthy lifestyle habits far more emphatically in medical settings. Nutrition and exercise specialists should be part of any primary care team. This was the model I helped develop in the Department of Family Medicine at Eastern Virginia Medical School and at All Saints Health System in Forth Worth, Texas, and one I have implemented in my own medical practice. It helps people, and it can be cost effective.

Let's look at some of the gender-specific issues and needs for women who are making the transformation from overfat to fit and leaner!

Research on Men Doesn't Necessarily Apply to Women!

Since estrogen and progesterone are both involved in regulating metabolism, blood glucose, and body fat storage, you'd think that researchers would have paid more attention to the "female factor" in obesity research. But, once again, most of these investigations have been done on males, assuming that information learned would apply to women as well. If you and your husband or boyfriend have ever gone on a diet at the same time, you have experienced first hand that weight loss is very different in men and women! A few years ago, when we both went on a spa vacation, I watched my husband peel off the pounds, while I struggled to get a *quarter* pound lower on the scale, and he even got to eat more calories than I did! Not fair! From an evolutionary perspective, it makes sense that females would be more efficient at storing (and keeping) body fat, since we are the ones endowed with carrying pregnancies to perpetuate our species. Now we live in a culture that *esteems thinness* and at the same time makes *eating* the predominate social activity and puts "fast food" options on every street corner! What insanity. Our bodies have not had several million years to adapt to the sudden availability of excess food!

Sugar and fat are two examples. I lived in Williamsburg, Virginia, for many years, and I was surprised to learn that in colonial American homes, sugar was such a rare and very expensive "delicacy" that it was often kept under lock and key! Today, we really live "la dolce vita" (the sweet life) when we put sugar in practically everything, even ketchup. Pounds of it, in fact. Today the average American consumes on average 125 pounds of sugar per person per year. That's incredible. Much of the sugar we eat is hidden. It appears in processed foods of all kinds, including soups, condiments, salad dressings, frozen dinners, and the obvious sources: desserts and soft drinks. It's been calculated that the average American eats *24 percent of daily* calories from sugars in various forms, mainly refined sugar (sucrose).

Then comes the FAT. Americans consume, on average, *40 to 43 percent* of daily calories from fat. That means *64 percent* of the calories you eat *every day* come from *fat* and *sugar!* No wonder Americans have more obesity and obesity-related diseases than any other country in the world. Since sugars and fats have no nutritional value except providing energy, that means that most Americans have to get the essential nutrients from only 35 percent of their food intake. It's clear that sugar and fat calories are crowding out the nutritious food groups from our diet. And for women, sugars and fats pack a double-whammy: eating them tends to create a vicious cycle of craving them, and our hormonal changes each month affect not only how our bodies metabolize both sugars and fats but our cravings for them as well. I will talk more about these "vicious cycles" further along in this chapter. But first, some metabolism basics as related to women's bodies.

Fat storage is one of our adaptations to the scarcity and unpredictability of food supplies before humans evolved to cultivate food on a steady basis. Humans who were more efficient at storing body fat were able to better survive the periods of famine. Females in particular needed to be able to effectively store fat in order to survive and to also provide the nourishment to sustain a growing fetus for nine months.

Estrogen helps to regulate blood sugar to keep levels steady, and it also functions to enhance storage of fat around the hips, thighs, and buttocks, which provides "fuel" able to sustain a pregnancy. Progesterone causes increases in appetite and metabolic rate, and alters insulin secretion in a way that *increases cravings* for sweets. This encourages a pregnant woman to eat more, which results in better nourishment for the fetus. Recent research has confirmed what women have always suspected: we get hungrier premenstrually due to hormonal influences! Appetite and metabolic rate increase about 12 to 15 percent in the second half of the menstrual cycle. If you ignore this increase in appetite because you are dieting, you may find that the sweet cravings become uncontrollable, leading to the "binge on sweets, feel guilty, starve again, binge cycle. If you eat fruit and whole grain breads high in complex carbohydrates, you provide the fuel needed to sustain blood glucose through the increase in metabolism but without adding excess fat, which is the main culprit in adding excess pounds.

Compared to men, women also have more of the *lipogenic* enzymes that help the body store fat instead of the *lipolytic* enzymes that break down fat so it can be used as fuel. Many of our female tendencies to gain weight and to crave sweets (instead of meats, which men tend to want) have strong hormonal influences, which as you can see, has an adaptive advantage for our species. Unfortunately, our biochemical makeup just doesn't fit well with our current cultural obsession with women having to be rail-thin to be considered sexy and attractive. It helps to understand these basics so you don't fall into the psychological trap of beating yourself up mentally because of your body size. You can help improve the ratio of lean muscle mass to fat mass by exercising regularly and eating healthy. As you read further, I will explain ways of achieving a better balance in what and when you eat, the difference between body *weight* and body composition, as well as the ways female hormones interact with appetite regulation.

Eating for "Wellness of Being"

I am not perfect. I have been FIT. I have been FAT. I have probably in my lifetime tried almost every diet that came out, until I learned about ten years ago that *diets don't work*. What works, plain and simple, is healthy, low-fat eating and regular exercise. Do I always do it? Not always. I'm just like most of you, too many things to do and too little time to do them. Until 1989 and the last round of surgeries on my neck, followed the next year by my hysterectomy, I had been really diligent about keeping up with exercise and maintaining my healthy body composition. I have to admit, the last few years have been much harder, and the many months of recovery from surgery got me out of my exercise routine so long and contributed to enough weight gain, that I have had a very difficult time reestablishing a consistent exercise program that works as well as what I did in the past.

I really do understand the frustrations and difficulties my patients describe in reaching their goals, since I'm right in there fighting the same battles. I do keep up with aerobic walking several times a week, even though for me it is not as exhilarating as the jogging I did regularly for many years. I also make an effort at work to walk up stairs instead of taking elevators a few floors, and I look for ways to walk more during daily activities. Every little bit helps.

But I will say this: over the last fifteen years, in an effort to better practice what I preach and to be healthier myself, I have made some pretty drastic changes in the way I eat. I have truly eliminated saturated fats. I don't use butter or margarine, or even much vegetable oil anymore. I used to make homemade mayonnaise, I enjoyed it so much. Now I prefer using nonfat yogurt in place of mayonnaise. I have red meat maybe once a month. I cut out colas (even diet ones) and other soft drinks with phosphates. I rarely have any alcohol, maybe three or four glasses of wine *in a month*! (A far cry from the days of William and Mary parties with lots of cocktails flowing!) I have cut out added salt and pick low salt options when I eat out or buy a prepared frozen dinner. I don't snack on sweets regularly like I used to do. I eat more fresh fruit. I eat whole grain bread. I only eat *plain* popcorn, no butter and no salt. I don't go to work without a good breakfast anymore. I make sure I keep up with my skim milk for calcium without the fat of whole milk. I pay attention to taking magnesium supplements and a multivitamin every day. My cholesterol is 136 and my HDL is 75. Taking this inventory really helped me to affirm the positive changes I have made. You might do the same.

Take an honest look at what you eat every day. **Can you find some healthy changes you have already made? Good. Now, (just as I will do) add to your list three or four *new ones*, changes you are ready to make *NOW*.**

Sorting out the Fads

As we baby boomers age, one thing is clear: we are getting fatter. Entrepreneurial types have quickly figured out that there is a huge market here and lots of money to be made with diet products of all types. The hype is everywhere, and there are figures to show we are buying into the hype: Americans spend close to $40 billion annually on diet and diet-related products. The sad part is, 95 percent of people who are buying all these diets will regain the weight. This creates the marketing opportunity of the millennium: selling the same product to the same people over and over again!

Fads in food abound. Fads in diets crop up faster than the weather changes! New diets sell products: books, tapes, flash cards, videos, cookbooks, supplements, special foods, prepared meals, you name it and there will be a product designed to go with the newest "diet-of-the-day." There's a diet to suit every taste and every food craving. High fiber, low fat. High fat, low fiber (for anyone who likes being constipated). High protein, low carbohydrate is in. No, it's out. High carbohydrate, low protein is the way to go. Don't mix protein and carbs at the same meal. Don't mix fruits and vegetables at the same meal. Don't mix protein and fat at the same meal. Don't mix protein and fruits and vegetables at the same meal. Eat grapefruit at each meal to burn fat. Don't eat grapefruit, it will cause acid stomach. It seem like it would be less confusing to just not eat. 1980: Margarine is OK, butter's bad. 1990: Margarine's bad, butter's better. What's a person to do?

How do I make sense of all this? (My suggestion: don't try! It doesn't make sense, *it just sells*). How do I sort out fads from facts and find something that works for me? I will hit the highlights here, but if you want more specific information, I highly recommend the books in the resources section of this chapter. I selected these few really good ones out of the many I have reviewed (of the dozens on the market) because I think these are the best and most relevant to women's needs. Each one is readable, practical, up-to-date, and contains good solid information with a focus on a healthy balance for lifetime living well with food.

Food as Fuel for Your Energy and Zest

"Carbs"—you've heard the term a lot in recent years. It used to be that all the magazines talked about cutting out the "fattening" carbohydrates. It turns out that the "carbs" aren't the bad guys at all, it's been *all the fat* we put on them, the sour cream, butter, oils, and mayonnaise. A plain baked potato has only about 100 calories, and is loaded with fiber, vitamin C, minerals, and lots of energy.

Carbohydrates are the body's primary fuel and are converted into glucose, which is the only fuel the brain can use. If you aren't getting enough carbohydrates in your daily food intake, it leaves you feeling "foggy-brained," because the brain isn't being properly supplied with the fuel it needs to function optimally. Clearly these macronutrients are a crucial element of a plan for "eating well" to maintain your energy throughout the day. Carbohydrates provide 4 calories of energy per gram (half as calorie dense as fat), but they actually require the body to expend more energy to utilize them as a fuel source. Complex carbohydrates—such as whole grains, vegetables, fruits, breads, pasta, cereals—should ideally make up about 55 to 60 percent of your daily food intake, which will provide more fiber, better stability in your blood glucose, and a healthy feeling of fullness so you won't have the desire to overeat.

Proteins provide 4 calories per gram as energy for the body and help keep blood sugar levels steady over several hours, compared to the shorter interval sustained by complex carbohydrates. A healthy balance of protein—about 20 to 25 percent of your daily food intake—is needed for building tissue, repair processes (such as muscle repair needed every day, particularly as you increase your exercise), and maintaining the blood proteins needed for immune function and others. Protein foods—meat, fish, chicken, eggs, cheese—are important elements in eating well, but watch out, since these foods also contain higher amounts of fat compared to carbohydrates. Your goal is to select those protein foods that are lower in fat: lean meats, low-fat cheeses, poultry without the skin, etc. Actually, I find that if I just use the fat content of my protein sources and don't add any more fat to what I eat, I'm generally pretty well on target with the 20 percent fat goal.

You don't need butter or margarine on your grilled cheese sandwich, the cheese has more than adequate fat content on its own! Aiming for a balance of carbohydrate, protein, and fat at each meal provides stability in blood sugar for your brain and body functions. I also recommend having a healthy snack in the late afternoon, about 4 P.M., when blood sugar normally hits the "afternoon slump." This really helps keep you from coming home from work ravenous and eating everything in sight.

Finding the Fat, Cutting It out

One of the easiest ways to reduce total calories if you want to lose weight or to maintain your healthy weight, is to cut out excess fat in your diet. Most people don't realize that **all fats** (whether vegetable oil, butter, margarine, or lard) **have twice as many calories per gram as carbohydrates and protein.** Fat is the most calorie-dense type of food we eat, but high fat foods don't take up space in the intestinal tract like high-fiber foods do, so we often don't realize how *much fat (and calories)* we have eaten! It is dramatic how much *more dietary fat* Americans eat now than was true at the turn of the century:

1900: 28 percent   vs.   1994: 45 percent

You may say to yourself, "but I don't eat much fat, I don't use butter or even margarine anymore." Unfortunately, that's not the primary source of dietary fat for most Americans. It's the *hidden fats* in foods that sabotage our best efforts. The new food labeling will help you detect these hidden fats, but you really have to stay alert to where they are. Watch out for the hidden fats when you eat out: the salad dressing on your salad, the cream sauce on your pasta (marinara is lower in fat), the olive oil for dipping your bread, fish cooked in butter, donuts at the morning coffee break, pizza dripping with cheese and pepperoni, French fries, those big yummy-looking "bran" muffins (there's probably a day's worth of sugar and fat in each one and not much bran!), the sauce glistening on your steamed vegetables, the list goes on and on. It helps to learn where the fats are hidden in various foods and gradually cut back *every day*.

I have included several helps lists and resources in the Appendix to illustrate common culprits for those lurking fat grams. There is also a worksheet for you to determine how many fat grams are needed each day to provide about 20 percent of your calories from fat, depending on your day's total calories. Take time now to do this homework and determine your daily calories and fat grams. Most women haven't the foggiest idea that they consume so much fat every day. It can be quite an eye-opener to count actual fat grams in you foods for a few days. You may find it helpful to buy a small paperback guide to counting fat grams, since there are now several good ones available. As you make these changes, tell yourself all the wonderful things you are doing for your body, now and down the road. You'll also notice you don't feel as sluggish. High-fat diets slow down the gastrointestinal tract motility, contributing to more constipation, distention of the tummy, and feeling generally fat and miserable, especially the second half of the menstrual cycle.

Depending upon the number of calories you need each day for a healthy nutritional balance, this chart gives you the desirable number of fat grams for a 20 percent fat meal plan.

20% Percent Fat Intake Guide		
IF CALORIES/DAY *Should Be:*	FAT CALORIES *Desirable Goal:*	FAT GRAMS *Desirable Goal:*
1200	240	27
1400	280	31
1500	300	33
1600	320	36
1800	360	40
2000	400	44
2200	440	49
2400	480	53
2600	520	58
2800	560	62
3000	600	67

You may ask, why is it important to keep daily fat intake at about 20 percent of daily total calories? Remember, this is the level at which there was a *drop* in the *rates of breast, colon, and possibly ovarian cancer*, as well as marked *decreases* in heart disease, hypertension, and diabetes. So, this 20 percent target for your fat grams has some important reasons for paying attention and working to achieve it.

While I am on the subject of dietary fat, I want to comment about a disturbing trend I have seen in women's health habits as I consult with individual women and speak to groups around the country. I encounter more and more women who tell me they have *cut out dairy products*, especially milk, *for fear of the fat* content. What do they replace milk with? Typically, it's soft drinks, whether regular or sugar-free and caffeine-free. Whatever type, they pose unique problems for women who want to be healthy and maintain optimal body composition and bone density.

All soft drinks contain high levels of phosphates, which attach to the calcium ions in the digestive tract and increase the loss of calcium from the body. Calcium then moves from the bones to maintain adequate blood calcium, needed for normal nerve and muscle function. So the more soft drinks you consume, the more calcium you lose. Regular soft drinks not only leach calcium from your bones, they are also loaded with sugar. A twelve-ounce non-diet soft drink contains about seven to eight teaspoons of sugar. This becomes a real problem when you drink five or six sugared sodas a day, because you end up with almost *half* your total daily calories coming from a source *without any nutritional value*! Think about it. Low-fat milk has about the same *calorie content* as a regular soda, *and it provides much needed calcium.*

Body Weight versus Body Composition

Most women I talk with are absolutely obsessed with the scale and what they *weigh*. Body weight has become the number one statistic women talk about, certainly in large part due to the cultural brainwashing that to be thin is to be desirable and acceptable as a woman. I want to emphasize that we really should be looking at body **composition** rather than body **weight**.

Body weight can vary immensely depending upon how much muscle mass you have built up and what your body build is. Someone who has a heavier bone density, for example, and more lean body mass may weigh twenty-five pounds more than a smaller boned person who has not been exercising, and yet both could have the same percent body fat. A patient of mine now is a young petite, thin woman (size 4) who is sedentary, and she has *34 percent body fat*. According to the current guidelines, she is in an unhealthy "at risk" range. Another patient, who is stockier in appearance and is a size 14, but exercises regularly, has *25 percent body fat* and is in a very healthy range.

The way to really determine an optimal weight for you is to have a body composition done, which will measure the percent body fat. For women the optimal ranges are between 20 percent to

30 percent body fat. The "at risk" range is greater than 33 percent. If you're over age thirty and you're trying to get down below twenty percent body fat, you really do increase your risk of osteoporosis. This is because you're losing enough body fat to lose some of the natural estrogen that's present in body fat tissue, and you begin to actually have some negative effect on your overall health.

Research at the Cooper Clinic, from the National College of Sports Medicine, and other investigators studying optimal healthy ranges, has found that when women get too low on percent body fat, they stop menstruating normally, have declining hormonal production, and begin to lose bone more rapidly. I really strongly encouraging women not to go below the 20 percent body fat level. Actually, if you get down *below about 15 percent*, you lose menses. That's when women become even *more at risk for osteoporosis*.

Those of you on a weight-loss regimen, and who are exercising several times a week, should focus on body measurements once a month, and not be obsessed with body *weight*. Your weight is not going to be an accurate indicator of the loss of fat tissue (which weighs about 1/6 as much as muscle tissue). It is much more accurate, and helpful, to focus on how your body is changing in the way of inches. This gives you a much better picture of the amount of *fat loss*. As you exercise you *increase* the *lean body mass*, so by only using weight measurement you won't realize that you're losing "lightweight" body *fat* as you build up *heavier muscle mass*. I usually recommend to women that they take their body measurements about once a month, and try not to weigh on the scale any more than once every other week. Focus on what's happening to the health of your body, not on the number of pounds! You can go tomorrow to your local health club and have your body fat percentage measured! Throw the scale away, buy a tape measure and use it once a month to check your progress.

Vicious Cycles: Food Cravings and the Menstrual Cycle

Over my years of clinical practice, I would say that about 75 to 85 percent of women patients have described cyclic food cravings that are clearly related to the second half of the menstrual cycle. And these cravings are the kind of intense urges which override rational awareness that junk foods aren't healthy! Women have even described going out late in the evening to a store to buy chocolate (or something salty or whatever) because the craving was so strong. I have to admit, I did that myself on occasion when the premenstrual "have-to-have-chocolate" urges hit! Why is this? And why is it that I have *never* had a *male* patient describe cravings for **chocolate** the way women do. Yes, I have had male (and female) patients who were alcoholic describe cravings for alcohol, but I see that as a different physiological issue and mechanism.

I think there is a key *hormonal* factor which affects women and contributes to these cravings: *the rise and fall in progesterone during the second half of the menstrual cycle.* How does this work? Progesterone alters the normal insulin response, which regulates blood glucose ("sugar" levels in the blood). Women then experience a greater tendency to have lower blood glucose levels, and more episodes of "reactive" drop in blood glucose following food intake, especially if the food intake is primarily sweets or other simple sugars. This tends to set up the vicious cycles that I have drawn in the diagrams below. Take a look at **"The Vicious Cycle"** and **"Another Vicious Cycle"** and see if you recognize yourself! Then read on about what is happening as your body cycles hormonally each month.

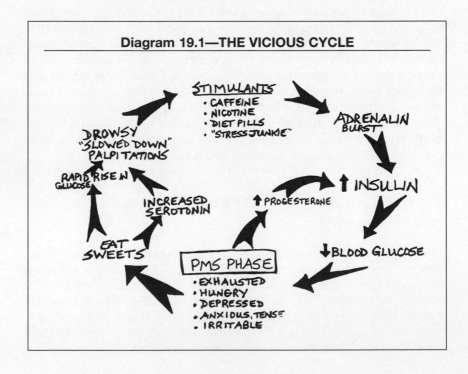

Diagram 19.1—THE VICIOUS CYCLE

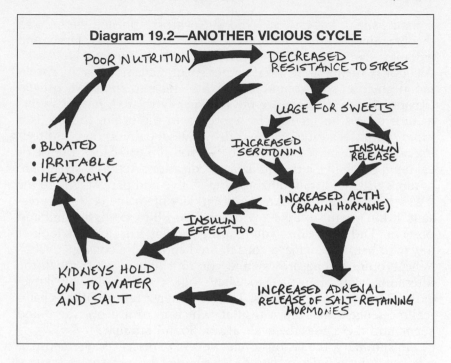

Diagram 19.2—ANOTHER VICIOUS CYCLE

Not too long ago, I came across a newspaper notice in bold letters, like this:

> **THE NUMBER ONE**
> **CAUSE OF**
> **KITCHEN DEATHS**
> **IS EATING AN**
> **ENTIRE TUBE OF**
> **CHOCOLATE CHIP**
> **COOKIE DOUGH . . .**
> **RAW!**

I howled with laughter at this. And so do audiences of women when I give a talk and show this slide. Most of us who have ever craved chocolate can relate to this, especially premenstrually!

Do any of you have cravings for chocolate premenstrually? I know I certainly have lived with that for a lot of years. Chocolate contains sugar, fat, and the "mood-elevators" phenethylmine and theobromine. When you are feeling exhausted, hungry, tense, and irritable, one thing that's quick and easy to turn to is *sweets*. Alcohol is metabolized as a simple sugar, causing a rapid rise in blood glucose, so alcohol cravings also tie into the premenstrual cravings for sweets that are physiologically related. Eating sweets in turn causes an increase in serotonin in the brain. If there is a *rapid* rise in serotonin, it causes drowsiness, palpitations, and feeling nervous. A more *gradual* rise in serotonin can cause a sense of calming, much like a tranquilizing medication. Actually, sweets are nature's original "tranquilizing drugs." I've had patients say to me "Well I don't want to take an antianxiety medicine or antidepressant. I don't want to take any drugs." So I'll turn this around and observe "Did you realize you're using *food* as a drug? Let's look at a way to help you achieve your desired ends more constructively," When you're feeling drowsy and you're trying to get through the afternoon, you often turn to what's quick and readily available: caffeine, nicotine, and sweets. These all trigger release of the chemical messengers that affect insulin, which in turn drops the blood sugar, and there goes the cycle again. Sound familiar?

In summary, the **vicious cycles** you've experienced premenstrually are *physiologically based, aggravated* by external stressors, and *intensified* by the wrong food choices and **lack of exercise**. Then we get into the vicious cycle of poor nutrition, which in turn affects our body's resistance to stress, which in turn increases our craving for sweets, which affects the serotonin and insulin levels, which in turn affects one of the brain hormones that regulates fluid balance. So there's more fluid retention, which is also an effect of insulin; the kidney holds onto water and salt; and you feel bloated, headachy, and irritable. Sound familiar?

Perhaps you are now seeing some places in the "vicious cycle" where you can make a *choice* for types of food or exercise that will *break the cycle*, not intensify it. But, if you *don't know* the vicious cycle is there, and how it works, then you can't deal with it constructively. That's my fundamental message: knowledge of what is happening gives you the power to make new and healthy choices. Be aware that when you're feeling bloated, irritable, and headachy, you don't feel like going out to exercise, yet *that's the very time you need it the most*. You also don't feel like fixing or eating a nice balanced meal with lots of steamed vegetables, but again, that's exactly what you need. **You have the power to perpetuate the vicious cycle or break it!**

It has been described since the 1930s, and perhaps even earlier, that women have altered glucose regulation in the luteal (progesterone-dominant) phase of the menstrual cycle. There are many complex metabolic effects of the hormonal shifts and complicated interactions of the various neuroendocrine "regulator messengers," that control body weight, fluid balance, appetite, food cravings, and other functions. In this discussion, I have presented a *very simplified* overview of some of the key factors. There are a number of good books, particularly those by Wayne Callaway, M.D., and by Debra Waterhouse, M.P.H., R.D., which go into more detail on these metabolic influences for women. I encourage you to read those.

I have for many years been interested in the connections between physiological changes such as blood glucose, and hormones, and so on, and the kinds of physical and behavioral responses that such physiological fluctuations can trigger. I have done five-hour (and sometimes six-hour) glucose tolerance tests (GTT) on many women with PMS during the past twelve years, and have found a strikingly consistent pattern of an abnormal response to glucose *if this testing is done in the mid to late phase of the second half (luteal phase) of the menstrual cycle.* Many doctors have said to my patients "You don't need to do glucose tolerance tests, we don't do those anymore to diagnose diabetes," or "It doesn't matter when in your cycle you do a glucose tolerance test, it's all the same."

Well, I disagree with both aspects. First of all, I am not simply looking for diabetes, I am looking for objective laboratory data to show changes in glucose levels which correlate with my patients' mood swings and physical symptoms and which could help explain the pattern of food cravings. Second, it is clear from *listening* to the patients that there is a definite *cycle-specific* characteristic to these cravings, and If I don't do the testing at the time when the women have the cravings, then how will I discover potential physical and hormonal factors involved in triggering these cravings?

Physiologically, the luteal phase of the cycle is when the hormone shifts have the most dramatic impact on the insulin-glucose regulations. If a glucose tolerance test is going to be done *in a female patient*, it is crucial to do it at the right time of her menstrual cycle to get the right information. The GTT should be done three to five days before the period is due. Timing of the GTT with the late luteal phase allows the best opportunity to pick up the way in which the hormonal shifts affect blood glucose regulation. This in turn helps me to individualize a dietary approach for that person, specifically *when* food is eaten and the *balance* of carbohydrate, fat, and protein that will best help that person.

If any of you have ever had a GTT to test for either diabetes or hypoglycemia, you know that patients usually go to the laboratory for the testing. No one except the laboratory technician observes the patient, and then the results (as numbers) are sent to the physician. Typically the physician looks at the individual numbers for each hour of the test, and if the numbers fall into the "normal" range, the patient is told "everything's normal" regardless of how the patient may have felt during the test. Most patients are never asked if they had any symptoms during the GTT! It seemed to me that this process overlooked the most crucial information: what the patient had to say!

I developed a different way of studying this when I first joined the faculty at Eastern Virginia Medical School (EVMS) in 1983 and have been using this method since that time in evaluation of women with these types of problems. I have the patient come to the office for the GTT, and she (occasionally it has been appropriate to do this for men, too) is shown how to keep a timed symptom log of everything she experiences throughout the test. My staff also makes written observations of the patient during the test and frequently also does a short cognitive assessment (to check memory, attention, concentration, etc.) at each blood draw. These combined objective and subjective observations are kept in the medical record and are reviewed in detail at the follow-up appointment when the "number" results are also discussed. This integration allows both the patient and me to correlate her pattern of body changes with the actual fluctuations in her blood glucose levels. It has been remarkable what has emerged from this approach, both in terms of hidden problems being properly identified, and in terms of the patient learning how her body responds, what's contributing to the sensations she experiences, and what to do to constructively correct the problem. Nine times out of ten, this process leads to the correct dietary modifications needed to turn things around. It gives the patient, and the nutritionist, important data to take into account in meal/snack planning. My approach is fairly basic in concept: observe the patient, listen to what she says, pay attention to body physiology and hormonal effects, and figure out how to put it together into a cohesive whole.

There is also another whole dimension to the way hormonal changes in women affect insulin regulation, which makes the syndrome of **insulin resistance** much more common in women, especially as they grow older. *Insulin resistance* refers to the phenomenon of having high levels of both circulating insulin *and glucose* in the bloodstream, but the insulin molecules can't bind properly to the insulin receptor sites on the surface of the cell to allow glucose to enter the cell and be used for energy.

This occurs when women (and men) gain weight; the fat cells become distorted in shape with increased fat storage, and the "lock" or receptor site for insulin is "warped" out of proper alignment, so the insulin molecule "key" no longer fits in the receptor. Insulin resistance makes it harder to lose weight, since the cells are not getting enough "fuel," you continually perceive you are hungry even though there is plenty of fuel circulating in the bloodstream. It also causes rising blood pressure and problems with "reactive hypoglycemia" (low blood sugar) when the excess insulin suddenly works, glucose rushes into the cells, and your blood glucose plummets. This sequence creates intense sweet cravings, and the whole cycle starts over; you get fatter, become more insulin resistant, and so on.

Such marked glucose swings contribute to feeling lethargic, sleepy, and having trouble concentrating when the glucose levels are rising, and then feeling sweaty, anxious, irritable, or weepy when the glucose levels are falling quickly. You may notice significant changes in how you feel and function relative to the time since your last meal or what types of food you eat. Insulin resistance is one of the "deadly four" that increase heart disease and diabetes, along with truncal obesity (waist area instead of hips), high blood pressure, and high cholesterol/triglycerides. When doing a GTT it is a simple matter to test for insulin resistance by checking insulin levels each time a glucose level is drawn. The GTT is more expensive when the insulin levels are added; yet, if the insulin resistance risk factors are there, I think it is important to do. Evaluating such an important risk factor in a systematic way, timed with the menstrual cycle, allows for early identification of women for whom this is blocking progress in weight loss and adding to the likelihood of developing diabetes and heart disease.

Moving the Body in Spite of Limitations

I have to be candid. There really are very few people who are so physically limited that they cannot exercise at all. With creativity, and guidance from physical therapists or trained exercise specialists, I have been impressed that there's exercise appropriate for (almost) everyone. Even when I was in a neck brace and could only walk about ten yards, the physical therapist gave me two ways of exercising aerobically to begin regaining my strength and stamina. Take a look at the picture.

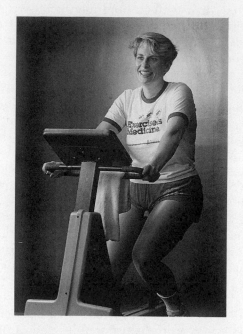

I have to admit, I made a pretty ridiculous sight, **but it worked!** The other exercise my physical therapist suggested was treading water, and I wore my neck brace in the water. Listening to music helped to stave off the boredom and keep up the pace. When I started out, I didn't have the stamina to last more than a few minutes. By the third week, I had progressed to being able to tread water for forty-five minutes, and I had made great gains in my leg, back, and arm strength. This experience was humbling, since I had been quite a swimmer in the past. It was at first very discouraging to find I didn't have the strength to do more than a few minutes in the water. But what a sense of accomplishment when I had built up my endurance! I continue to enjoy swimming and treading water for exercise, yet I have to admit I often find that it's easy to let my schedule demands keep me from getting in the pool as often as I know is healthy for me to do. Each of us needs to find ways to increase body movement in all of our daily activities, particularly if the "exercise workouts" may only be three times a week.

I sincerely feel that if you have never exercised regularly in your life, there is *nothing* better you can do for yourself that will boost your self-esteem and pride in accomplishment as much as seeing the progress you can make once you start and keep at it. In addition to making you feel good about yourself, exercise, even simple walking, is the one wellness activity you can do that has so many profound effects on your total brain-body health and can prevent so many chronic, debilitating conditions and diseases. I have learned a great deal about the role of exercise in health through my own back surgeries and rehabilitations. I still miss the exhilaration I felt running, but I am grateful to have the strength and movement back that I have regained through exercise as a major part of each recovery process. I have included some excellent resource books on exercise in the Appendix. You may also find it worthwhile and very helpful at the beginning to hire a personal trainer to get you started and keep you on the right track for a month until your new exercise habits are well estrablished and you know how to do the exercises properly.

Osteoporosis: A Case for Preventive Medicine

Osteoporosis is a disease that begins many years before actual menopause, and can be largely prevented with proper attention to what you eat, what type of exercise you do consistently, and checking with your physician to evaluate hormonal status. Osteoporosis occurs when bone becomes more porous, or soft, through loss of the normal bone spicules and cross-links which provide its structure and strength. In your home, this would be analogous to termites eating away at the foundation, even though the house (i.e., your body) may look fine on the outside. The problem with both termites in your house, and bone loss in your body, is that these are **silent** until there has been structural damage, and areas collapse (or fracture). I find women are far more fearful of breast cancer, even though osteoporosis is much more common. Your lifetime chances of having a hip fracture are greater than your chances of breast, uterine, cervical, or ovarian cancers combined!

Potential consequences of osteoporosis can be devastating. We do not have any way that biotechnological medicine can fix the bones once the collapse and breakage process has begun. Hip fracture is not a simple thing. If we look at the number of hip fractures in this country on an annual basis, the cost to society, in actual dollars, and in individual pain and suffering, is staggering. Dollar estimates run between 7 and 10 BILLION dollars annually.

Osteoporosis has an enormous adverse impact on the mobility and independence of older women and it is one of the most common reasons that older women end up having to go into a nursing home. Even more tragic is that up to twenty percent of women *die* within three months of a hip fracture due to the complications. So, although you hear "just get a hip replacement" bandied about rather lightly, it's not that simple. Surgery this major requires a long and frequently painful recovery, along with hard work to regain your mobility. If there is significant bone loss, it makes some of the treatment avenues rather limited, since hip replacements can't even be done unless there is healthy bone to support the prosthesis attachment. Now you see why I am concerned that we need to help more women be aware of the preventable nature of this disease.

My goal is to help women understand, and implement, ways of keeping bone loss from starting and then look at ways to help maintain adequate bone density so that you're not in the position of needing to be fixed. Bone loss occurs even before menopause in women with risk factors such as:

- cigarette smoking (smokers also become menopausal 5 to 7 years sooner than nonsmokers).
- daily and/or regular alcohol intake
- heavy caffeine intake (coffee, tea, soft drinks, etc.)
- chronic dieting, anorexia, and/or bulimia
- poor calcium and magnesium intake (the average woman in the U.S. gets only about a third of the needed calcium in her diet, and less than a third of the necessary magnesium each day).
- diet high in phosphates, which bind calcium and carry it out of the body (the biggest source for American women is *soft drinks*).
- genetic factors: ethnic group (Black women typically have denser bones than Caucasian or Asian women), family history of mother, sister, or grandmothers with osteoporosis and/or early menopause.
- missing menstrual periods longer than six months at any time after puberty (except when pregnant).

I have been disturbed by the increasing numbers of young women who already have the beginnings of osteoporosis due to anorexia or chronic dieting which has stopped their normal menstruation. These young women don't develop peak bone mass and so will reach menopause at even greater risk.

Significant and sustained life stresses add to early decrease in ovarian hormone levels, which in turn contribute to earlier bone loss *before* your periods stop. Our female hormones play a critical role in bone growth; they deposit proper minerals into the skeleton for strength and keep the bone breakdown process from overcoming new bone formation. Estrogen helps absorb dietary calcium and magnesium from the intestinal tract and deposits these minerals into bone. Estrogen "primes" certain bone cells to respond to progesterone and stimulate new bone formation, while also helping to block the process of bone breakdown.

Progesterone helps stimulate new bone growth if there is adequate estrogen present. Testosterone stimulates new bone growth, increases bone density, and enhances bone strength. You may not need to add hormones from an *outside* source to have enough circulating hormones to prevent bone loss. The problem is, you won't know whether you need supplemental hormones or not until you measure bone density and hormone status.

It is important to keep in mind that worldwide research over the last three decades has clearly shown that there is much less bone loss in the women who are taking estrogen after menopause. We now have additional research to show that the threshold blood level for estradiol to prevent bone loss is about 60 pg/ml (less than half the average levels of the normal menstrual cycle), which is higher than doctors have previously been taught is needed for postmenopausal women. This is another reason the blood level is so important for you to know.

Women on ERT have significantly greater bone density at all ages after menopause, even compared with women who exercise and consume adequate calcium. Recent studies have definitely shown that the **combination** of hormones *plus* calcium-magnesium supplements *plus* exercise has a greater bone protective effect than either calcium alone, exercise alone, or exercise and calcium without hormone therapy. In women with marked bone loss, adding testosterone and possibly progesterone provides even greater benefit.

How do you tell if you are losing bone? There is no *reliable* measure of bone loss other than having a test of bone mineral density. Knowing your risk factors helps, but even taking into account the best risk factor assessment, doctors can still only identify about 30 percent of the women who are actually losing bone. That means if we *just go by risk factors, we miss 70 percent of women with bone loss*.

And there really are not many observable symptoms of bone loss before a fracture occurs. The earliest change *you* can measure is a loss of height. With loss of bone in the vertebrae of the spine, the vertebrae collapse onto each other resulting in diminished height and increased spinal curvature. Women not on hormone therapy lose an average of two and a half inches of height over the years after menopause. A loss of more than 1/4 inch in height is considered a reliable sign of spinal bone loss. At the time of your annual physical exam make sure that the nurse *measures* your height (don't just tell the staff what you think or wish your height is!) and then tells you what it is, so you know whether it's changing. Always make sure the nurse tells you your height and blood pressure. Most women are more concerned about their body weight, which is less of a health risk than what's happening to their height and blood pressure. I encourage you to keep track of these various health measures, and write them down so you can compare the results of what is happening to your body each year.

Another indicator of possible bone loss is urinary calcium excretion. If you want to know whether or not you're in a negative calcium balance, you can ask your physician to do a twenty-four-hour urine test for calcium excretion. There are two things I look at with this test: (1) if the urinary calcium is very low, it tells me you're not absorbing calcium very well and may need additional calcium in the diet, a better estrogen balance, or additional tests to find out why the calcium isn't being absorbed properly; and (2) if the urinary calcium is very high, it tells me you are excreting more than you are absorbing, which typically occurs in women who are too low in their body estrogen.

Dual energy X-ray absorptiometry (DEXA) is an extrememly helpful and simple way to reliably measure your actural bone mineral content, but I think we are waiting too late in life when these tests are done at menopause or afterwards. I recommend that women have measurements of *bone mineral density* by age 35 to 40, or earlier if you have many risk factors. DEXA only takes a few minutes to do, is less expensive, and uses less radiation than CAT scans of bone density. Three companies make the DEXA equipment and it is now more widely available at hospitals and osteoporosis centers around the country. If bone density testing is done at a younger age, we have a crucial "window of opportunity" for a premenopausal woman to help her decide what steps she must take to reduce further bone loss. It is not enough just to say "take hormones." If a woman is losing significant bone before menopause, she will probably need hormones *plus "anti-resorptive" medications* such as etidronate (Didronel) or the new one now being used in Italy and Mexico called alendronate (Fosamax) to prevent bone breakdown. The types of approaches needed for you as an individual woman will be determined by the results of your present bone density, risk factors, and your homone levels.

You may have to be assertive about getting a bone density test done. I have had patients tell me they asked for it, and were told "you don't need it, you're too young, and you look healthy." I emphasize again: You cannot tell a woman's bone density by how she looks, any more than you can see termite damage in a house by only looking at the outside. Some insurance plans still don't cover this important test for women. You may have to bite the bullet and pay out of pocket so you can have the information to guide you in your health management decisions. It is an important investment in your good health for the future.

We read and hear a lot about the role of **calcium** in maintaining bone. The sad part is that with as much emphasis as there has been on calcium in this country, the average calcium intake for women is still only 450 milligrams a day. The recommended amount for premenopausal women is 1000 to 1200 mg daily, and for post-menopausal women not on estrogen, 1500 mg daily. Women have decreased their consumption of dairy products in an attempt to lose weight, and their dietary calcium intake has decreased. At an average of 450 mg daily, we are far off the mark. We have not paid enough attention to the importance of magnesium in the diet; another mineral crucially important to bone growth and maintenance of healthy bone. The average American woman only gets about 100 to 200 mg a day of magnesium from her diet, and the RDA for magnesium is 400 to 600 mg daily. The 2:1 ratio of calcium intake to magnesium intake is important for proper body balance.

Magnesium is a also a critical mineral for nerve cell conduction, muscle contraction, and it has a strong independent role in regulating blood pressure. It appears to be an important factor in preventing heart attacks, probably because it helps prevent spasms of the blood vessels throughout the body but especially in the coronary (heart) arteries. Magnesium also helps maintain normal structure and contraction strength of the heart muscle itself. In the brain, magnesium is a cofactor in the production of the important mood-regulating chemical messengers such as dopamine. It is thought to be an important mineral in helping to prevent, and possibly relieve, such mood changes as those that occur with PMS and milder forms of depression. I urge my patients (and I do it myself) to take 200 to 250 mg of magnesium supplement *every morning* and 200 to 250 mg *every evening*. Taking magnesium and calcium two times a day provides better absorption and more even levels throughout the twenty-four hours.

It is never too late to start exercising: significant improvements in aerobic power, muscle endurance, and bone density have been demonstrated in women over age seventy with exercise therapy. One study evaluated women in nursing homes with an average age of eighty-one. Remember, I said at the beginning of this section that almost anyone could do, and benefit from, an exercise program. The study participants were taught to do various exercises involving a chair; this increased their midshaft bone mineral density in the exercise group by close to 2.5 percent. Those who did not exercise continued to lose bone density. Exercise is a major component of maintaining adequate bone mineral density. Make sure that you have weight bearing and strength training exercise. It is the resistance across the joint, pulling on the bone, along with the impact of weight-bearing exercise, that helps to increase bone formation.

Studies have demonstrated that significant improvements in bone mass accrual, lean body mass, aerobic power, glucose tolerance, and mental well-being occur among postmenopausal women who exercise. Studies of the effect of exercise in humans have shown that exercise leads to higher blood concentrations of catecholamines and beta-endorphins, which are believed to contribute to mood elevation. Thus, regular physical exercise may help to prevent or reduce many physical and emotional symptoms that affect climacteric women. Newly reported data suggests that there also appears to be a lower incidence of cancer among physically fit women. I have been doing individualized exercise prescriptions for my patients for the last decade or more, and they are some of the most important prescriptions I give my patients! I agree with Morris Notelovitz, M.D., Ph.D. of the Women's Medical and Diagnostic Center and The Climacteric Clinic, Gainesville, Fla., who has said "physicians need to prescribe exercise just like ERT. The physical and mental health of climacteric women can be enhanced by prescribing aerobic and muscle-strengthening exercises with, or without, hormone replacement."

In summary, osteoporosis prevention is like a three legged stool, which needs all three "legs" for balance and stability: (1) Adequate calcium/magnesium, (2) adequate weight-bearing (low to moderate impact) exercise, and (3) being hormonally complete. If any one of these "legs" is missing or wobbly, balance and stability is compromised or lost. I've had a number of women who have said, "I really prefer not to take estrogen. I'd like to monitor this and see whether or not my fitness and my diet and my calcium and all of those things are taking care of my health and my bone mineral density." That's fine. Just do it from the standpoint of knowing what your bone density is *now* by having the objective measure of the dual energy X-ray absorptiometry, and then recheck it in a year or two to be sure you are maintaining the desired bone density.

One woman that I was following over a period of a couple of years had lost 10 percent of her bone density in spite of her very healthy lifestyle. So in giving her that information, I just said, "you might want to rethink your decision in light of this new information. Or certainly make sure you recheck the bone density in another year and if the negative trend is continuing you may want to rethink your decision about estrogen." I find that having the definitive information on bone density is the *single most important* piece of data that can help women make the important decision about adding, or not adding, hormone supplements to exercise and dietary approaches.

For women who have already lost bone, another treatment option is the use of medications called *anti-resorptive agents*. Etidronate (Didronel) has been available in the U.S. for Paget's disease. It is given in three-month cycles to halt further bone loss. A number of my patients taking Didronel have actually shown modest *increases* in bone density. Its use has been somewhat limited by the fact that it must be monitored carefully, can only be given for two weeks at one time before taking a "drug-free" interval of three months, and has a lot of side effects.

Alendronate (Fosamax), which was discovered in Italy, is a promising new drug for prevention and treatment of osteoporosis. Alendronate inhibits bone resorption (breakdown), which reduces the effects of estrogen loss on the skeleton and results in increased bone mass and bone strength. Recent studies from Australia showed that women receiving 10mg daily of alendronate for three years increased their bone density at the lumbar spine by an average of 6.8 percent, while women on placebo had an average *decrease* in bone density of 0.6 percent. The women in the study who received active drug (alendronate) showed an average of about 6 percent increase in bone density at the hip sites as well, which is exciting news for women at high risk of hip fracture. The new bone formed at the hip and spine sites was normal quality and well-mineralized, an improvement over previous treatments for osteoporosis. Women receiving only placebo continued to lose bone at the hip sites. Alendronate produced few side effects in the studies to date and can be taken daily rather than in the "on-off" cycles needed with etidronate. I hope this medication will be approved by the FDA for use in the United States soon. It is already being successfully used in Italy, Australia, and Mexico.

I am seriously concerned about the current spate of misleading advertisements and articles that suggest that low dose progesterone skin creams *alone* are enough to protect you from bone loss. They are not. You are gambling with an irreversible health problem if you ignore the overwhelming, well-documented studies that demonstrate estrogen's role in bone preservation. I think it is crucial that we get a more balanced picture across to women. This business of accusing physicians of "medicalizing" menopause is hogwash, in my opinion. The reality is that the very medical research women have been asking for, and deserve, has overwhelmingly demonstrated the *physiological reality* of the profound consequences to women with many years of estrogen loss.

Call it what you like: medicalization, physiology, or whatever; what *cannot be ignored* is that *bone loss is real*, and it *accelerates rapidly as estrogen declines*. I feel that one of the real tragedies is that osteoporosis is potentially so preventable, yet 80 percent or more of postmenopausal women aren't getting the message about the importance of maintaining a normal balance of the hormones that maintain bone. In this country still only about 15 percent of the postmenopausal women who might benefit from it are getting any estrogen replacement therapy. The problem is there's been so much negative information that the resulting imbalance in the press has frightened women away from options with hormones that might help them reduce their risk of bone loss and later debilitation.

I still believe that with careful attention to diet, exercise, calcium and magnesium supplements, and hormonal balance, we can do a lot more to help pre-menopausal women prevent bone loss which increases the risk of fractures in later life. For women who have already lost significant amounts of bone mass, these new treatment options offer a lot of hope for halting the progression of this debilitating illness. Ultimately, the decision about *which* approaches to use is up to the individual woman. I urge you to make your choices from a basis of knowledge, not fear! Most important: just do something postive to protect your bones.

As Will Rogers said, "Even if you are on the right track, you will get run over if you just sit there!"

CHAPTER 20

Take Charge! A Woman's Guide to Optimal Health and Well-Being

I first used this title for a talk on women's health in 1985, and it summarizes the process I have described throughout this book. In previous chapters, I have talked about the importance of caring for the physical aspects of your health: knowing your height, blood pressure, cholesterol/HDL, body composition, hormone levels; taking time to provide your body with healthy fuel; taking time to move the body in exercise; having the appropriate preventive medicine check-ups and screening tests. All of these steps are basic to healthy aging. I have focused primarily on the overlooked hormonal connections in women's health because there is so little integrated information available for women to find answers to their questions. I do not want to suggest, however, that your *physical* health is the only dimension I think is important.

I have a profound belief in, and respect for, the power of the mind and spirit in all aspects of health, disease, and the healing process. Indeed, these dimensions may be the most critical of all as we seek the *wellness of being* that is at the core of our human quest, instead of the cultural emphasis on *doing and achieving*.

I want to share with you some of my thoughts on these aspects of health. And, as a dragonfly skitters over a pond, I recognize that I am just touching on the surface of these dimensions. There are many beautiful and inspiring books that are available to guide you to greater depth on these subjects. I encourage you to seek out the ones that call to your heart and soul as you travel further on your journey of self-exploration and spiritual growth.

Quiet Time: Reflection, Journaling, Meditation

*Getting to know yourself takes **time** being with yourself!*

This statement seems so obvious, and yet how often do we as women take the time to do it? We are giving to others day in and day out—as the twenty-four hour a day mother, the attentive wife, the dutiful daughter, the dedicated community volunteer, the care-taker of the ill, the teacher of children at home-school-church-synagogue-day care, the political activist. No matter what your particular roles, if you stop to count them all, you will discover (sometimes with amazement) they are many.

Women are constantly "switching hats" as our multiple roles require that we dip into diverse areas of skills-insights-wisdom when new demands emerge. A man may have one primary career focus for his entire life. Women typically have several. I know you have heard these ideas and observations before. So when are you going to do something for *you*? Janis Joplin said, not long before she died of a drug overdose: *"Don't compromise yourself. You are all you've got."*

Do you really know who YOU are and what you want for yourself out of life? Have you looked within to find out? If not, when do you plan to do it? Why not take time *right now* to write down the first six things that come immediately to mind as you read the following:

If you were told you had four months to live, what do you most want to accomplish in that time? How do you want to spend those days?

Only you can see that you begin **now** to make time in your life for those meaningful activities or ways of being that you just wrote down.

Start some form of journal to give voice to this *inner you*. She deserves your time too! Use whatever form is helpful and useful to you: write down your thoughts and feelings; if you don't like to write, make a collage of your feelings by gathering images and words that "speak" to you from magazines and pasting them on a piece of paper with the date; collect quotes and jot down how they affect you; use crayons and "doodles" to express your mood and feelings; write a song, poem, or story. Use your imagination! What's important is that the spontaneous part of you has some time set aside for your *undivided* attention! Clarissa Estes, Ph.D.

calls this part of us the "Wild Woman," and says *"Wild woman whispers the words and ways to us and we follow."*

.... FIRST, WE MUST <u>LISTEN</u> TO HER WHISPERS. SHE is the voice within you *Screaming to be HEARD! Give her a commitment of some of your time to listen..................just L—-I—-S—T—-E—-N..........listen.*

Food for the Soul—Women's Spiritual Needs

In the 6th century B.C. Pythagorus described the physician's task: "The physician's task is to teach men and women the *physical and spiritual* laws of life and to live in accordance with God's purpose for them." In the ancient healing arts of all cultures and in the tradition of the physician as "healer," the person who practices the art and science of medicine, the emphasis has traditionally been on the *whole person*. This included addressing spiritual needs as well as physical and emotional needs. Healing traditions through the centuries have also encompassed healthy lifestyle approaches in treating physical illness and emotional-spiritual pain.

Alexis Guirdham, Nobel prize winner, said *"We cannot fragment our healing efforts by declaring them spiritual or medical, but recognize that only the total synchronizing process of healing, for the goal is wholeness and harmony."*

I think for us as women, this statement has a particularly powerful message, since many of us live our lives in a medical model and culture that tends to fragment us into body parts and different roles. With such fragmentation and increasing high-tech (and often impersonal) approaches to *medical* care, women seeking *health care* (caring) are turning in droves to alternative practitioners. They typically emphasize time for communication; self-empowerment; healing approaches that are seen as more natural, more gentle, and more "high-touch;" and create a better feeling of being "listened to" *and heard* in person-to-person encounters. Many women have expressed a desire to have health care approaches that address them as a "whole" person, not just body parts.

We must take into account the role of the spiritual nature of human beings as an important dimension of healing. In using the term "spiritual" I am not referring to a person's religion. To me, one's spiritual connection with life and this universe is a personal, deeply held individual experience. It is having a sense of meaning and purpose to your life. Religion, in my view, refers to being a part of an organized group with a defined set of core beliefs. You may be deeply spiritual, yet not belong to an organized religion. I have also encountered people who are very active in their religion who are not particularly spiritual. Clearly, there are people who are both, and people who are neither. I think the unheard cries of the soul, however we may define them, are a critical dimension of the pain present in the lives of many women and men today.

I find that the more I ask patients about the role of faith in their lives, the more I hear stories of the pain from feeling a void in their spiritual lives, a sense of emptiness and meaninglessness. This has such a profound impact on one's overall health. I was taught in my formal medical training that physicians should not discuss these issues with patients, but I have found over the years that many patients who are in spiritual pain have no one else with whom they can discuss their concerns. These are frequently patients who have been traumatized by earlier church experiences or have not had a particular religious focus in their life experience. More often than not, they have been grateful that I asked about this dimension of their lives.

I find this especially true for women. Many traditional religious institutions have left women feeling invisible because of the patriarchal emphasis on God and His earthly representatives as male. I grew up attending the Presbyterian Church. I never realized how much I had been affected by not seeing women as role models in the worship services of the church until as an adult I went to a Presbyterian church in Norfolk that had a woman associate pastor.

For the first time in my life, I heard a woman minister give the sermon and watched *women* elders serving communion. I was truly overcome with emotion as the impact of women being part of the service hit me fully. Here I was almost forty years old, and this was the first time in my life I had seen women in these roles! What kind of subtle, and not-so-subtle, messages have we given little girls all these years about their worth, when all they see are boys and men participating in the services and hear God always referred to as male. The soul pain with this realization was immense. I was not prepared for the impact I felt sitting in that service and listening to The Rev. Katherine Cameron present the lessons through the eyes and experiences of a woman.

Women have not always been so invisible in religions of the world. Cultures we have called "primitive" have long included the feminine qualities of the Creator as being an important dimension of balance and harmony. The ancient Chinese philosophy of Yin and Yang reflects this blend of the masculine and feminine energies and qualities. Since coming to Tucson, I have been privileged to be able to participate in Native American prayer ceremonies. The depth of spiritual commitment of these people, and their deep reverence for all life in its masculine and feminine forms, has enriched me greatly. Healing the deeper spiritual wounds for women is also part of health and wholeness. We physicians neglect this at our patients' peril. We must weave together all parts of the human experience in our search for health and well-being. I feel it is important to respect individual beliefs, and I believe we can do this at the same time we create healing environments that encompass the spiritual dimensions of life.

Our bodies and minds change; our spirit grows in new directions; and we move onward in our journey, sometimes looking back with regret, sometimes looking back with pride; sometimes looking ahead with excitement about what lies out there, and sometimes looking ahead with fear. It seems to me much like what Ingmar Bergman must have meant in this statement: "Old age is like climbing a mountain. You climb from ledge to ledge, the higher you get the more tired and breathless you become. But your views become more expansive."

As we get older and wiser we have learn to cherish the considerable skills, insight, and wisdom we've accumulated adapting to all of the changes that have occurred throughout our lives. We have woven these experiences into our own unique tapestry, which we may then share with those around us. This is part of the *transcendence* of life that gives it meaning and purpose. I think it is important for each of us to search out the parts of our life that have a sense of meaning and purpose. Then, no matter how busy you are, *make* time for that dimension of your life. Your very survival, at a spiritual and physical level, may depend upon your listening to this inner voice which screams for you to listen. Take heed and act on its message.

As a woman at mid-life and beyond, you are moving from creating *new* life to creating *your own life*. For many women, there is a sense of uncertainty as their roles change. "Who am I" What do I want to accomplish? Who do I want to be? These existential questions do not have easy answers. Yet, your sense of self-worth and feeling of direction in your life is enhanced greatly by the time you set aside to explore what responses to these questions are meaningful for you. Clarissa Pinkola Estes writes in *Women Who Run with the Wolves*:

Creativity is the ability to respond to all that goes around us. To choose from the hundreds of possibilities of thought, feeling, action and reaction and to put these together in a unique response, expression, or message that carries moment, passion and meaning a woman's creative ability is her most valuable asset. For it gives outwardly and feeds her inwardly at every level, psychic, spiritual, mental, emotive, and economic.

To create is also to *change*. As women we face many changes throughout our life journey: physical changes, role changes, emotional changes, spiritual changes. How we view *change* is a significant part of the challenge we face. Is change a *crisis* to you, or do you see change as an *opportunity*? Do you feel overwhelmed by changes in your life, or are changes exciting to you? Do you enjoy new challenges, or do you view them as threats? One woman, moving from Norfolk, Virginia to New York City on her own, described her feelings about this major change in her life: "I feel a sense of *petrified excitement!*" WHAM! THAT said it! In two words, she captured the essence of the mixture of emotions that often hits us when we have signi...nt changes in our lives.

How we view change is a big part of its impact on us. Even positive changes create a stress response in our bodies as we adapt, but the *degree* of impact on our body health is dramatically intensified when we perceive changes in our lives as negative ones. All of us are going through biological-psychological-social changes all the time. It's how we *perceive* these changes, what we *do* with them, and how we *use* them in our lives that makes a difference in our psychological hardiness. When we use such changes as opportunities to improve ourselves, to have an impact on others, to better the conditions around us, we create more feelings of control in our lives.

I grew up near the water in Virginia, and I loved sailing. I learned the hard way that there is no way to control the wind. I could plan a weekend sailing get-away down to the last detail, except I had to face the inevitable: no matter how much I might want to, *there was no way I could control the wind*. What I had to learn to do was *adjust the sails* to take advantage of the way the wind was blowing and just accept that sometimes it wasn't! There were plenty of days when the wind just died, and I'd be stuck, unable to reach my destination that day! No matter how frustrated and in a dither I got, I could NOT, by force of my will, make the wind pick up. So it was a great lesson in patience, practice, and learning when to just flow with whatever was happening.

Over the years, I have come to realize what a great experience those sailing days were in teaching me a useful metaphor for life.

Think about this for your life. How do you view yourself? Are you kicking and screaming trying to *make* the wind blow? Or are you learning from experiences and figuring out ways to *trim the sails* to take advantage of whatever wind there is, or even just learning to kick back and *flow* with circumstances until the wind picks up again? Each of us, based upon how we view ourselves and how we experience our inner sense of power and control, has the ability to increase our self-confidence, self-esteem, and feelings of accomplishment in our lives. And that in turn enhances the *spirit* of the inner self, creating the individual woman who is *psychologically hardy.*

HARDINESS = CHALLENGE

HARDINESS = CONTROL

HARDINESS = COMMITMENT

Keep these words on your mirror or your refrigerator door, and remind yourself each day:

1. Changes are *challenges and opportunities*; they do not have to be experienced as threats unless you choose to experience them that way.
2. You have *control* in your life, no matter what the situation. You can control the choices you make, even if you cannot control the situation itself. An internal sense of control,—"I have the freedom to choose my mental outlook, even in the worst adversity"—creates a strong sense of self. It is the opposite of powerlessness, the opposite of being a victim of circumstance.
3. *Commitment* is the belief that your life has meaning and purpose. Commitment is the opposite of *alienation*, the opposite of isolation and just drifting through your life. Decide what means something to you and then look for the resources around you to help you achieve it.

In thinking about all of this, remember that if you focus on *daydreaming* about the person *you would like to be*, you end up wasting the time to enjoy being the person you are now. So focus on your gifts and abilities and talents now and celebrate what is right, good, and wonderful about you as a person.

I moved to Tucson in 1992, having spent my entire life on the East Coast and very much a water-oriented person. Yet, something kept pulling me to the desert and to this land, the sky, and the mountains. The mountains here have a very different form and feel than the ones back East. They feel closer somehow, more *right there*, as if I could reach out and touch them. And the form is a feminine one, the rounded rocks visible to the very earth itself, not covered by the trees as the Eastern mountains and the Rockies are. There was something primordial and powerful tugging at my spirit whenever I sat and watched the sunlight and clouds playing over the faces of the Catalina mountains. I came across this poem in 1994, which to me captured this ancient connection:

Of Mountains and Women

The hearts of mountains
    and the hearts of women
Are both the same. They beat to
    an old rhythm, an old song.

Mountains and women
    are made from the sinew of the rock.
Mountains and women
    are home to the spirits of the earth.
Mountains and women
    embrace the mystery of life.
Mountains give patience to women.
    Women give fullness to mountains
    Celebrate each mountain, each woman.
    Dance for them in your dreams.

The spirit of mountains and of women
Will give courage to our children
Long after we are gone.

—Nancy Wood, *Spirit Walker*,
Doubleday/Delacort Press, 1993

Each time I came to Tucson to visit over the years, I continued to hear the call of that inner voice pulling me to these mountains, even though my mind kept saying "But you can't leave your family, friends, patients, and professional ties in Virginia. How are you going to start over *now*?"

I finally listened to the call of my soul and took the leap into the unknown and the uncertainty of a new beginning. Moving from a high rise in the city of Norfolk to a one story stucco house in Tucson, I felt a strong sense of coming *home* to this land—this land of mountains and sky, of earth and rock; this land of incredible diversity of plants and animals adapted to the harshness of the desert terrain.

In the desert, I have found the connection with the earth, the mountains, and the sky, and in the quiet of the soft breeze I have reconnected with the inner voice that guides me along the path of creative change one small step at a time. I am learning to let go of a focus on "perfection" and "completion." My goal has become *experiencing* the process, experiencing the feelings—joys and pains—of the journey, knowing that with every change I make, I am becoming more *whole*.

The Physician Becomes Patient... Again

March 27, 1989 was a day of immense despair, pain, and hopelessness in my life. I could not recall ever feeling like I was in such a bottomless dark hole. Previously an energetic, independent, healthy woman in her early forties who had been jogging regularly three to four miles a day, I was now being discharged from Johns Hopkins after my third hospitalization and second spine surgery in three months. The two cervical spine surgeries had been only about six weeks apart, hardly enough time to recover from the first before unexpectedly being faced with a second, which was caused by a bad fall from the physical therapy table during treatment after my first neck surgery.

The last surgery had been more complicated and required a fusion of two neck vertebrae using a bone chip from my hip. I was now faced with eight months in a steel two-poster neck brace from chin to chest. My neurosurgeon had just told me the *good* news that I didn't need any more surgery. The *bad* news was the discs throughout my spine had been damaged badly in the fall and now compounded the difficulty recovering. I was able to walk only a few yards and had such little arm strength I could not even lift a full water pitcher or put on the cumbersome neck brace. The back pain was constant, debilitating, and draining, and I frequently felt exhausted in the morning, even after eight or nine hours in bed.

All of a sudden here I was, a woman who had been in such good health and had felt so in charge of her life and career, blind-sided by a tornado, out of control. It was definitely not a feeling I liked or wanted. I was supposed to be the one in charge, not the one on the receiving end of this bad news discussion! The neurosurgeon had told me I would need to go into a rehabilitation program for another five to six weeks to strengthen my legs, back, and arms enough that I could return to work later that spring or summer.

It was a devastating blow. I had a sinking feeling as I realized what an impact this would have on my family and business. There was no choice. I either took more time out from work now for the full recovery from both surgeries, or I faced having long-term limited mobility and pain. I had a sense of being outside of myself watching as I fell deeper and deeper into a seemingly endless black well of despair.

I knew enough to recognize that I desperately needed a healing environment, a place where I could get the help I needed from medical and complementary therapies, which could provide the mind-body work I needed. I was also concerned about finding a setting where healthy food could help me start to lose the excess weight from recent months of inactivity and steroid therapy. But where could I go? My fall had occurred in a hospital program in my own town; I obviously did not want to go back there. I wasn't severely injured enough to qualify for *inpatient* rehabilitation programs; besides, I knew those programs would not have the kind of massage therapy and other approaches I knew I needed. Yet I really couldn't go to a health club setting in a wheelchair and a neck brace.

What to do, and how to find help? I remembered a place of healing in the Southwest desert, where I thought I could put together the program I needed. My body wisdom knew this was what I needed; yet the rest of my mental processes were so overwhelmed, I could not even think straight and deal with the enormity of the decision. I didn't have the strength or energy even to begin to think about how I could possibly get there or be able to pay for it, since I had been out of work so long.

The inner me *knew* what I needed to recover, but I hadn't yet learned to listen completely to my body wisdom. My family, my minister, and my friend-business attorney had the clarity of thinking and insight I lacked at this point. They sorted out the issues and pointed out that I could not take care of anyone or anything else unless I first got well. They helped me make the only decision that could help me survive and begin to heal again. I simply *had* to get away from the overwhelming stressors at home and into a healing environment where the treatment I desperately needed could be available in one place, even if it meant going into debt and taking a long difficult journey to get there.

There simply was no alternative. But my intellect kept saying, "wait a minute, I can't leave, I have obligations." Of course, it was apparent to *everyone else* that I couldn't meet those obligations anyway, even if I stayed at home. I was in such bad shape I *couldn't* work! I just could not see with the clarity they did. I finally accepted that they were right.

What a scary leap it was. I had to trust my body wisdom, I had to let go. I teetered on the edge. Then, at one moment, I knew I wanted to get well. I wanted to survive this ordeal and come back strong again. I had to take the leap of faith and put myself in the hands of gifted people from many fields who could help me heal. I agreed to go. I made the choice of *life*. My soul began to feel like flying again. Well, not exactly flying I guess, when I couldn't even *walk* ten yards! But I did feel instantly "lighter" in spirit once I had turned the corner and made the decision my inner self knew was necessary and *right for me*. Mind, body, spirit: all parts of me needed help to get me back on my feet. Supportive, capable people, a healing environment, the needed facilities in one location. It was time to start the journey.

Competent and compassionate people in massage therapy, hydrotherapy, physical therapy, nutrition, exercise physiology, hypnotherapy, biofeedback, acupuncture, medical, nursing, gynecology, and endocrinology all combined their talents to help me get headed back in the right direction and regain my strength and vitality. The healing presence of nature and her beauty, the sunshine, the mountain air, and soft breezes all soothed my body and my weary psyche. My soul was revived. I felt close to my Creator, grateful to be alive, to have loving people in my life to give my courage a boost. I felt and experienced the recuperative power of combining the best of Western medicine with all that complementary modalities can offer in the healing process. It was a *transformational experience* in my life. I now know that it was a crucial part of my process and preparation to continue my role as a physician, healer, and teacher of other health professionals.

In times of real crisis in your life, I am sure that each of you has felt a certain clarity about what "ought" to be done. Finding the courage and strength to carry out what "ought" to be done is another matter. Many times we are afraid to accept that insight because of all the "what ifs" that might happen, or the gamble that we might be taking on a bad choice. Oftentimes we are so confused or disoriented by the darkness of the "hole" we have been sucked into, the hole in which we see ourselves trapped or forced, that we need someone to shine a light in the hole for us to see things more clearly and be able to find a way out. Each of us have these "lights" in our lives, but many times we forget to use them, or to ask people close to us to share *their* light with us to guide the way.

I realize now that a significant part of the reason I was drawn to Tucson in 1992, in making such a major change in my work setting, was that the desert had been a healing place for me personally. It had also been an environment in which I had *experienced* allopathic medicine to be more accepting of a broad view of the whole person and more accepting of the use of alternative medicine modalities than the traditional medical-surgical model I was part of on the East Coast.

For many years, I have sought information and approaches that traditional medicine has overlooked or left out, and I have wanted to blend them with what I learned in medical school. My philosophy has been "let's find out why," instead of being bound by traditional mindsets that say "no that can't be." I am more aware now that my intuitive knowing of what needed to be included in Western medicine had found its home in Tucson, and my mind simply needed to heed the soul's call. I am still in the process of weaving my life tapestry. While the *pattern* of the tapestry will ultimately be different for each of us, many of the threads and colors we will use for weaving are similar. I hope that you will find ideas and encouragement for your own journey towards being whole as you read and reflect on my story.

You have the power to be a major influence on the course of your life. Albert Einstein, who had difficulty passing in school, said:

Great spirits have always encountered violent opposition from mediocre minds.

Don't let negative, mediocre minds get in the way of what you want to be and accomplish. Be the "great spirit" that you can be, and take charge of your life and well being.

The moment of YOUR power and strength is NOW.

LISTEN to what lies within you; make the most of the beautiful and unique person you are. Take a step NOW to *claim* your life for what is important and meaningful to YOU.

SCREAM if you need to.

BE HEARD! Your health, indeed your very soul's survival, depends on it.

It's never too late to be who we might have been.
—George Elliot

Glossary of Terms

This is a glossary of the medical terms used most frequently in this book. If you are going to take charge *of your health*, you will need to become informed about what these terms mean, so that you understand terms used by your physician to explain what is happening to your body.

ADRENAL GLANDS: Two small glands situated on top of the kidneys, which secrete steroid hormones (cortisol, aldosterone, DHEA) and the stress hormones epinephrine and norepinephrine (sometimes grouped together in common usage and called *adrenaline*).

AFFECT (AFFECTIVE): A term used to mean "mood" or range of emotional expression. "Affective" refers to emotional content or to disorders of mood.

AIDS: Acquired Immune Deficiency Syndrome, a sexually-transmitted viral disease with a long incubation period; usually fatal.

ALOPECIA: Loss of hair that is excessive and abnormal. There are many medical, dietary, and lifestyle causes. Anorexia, bulimia and decline in ovarian and thyroid hormones are common causes in women.

AMENORRHEA: The absence of menstrual bleeding in a woman who has not gone through menopause; may be due to prolonged stress, thyroid disorders, excessive exercise, eating disorders, premature ovarian failure and others.

AMINO ACIDS: Chemical molecules found in foods that serve as the "building blocks" for the body to make its proteins. **Essential amino acids** are those that the body cannot synthesize and that must be included in the food we eat. Dietary protein containing all of the essential amino acids is "complete protein" and can be obtained from animal/dairy products and also by combining any three of the following: nuts, grains, seeds, or legumes at one meal.

ANABOLIC STEROIDS: Hormones that stimulate the growth of bone and muscle (lean body mass) and have male ("virilizing") effects on body chemistry and shape.

ANDROGENS: A group of hormones that produces masculine effects on the body. This group of hormones is produced by both the adrenal glands and the gonads (testes in males and ovaries in females) but in much smaller amounts in women. After menopause, the levels of androgens in women are higher and produce the characteristic body changes seen in older women.

ANDROGENIC: Describes substances (natural or synthetic) that produce masculine changes in the body: stimulating hair growth in a male pattern, oily skin, acne, deepening of the voice, increased appetite, increased muscle mass, and increased total cholesterol with lower HDL.

ANGINA: Pain in the arm, neck, or chest caused by lack of blood supply (ischemia) to the heart.

ANTIOXIDANT: Substances such as vitamins A, C, and E, beta-carotene, and selenium, which protect the cellular structures from oxidative damage caused by free radicals.

ATHEROSCLEROSIS: Artery-clogging deposits formed by cholesterol, fibrin and "sticky" platelets; a major cause of heart attacks, strokes, angina, and other cardiovascular disease.

ATROPHY: Wasting or thinning of tissues or organs.

BENIGN: Noncancerous or nonmalignant.

BIOFLAVINOIDS: Substances found in plants along with vitamin C that exert a beneficial effect upon the walls of the blood and lymphatic vessels.

BODY MASS INDEX (B.M.I.): A scientific way of determining body composition. It is calculated according to the formula B.M.I. = weight (kilogram)/height squared (meters). The normal B.M.I. for women ranges from 20 to 25 kg/m^2 and many hormonal and menstrual problems can be overcome by keeping weight in the normal range.

BREAKTHROUGH BLEEDING (BTB): Irregular vaginal bleeding or spotting occurring in women when they are taking oral contraceptives or postmenopausal hormone therapy.

CANCER: A malignant growth/tumor with rapid multiplication of abnormal cells which may spread to and invade distant body parts.

CARDIOVASCULAR DISEASE (CVD): Disease of the heart and/or arteries, veins, and capillaries that make up the circulatory system.

CAT SCAN: A computerized X-ray of consecutive sections of the body, which is used to look for tumors, masses, and other abnormal structural changes inside the body.

CELLULITE: Fatty deposits resulting in a dimply or lumpy appearance of the skin. It is gradually lost with proper fluid intake, exercise, and overall weight loss.

CERVIX: The opening of the uterus that projects into the vagina. It is also called the mouth of the womb.

CHLAMYDIA: A sexually-transmitted bacteria that is a common cause of pelvic infection and infertility.

CHLOASMA: Brownish pigmentation of the face that can occur in pregnancy (may also be caused by some types of hormonal imbalance).

CHOLESTEROL: An important body molecule that is the precursor for the body to make sex hormones, adrenal hormones, and other molecules. It is found in the blood in three forms: (1) High Density Lipo-protein (HDL), which *protects* against plaque formation in the arteries (atherosclerosis); (2) Low Density Lipo-protein (LDL), which *promotes* plaque formation (atherosclerosis); and (3) Very Low Density Lipoprotein (VLDL), also a plaque promoter. Cholesterol is a component of all animal fats and oils.

CLIMACTERIC: The span of years in a woman's life when hormone levels are gradually decreasing, leading to changes in body shape and function ultimately ending in the last menstrual period.

CLITORIS: The female equivalent (embryologically) of the penis. It is a small bulb found at the top of the vulva, just below the pubic bone, and is covered by a hood of tissue. It contains erectile tissue and nerve endings that are very sensitive to stimulation and enhance a woman's sexual arousal and orgasm.

CLUSTER HEADACHE: A severe and intense headache, more common in males, which lasts several hours and may recur frequently over a six- to eight-week period.

COMBINED ORAL CONTRACEPTIVE PILL (OC): A contraceptive pill containing the female sex hormones estrogen and a synthetic progestin. There are also progestin-only contraceptives (Micronor is an oral tablet; Norplant and Depo-Provera are long-acting implants/injectables).

COMPLEX CARBOHYDRATES: Carbohydrates occurring in an natural unprocessed form, "complexed" with fiber, minerals, and other nutrients. They are more slowly absorbed and utilized than processed or refined carbohydrates. Examples: beans, pasta, cereals, grains, fruits, vegetables, whole grain breads.

CONCEPTION: The fertilization of the female egg by the sperm.

CONSENT FORM: A legal document that you are required to sign, thereby giving your consent, before undergoing a surgical operation or before taking some medications.

CONTRAINDICATION: A medical condition that makes it inadvisable to use a certain medication, e.g., the presence of breast cancer would contraindicate the use of exogenous estrogen; cigarette smoking is a contraindication for using the oral birth control pill.

CORPUS LUTEUM: The yellow-colored, progesterone-producing sac that is formed within the ovary from the remains of the follicle after it has released its egg at ovulation.

CORTISONE: A steroid made by the adrenal glands and also synthetically in laboratories for use as a drug. It has a powerful anti-inflammatory effect, but may produce many adverse side effects.

CUSHINGS SYNDROME: A collection of symptoms and signs such as moon-shaped face, buffalo hump, and high blood pressure caused by excessive amounts of cortisone either produced by the adrenal gland or taken as medication.

CYSTIC ACNE: A skin disorder manifesting as blocked pores and pimples, many of which are blind cysts containing pus. It is a severe form of acne.

DEXA: Dual Energy X-ray Absorptiometry, a highly reliable means of measuring bone mineral density using very small amounts of radiation. Recommended for women with multiple risk factors for osteopenia/osteoporosis, or women who want a baseline measure before beginning menopause.

DIURETIC: A substance, whether synthetic or natural, that stimulates the kidneys to excrete salt (sodium chloride) and water, thereby relieving fluid retention.

DOPAMINE: A mood-elevating chemical messenger produced in the brain and body; it is also important in preventing Parkinson's disease, and as an inhibitory neurotransmitter preventing inappropriate milk secretion by the breast.

ECTOPIC PREGNANCY: A pregnancy implanted in an abnormal position, usually inside a fallopian tube; may cause severe pain, hemorrhage and infection if it ruptures into the pelvis.

ENDOCRINE GLANDS: Manufacture and secrete hormones.

ENDOCRINOLOGIST: A medical specialist in diseases of the endocrine glands and their hormones; Endocrinology is the study and treatment of disorders of glands and their hormones.

ENDOMETRIOSIS: The presence of endometrium (normally found only inside the uterine cavity) outside of the uterus, scattered about the abdomen and pelvic cavities. Endometriosis causes severe pain at the time of menses due to the cyclical bleeding of the endometrial tissue in abnormal locations where the blood acts as an irritant to other organs.

ENDORPHINS (ALSO ENEKPHALINS): Natural pain-relieving and mood-elevating compounds (peptides) produced in the brain, spinal cord, and body to produce a morphine-like analgesia.

ENZYMES: Proteins produced by living cells that function as catalysts in specific biochemical reactions but are not themselves consumed in the reactions.

ESSENTIAL FATTY ACIDS: Fatty acids necessary for cellular metabolism, which cannot be made by the body, but must be supplied in the diet. Suitable sources are fish oil, oils from nuts and seeds, and evening primrose oil.

ESTRADIOL (E2): The primary estrogen produced by the ovary before menopause. It is the biologically active estrogen at the estrogen receptors and is involved in over 400 functions in the body.

ESTRIOL (E3): The weakest of the primary human estrogens, it is produced in large amounts during pregnancy. It is barely detectable in the *nonpregnant* female body, so women do not normally have estriol present to a measurable degree on a continuous basis.

ESTROGEN: Three types of female sex hormones secreted by the ovary, that are responsible for the female characteristics of breasts, feminine curves, and menstruation.

ESTRONE (E1): One of the three human estrogens made by the ovary. It is the one found in higher amounts after menopause, and it is thought to be the primary culprit in increased risks of endometrial and breast cancers.

EVENING PRIMROSE OIL: The oil extracted from the evening primrose plant. It is a good source of the omega 6 fatty acids, in particular the essential fatty acid know as gamma linolenic acid (GLA).

FALLOPIAN TUBES: The tubes that carry the egg (ovum) from the ovary to the uterus. Fertilization of the egg occurs in the outer part of the tube.

FEMALE SEX HORMONES: Hormones produced by the female ovary: estrogen, progesterone, and testosterone.

FERTILIZATION: The union of the female egg (ovum) with the male sperm (spermatozoa), which occurs in the fallopian tube.

FETUS: A developing human from the end of the eighth week of pregnancy until birth.

FIBROIDS (FIBROMAS): Noncancerous growths of the uterus consisting of muscle and fibrous tissue. The medical term is leiomyoma, or sometimes just "myomas."

FOLLICLE STIMULATING HORMONE (FSH): A hormone secreted by the pituitary gland that reaches the ovaries via the blood circulation and stimulates the growth of ovarian follicles (eggs).

FOLLICULAR (PHASE): The first half of the ovarian hormone cycle leading up to the release of the egg at ovulation. Estrogen is the dominant hormone for this part of the cycle, and there is very little progesterone present.

FRIGID (SEXUAL): A negative term applied to women who are considered by their partner to be sexually unresponsive and disinterested. Hormonal, medical, and relationship factors may cause loss of sexual desire and responsiveness.

GALACTORRHEA: The presence of milk or milky fluid in the breasts when not breast-feeding. It is usually a symptom of elevated prolactin, which may be caused by medication or by hormone-producing tumors of the pituitary gland.

GAMMA LINOLENIC ACID (GLA): An omega-6 essential fatty acid that is used to synthesize prostaglandins. It has an anti-inflammatory effect in the body. Good sources: breast milk, evening primrose oil, borage plant oil, and black currant seed oil.

GLANDS: Body organs or tissues, generally soft and fleshy in consistency, that manufacture and secrete or excrete hormones, which then exert their effects on target organs elsewhere in the body.

GYNECOLOGY: Surgical specialty of medicine that provides surgical and medicinal treatments for problems related to women's reproductive organs.

HIRSUTISM: A condition of excessive facial and body hair (excluding hair on the scalp).

HORMONES: Chemicals produced by various glands that are transported around the body to exert multiple metabolic effects.

HORMONE REPLACEMENT THERAPY (HRT): Technically, the administration of any hormonal preparations (natural or synthetic) to replace the loss of natural hormones produced by various glands (thyroid, ovary, testes, etc.). HRT in common usage now refers to administration of female hormones (estrogen and progestin) after menopause.

HYPOTHALAMUS: The "master conductor" or "control center" situated at the base of the brain regulates body temperature, thirst, appetite, sex drive, and all other endocrine glands. Releases hormones that travel to the pituitary gland and stimulate release of pituitary hormones, which govern the other endocrine glands.

HYSTERECTOMY: Surgical removal of the uterus only. Commonly, women say "hysterectomy" when both the uterus and ovaries have been removed *or* when just the uterus has been removed.

IMMUNE SYSTEM: The defense and surveillance system of the body that protects against infection by micro-organisms and invasion by foreign tissues and substances.

IMPLANT: A chemical substance, hormone, or object in a capsule, that is surgically placed into a part of the body.

INFLAMMATION: A condition characterized by swelling, redness, heat, and pain in any tissue as a result of trauma, irritation, infection, or imbalances in immune function.

IUD: Intrauterine device, typically used for contraception, but may also be a means of delivering hormones and medications directly to the uterus.

LAPAROSCOPE: A long thin telescopic instrument utilizing a fiber-optic lighting system, which is inserted through a small incision in the abdominal wall. It functions like a hollow flashlight enabling the surgeon to view internal organs and insert operating instruments through its hollow tube.

LIBIDO: Level of sexual desire, sexual energy, or drive.

LUTEAL (PHASE): The progesterone-dominant second half of the menstrual cycle, from ovulation until menses begin. The primary hormone of this phase is progesterone. It is also the time of the cycle when PMS occurs.

LUTEINIZING HORMONE (LH): A hormone produced by the pituitary gland that triggers ovulation and the development of the corpus luteum.

MALE HORMONE: A hormone that promotes masculine characteristics in the body such as facial and body hair, acne, deepening of the voice, increased muscle mass, and increased libido.

MALIGNANT: Cancer, cancerous.

MANIC DEPRESSION (BIPOLAR DISORDER): A biological disorder of brain function that produces episodes of euphoria, delusions, and abnormally increased energy, alternating at variable intervals with severe depressions.

MENOPAUSE: The cessation of menstruation. The last period.

MENSTRUAL CLOCK: A specialized part of the hypothalamus regulating the cyclical timing of the phases of the menstrual cycle.

MENSTRUATION: Monthly bleeding from the vagina in women from puberty until menopause, caused by shedding of the lining of the womb if there is no fertilization of an egg.

METABOLIC RATE: The rate at which the body converts chemical energy in foods into heat (thermal) and movement (kinetic) energy.

METABOLISM: Chemical processes utilizing the raw materials of nutrients, oxygen, and vitamins along with enzymes to produce energy for bodily functions.

MICROSURGICAL TECHNIQUES: Surgery performed on small parts of the body such as nerve fibers, blood vessels, or fallopian tubes, requiring the use of the operating microscope.

NEUROTRANSMITTERS: Chemicals that transmit messages from nerve cell to nerve cell in the brain, and between the brain and the tissues and organs of the body.

NON-ANDROGENIC: Not causing masculine effects in the body.

NOREPINEPHRINE (ADRENALIN): A hormone produced by the adrenal gland, and certain areas of the brain, that helps the body prepare for and cope with stress. It also has a mood-elevating effect, but higher levels may cause feelings of anxiety.

OOPHORECTOMY (OVARIECTOMY): Surgical removal of the ovaries

ORAL: Indicating something is to be taken by mouth.

ORGASM: The physical and emotional release of sexual arousal tension; also called *climax*.

OSTEOPENIA: Loss of bone density that is not yet severe enough to be considered osteoporosis. Osteopenia will progress to osteoporosis if active measures are not taken to maintain bone (such as calcium, magnesium, exercise, and hormone therapy).

OSTEOPOROSIS: Loss of bone mass due to loss of bone minerals and reduction of the normal bony architecture that provides strength to the skeleton. Porous condition of bones.

OVARIAN BLOOD SUPPLY: The blood carried to the ovaries via the ovarian arteries, which branch off from the uterine blood vessels. The ovarian arteries run alongside the fallopian tubes and may be injured or damaged with surgical procedures on the tubes.

OVARIES: The female sex glands (gonads) located on each side of the uterus, which produce eggs and the female sex hormones (estrogen and progesterone), along with small amounts of testosterone.

OVULATION: The release of the egg from the ovary occurring around mid-cycle.

OVULATION PAIN ("Mittelschmerz"): Occurs at ovulation, may be sharp and severe; lasts from a few minutes up to twelve hours.

PARASYMPATHETIC NERVOUS SYSTEM: The part of the autonomic nervous system that regulates body relaxation and functions of growth and repair such as digestion. Its primary chemical messenger or neurotransmitter is acetylcholine.

PARENTERAL: A method of delivering substances (such as medications) directly to the bloodstream bypassing the digestive system and liver metabolism. Parenteral routes include: vaginal and rectal suppositories/tablets, sublingual tablets/capsules, transdermal (skin patch), subcutaneous (implant), intramuscular (IM), and intravenous (IV) injections.

PELVIC INFLAMMATORY DISEASE (PID): Inflammation of the pelvic organs, particularly the uterus and fallopian tubes, caused by infectious micro-organisms, typically occurring from sexually-transmitted bacteria, fungi, and viruses.

PERIMENOPAUSAL: The several years prior to menopause when menstrual periods start to be skipped and continuing through menopause to the first few years just after periods stop. It has a variable age of onset and is commonly accompanied by bone loss, cholesterol changes, sleep changes, hot flashes, and other phenomena. (See also premenopausal, etc.)

PESSARY: Oval-shaped object inserted into the vagina to support a prolapsed uterus or to deliver medications or hormones to vaginal tissue.

PHYSIOLOGICAL: Normal body processes and functions.

PITUITARY GLAND: A mushroom-shaped gland connected by a vascular stalk to the base of the brain. The pituitary gland manufactures hormones (FSH, LH, TSH, ACTH, and others), which in turn control other hormonal glands, such as the thyroid, adrenals, ovaries, and breasts.

PLACENTA: The hormonal organ that provides nourishment of the fetus and the elimination of its waste products. It produces the hormones to sustain pregnancy. It is formed in the uterus by the union of uterine mucous membrane with membranes of the fetus.

POLYCYSTIC OVARY SYNDROME (PCO): A hereditary disorder of the ovaries in which the usual female hormonal balance is altered, and there are excessive levels of male hormones accompanied by changes in body shape and irregular menstruation. It may also be triggered by stress or weight gain. In PCO syndrome, the ovaries have multiple small follicles or "cysts," which can be seen on an ultrasound scan of the pelvis. Other common features: truncal obesity, acne, glucose intolerance and insulin resistance, hypertension.

POST-MENOPAUSE: The years following the end of menstruation and decline in production of ovarian female hormones (menopause).

POSTNATAL, POST-PARTUM: The time period after childbirth.

PREMATURE MENOPAUSE: Cessation of menses and decline of ovarian hormones occurring before the age of forty-two.

PRE-MENOPAUSAL: The time leading up to menopause, characterized by hormonal changes and irregular menstrual flow. It may begin as much as ten years before actual menopause, but more commonly occurs about four to five years before menopause (see also perimenopausal).

PREMENSTRUAL SYNDROME (PMS): A collection of variable symptoms such as mood disturbance, headaches, abdominal bloating, etc. recurring on a cyclical basis in the week or two before menstrual bleeding (see also perimenopausal).

PROGESTOGENS: Natural or synthetic substances that have effects similar to the natural female hormone progesterone. Synthetic progestogens (called progestins) are commonly used in birth control pills and HRT to regulate menstrual bleeding. Examples are medroxy-progesterone acetate (Provera), norethindrone (Aygestin), norethisterone, norgestrel, and others.

PROGESTIN PILL ("mini-pill"): A contraceptive pill containing only a progestin such as norethindrone (Brand: Micronor). Not recommended for midlife women or for women with a history of depression, diabetes, hypertension or weight gain as it will aggravate all of these problems.

PROLACTIN: A hormone secreted by the pituitary gland that stimulates milk production in the breasts.

PROSTAGLANDINS: Chemicals manufactured throughout the body that exert a hormone-like effect and influence muscular (including the uterus) contraction, circulation, and inflammation.

PROSTATE GLAND: This gland is located just below the bladder in men and secretes fluid into the ejaculate of semen during male orgasm.

PSYCHOSIS: A severe biochemical disorder of brain function characterized by delusions, hallucinations, and abnormalities in thinking and reasoning. It may be due to many causes: schizophrenia, major depression, manic-depressive disorder, alcohol intoxication, severe endocrine illness, drug abuse (cocaine), and medication toxicity (such as atropine, lidocaine, digitalis, and others).

PSYCHOSOMATIC: Physical symptoms that are triggered by psychological and emotional causes and not due primarily to physical disease. This term is often misused when applied to women, as in "the cause isn't known so it must be psychosomatic, or stress."

PSYCHOTHERAPY: The process of using systematic "talking" approaches to treat stress-related problems, emotional issues, and disturbances in self-image. Many different methods may be used, depending upon the training of the therapist.

PSYCHOTROPIC DRUGS: Drugs that act primarily on the brain to produce effects on mood, thinking, sleep, and other functions. Examples are sedatives, tranquilizers (anti-anxiety agents), anti-depressants, anti-psychotics, analgesic, and anesthetic agents.

PUERPERIUM: The six to eight weeks after childbirth required to return the reproductive organs to their prepregnant size and condition.

SEBACEOUS GLANDS: Tiny oil-producing glands in the skin. If they overproduce oil and/or become obstructed, pimples or acne will result.

SEROTONIN (5-HT): A potent brain chemical that regulates sleep, mood, libido, appetite, pain, and repetitive thoughts and actions. Serotonin's chemical name is 5-hydroxytryptophan and it is made by the brain and body from dietary sources of the amino acid tryptophan (milk, turkey, whole grains, etc.).

SEX HORMONES: The male and female hormones produced from cholesterol by the testicles, ovaries, adrenal glands, and body fat: testosterone, estrogens, progesterone, androgens.

STEROID DRUGS AND HORMONES: The group of chemical substances consisting of multiple rings of carbon atoms. Cortisone (the drug), estrogen, progesterone, and testosterone (sex hormones).

STROKE: Brain damage resulting from a disturbance of blood supply (ischemia) to the brain.

SYMPATHETIC NERVOUS SYSTEM: The part of the autonomic nervous system that prepares the body for stress through effects of the stress hormones it releases (examples: by increasing oxygen to the tissues, increasing heart rate, blood pressure and glucose release, etc.). Its primary chemical messengers (neurotransmitters) are norepinephrine and epinephrine.

SYMPTOMS: Any physical or emotional change in the body that is perceived as distressing or painful. "Symptom" usually means a change which makes a person feel unwell. "Phenomena" is a word used to describe changes which do not necessarily cause distress.

SYNDROME: A group of signs and symptoms that collectively characterize a disease.

SYNERGISTIC: Helps or increases the effect of another substance.

TESTOSTERONE: The major male sex hormone produced in the testes and also in smaller amounts by the female ovary.

THYROID GLAND: The endocrine gland situated in front of the larynx that produces the major hormones of metabolism: thyroxine and tri-iodothyronine.

THYROID STIMULATING HORMONE (TSH): The hormone produced by the brain that regulates the production and release of thyroid hormones from the thyroid gland. TSH levels are **low** in *hyper*thyroidism, and **high** in *hypo*thyroidism.

TRIGLYCERIDES (TG): One of the blood fats that the body can use to make cholesterol; elevated TG (from diet, alcohol intake, lack of exercise, and some drugs) are a significant risk factor for heart disease particularly for women.

TRYPTOPHAN: An amino acid found in foods that is the major precursor ("building block") for the body and brain to make serotonin (5-hydroxytryptophan, 5-HT).

TUBAL LIGATION (BTL): The surgical procedure to cut or tie the fallopian tubes for the purpose of permanent contraception. BTL is considered permanent because it is difficult and expensive to reverse, with low probability of success.

TUMOR: An abnormal growth, that may be cancerous or benign.

UTERUS: The womb; the organ which carries and nourishes a growing fetus; rhythmic contractions of the uterus occur during orgasm (not all women feel this) and may enhance sexual pleasure.

UROLOGIST: A surgeon who specializes in diseases of the kidneys and urinary tract.

ULTRASOUND SCAN: A method of visualizing the internal organs, and and blood vessels, fetus. Ultrasound utilizes very high frequency sound waves (more than 20,000 hertz) that are above the audible limit to provide an image of organs; it does not involve radiation.

VAGINA: The genital (or birth) canal or passage leading from the uterus to the vulva; it is muscular and elastic, expanding to accommodate the penis during intercourse, or for delivery of a baby.

VAGINAL DIAPHRAGM: A soft rubber cap that fits snugly over the cervix and is used for contraception.

VASOACTIVE DRUGS: Drugs or substances (e.g., nicotine) acting on the blood vessels to cause either dilation or constriction of the arteries.

VIRILIZATION: The development of masculine physical characteristics due to male hormones.

VULVA: Female external genitalia. Also known as the lips of the vaginal opening.

APPENDIX 2

RESOURCES

I. SOURCES FOR NATURAL HORMONES, TEST KITS

Marla Ahlgrimm, R.Ph., Madison Pharmacy Associates 800-558-7046 Madison, WI.
Pioneer in compounding natural progesterone options for women with over 15 years experience providing assistance to physicians and patients; also provides individual compounding for other natural hormones including testosterone, DHEA, estriol. Publishes *Women's Health Access Newsletter*, and the *Women's Health America* catalog of reputable women's health products and services nationally. A good source for vitamins tailored to the needs of women with PMS and during menopause. Pharmacists are available to answer questions for physicians and patients on natural hormone preparations; an excellent information package is also available for consumers and health professionals.

Charles Hakala, R.Ph., Belmar Pharmacy 800-525-9473 Lakewood (Denver area), CO.
Specializes in compounding (to individual prescription) micronized testosterone, DHEA, progesterone, 17-beta-estradiol and sustained release thyroid (T3). Uses **hypoallergenic formulations: no dyes, lactose-free.** Provides a full-service pharmacy and is able to work with most health insurance plans.

The above resources are ones I have depended upon to provide individual prescriptions for my patients, and my family; we have been pleased with the results. These pharmacists are skilled, knowledgeable, and committed to providing quality service to you and your physician. Women have asked me "Are these hormones FDA approved?" The FDA requires rigorous testing and a formal approval before new medications are *manufactured* and distributed in mass quantities. Individual pharmacists operate within their training and licenses when they prepare ("compound") individual prescriptions based on your own physician's decision about dose and type of medication best for you. Since these individually compounded prescriptions are not *manufactured* in commercial quantities, the FDA does not require the same approval procedures. Many medications used to be compounded individually, but it is no longer advantageous to do so with the current quality of manufactured products widely available. Current use of individual compounding is typically for patients with allergies, marked sensitivities to dyes and binders in commercial preparations, those who need smaller doses, and in particular, women who want to take native human forms of hormones.

Natural ovarian hormones have been in widespread use in Europe, Australia, Canada, Japan and other countries for many years, generally with better clinical response and fewer side effects than the synthetic progestins, conjugated equine estrogens and synthetic methyltestosterone compounds used in the U.S. There are three brands of the natural or *native human estrogen (17-beta estradiol)* available in the United States which are FDA approved and made by ethical pharmaceutical companies: *Estrace* tablets and vaginal cream, *Estraderm* and *Climara* transdermal (skin) patches.

We do not have a major pharmaceutical company in the United States which has developed native human micronized testosterone or progesterone preparations approved by the FDA for widespread consumer use in menopausal and PMS regimens. As we understand more about the important differences between the native human forms for hormones and the synthetic or animal-derived ones, I hope the women of this country will have better options widely available. Until that time, you may ask your physician to work with reputable pharmacists, such as the ones above, to compound the natural progesterone and testosterone to suit your needs. **I have <u>no financial interest</u> in any of these pharmacies or their products. I provide this information as a service to you and your physician because such information has been difficult for the average consumer to obtain. I have seen over many years what a marked positive difference it makes when women use native human hormone options.**

HORMONE TEST KITS

Aeron LifeCycles Laboratories, Phone: 800-631-7900, FAX 510-729-0383
1933 Davis St., Suite 310, San Leandro, CA 94577
Well-established researchers in hormone receptor assays, Aeron LifeCycles has recently developed individual patient saliva test kits to measure salivary levels of progesterone, testosterone, estradiol and cortisol. Contact Gladys Warr, MT (ASCP) for further information and/or to order kits.

I. RESOURCES FOR INFORMATION: Books, Clinical Centers, and National Organizations

Chapter 1: Screaming To Be Heard!

1. **Woman As Healer**. Jeanne Achterberg, Ph.D., Shambhala, Boston, 1990. Dr. Achterberg examines the role of women and their pivotal roles in healing traditions in ancient cultures, as well as the loss of the feminine influences in the Western medical traditions. A profoundly moving and inspiring book which helps us understand women's vital contributions and influence in the past, and sheds more light on the problems in the world today, medicine in particular.

2. **Medicine Women, Curanderas, and Women Doctors**. Bobette Perrone, H. Henrietta Stockel, and Victoria Krueger, University of Oklahoma Press, Norman, Oklahoma, 1989. Presents ten Southwestern female healers from three cultures (Native American, Hispanic, and Western) and provides an in-depth analysis of alternative healing methods along with remarkable insights about the profound impact of the psyche/soul on physical illness. Inspirational reading.

3. **BACKLASH—The Undeclared War Against American Women** by Susan Faludi, Crown Publishers, Inc., 1991. Ms. Faludi makes a compelling case that whenever women make progress in their efforts for equality, an anti-feminist backlash strikes on all fronts—in the media, politics, fashion, and the workplace. Also relevant to understand why women's health needs have not been adequately addressed, and women's voices not listened to.

4. **Women & Self-Esteem—Understanding and Improving the Way We Think and Feel About Ourselves,** by Linda Tschirhart Sanford & Mary Ellen Donovan, 1984, Penguin Books. An excellent overview of issues affecting women, still relevant (perhaps more so) in 1995. Helps women understand cultural sources of low self-esteem, provides practical approaches for building an enhanced self-esteem; a valuable resource.

Chapter 2: Making "Holistic" Medicine Whole

1. **Woman's Body: A Manual For Life** Dr. Miriam Stoppard, Dorling Kindslerly, London and New York, 1994. Compiled by a team of health experts from many fields, illustrated with hundreds of color charts, graphs, photos, this is one of the most comprehensive and practical women's health books I have found. Covers physical and emotional concerns of women throughout the life span.

2. <u>Mind/Body Medicine: How To Use Your Mind For Better Health</u>. Consumer Reports Books, New York: Consumers Union of U.S., Inc., 1993 (by the leading authorities from the Nation's Top Medical Centers).

3. <u>The Wellness Book: The Comprehensive Guide to Maintaining Health and Treating Stress-Related Illness</u>. Herbert Benson, M.D. and Eileen M. Stuart, R.N., M.S., Birch Lane Press, New York, 1992. Competent overall look at wellness with practical how-to information.

4. <u>The Honest Herbal</u> and <u>Herbs of Choice</u> Varro E. Tyler, Ph.D., Pharmaceutical Products Press. Dr. Tyler is internationally known for his work on medicinal qualities of herbs, as well as their potential risks. He is the Lilly Distinguished Professor of Pharmacognosy at Purdue University School of Pharmacy and Pharmaceutical Sciences.

Chapter 3: Hormones

1. <u>Listening To Your Hormones</u> Gillian Ford, Prima Publishing Co., Rocklin, CA, due Fall 1995. An excellent review by well-known PMS and Menopause Educator, Gill Ford. Has over 200 references for those who would like to read originial medical articles. An updated version of Ms. Ford's well-received 1992 book below.

2. <u>Managing Contraceptive Pill Patients</u>. Richard P. Dickey, M.D., Ph.D., 8th Edition, may order from Essential Medical Information Systems, Inc., PO Box 1607, Durant, OK 74702-1607. A through review of all the oral contraceptives on the market, their side effects, potencies, and recommended uses.

Chapter 4: Hormones and the Brain

1. "New Perspectives on the Relationship of Hormone Changes to Affective Disorders in the Perimenopause" by Elizabeth Lee Vliet, M.D. and Virginia Lee Hutcheson Davis, M.S., NAACOG'S Clinical Issues Vol. 2, No. 4 October/December 1991, pp. 453–471

2. <u>What's Wrong With My Hormones?</u> by Gillian Ford, Desmond Ford Publications, Auburn, CA, 1992. May be ordered from Bajamar Pharmacy, St. Louis, MO.

Chapter 5: The Big Question

1. <u>Menopause and Midlife Health</u>. Morris Notelovitz, M.D., and Diana Tonnessen, St. Martin's Press, New York, 1993. Written by a pioneer in osteoporosis and menopause, this book presents accurate and

up-to-date information about managing your health, including the role of healthy lifestyle habits. Discusses hormone therapies, pros and cons of gynecological procedures, issues about breast cancer and other concerns of importance to women.

2. <u>Making Sense of Menopause</u>. Faye Kitchner Cone, Simon and Schuster, New York, 1993. Practical, common-sense advice and up-to-date information on mid-life health issues, hormone therapy, and alternative options. This is a good overview of the menopause transition with a positive focus, but it does not address newer insights about brain-hormone connections involved in mood changes, migraines, and pain syndromes.

3. <u>Estrogen: The Facts Can Save Your Life</u>. Lila Nachtigal, M.D., and Joan Rattner Heilman, Harper Perennial, New York, 1991. Accurate and balanced picture of estrogen benefits written by a leader in the field of hormone research.

Chapter 6: The Overlooked *Women's* Hormone

1. <u>The Magic of Sex. The Book That Really Tells Men About Women and Women About Men</u>. Miriam Stoppard, M.D. 1991, Dorling Kindersley, Inc., New York. Men and women approach love and sex with different expectations; they respond to physical love in different ways; and even when their responses are similar, they often happen at different times and are brought about by different stimuli. With beautiful photographs, <u>The Magic of Sex</u> covers this subject from both the man's and the woman's point of view. This is THE best, most comprehensive and beautifully written book on sex I have found, and I highly recommend it.

2. <u>The Art of Sexual Ecstasy: The Path of Sacred Sexuality for Western Lovers</u>. Margo Anand, 1989, Jeremy P. Tarcher, Inc., Los Angeles. A comprehensive and clearly written work on contemporary Tantric and Taoist practices adapted and made understandable to Western readers.

3. <u>Becoming Orgasmic; A Sexual and Personal Growth Program For Women</u>. Julia Heiman, Ph.D. and J. Lopiccolo. Ph.D. 1988. Simon and Schuster, NY. If you have any inhibitions about sex or want to enhance the pleasure you get from sex, the program presented will help you feel comfortable with yourself and your ideas about sex.

4. <u>Dancing With Myself: Sensuous Exercises for Body, Mind and Spirit</u>. K. dePeyer, 1991, Nucleus Publications, Willow Springs, MO. Intuitive approach to physical fitness which embraces mind, body and spirit; suggests exercises which enhance body/sensual awareness.

Chapter 7: PMS, Depression, or Perimenopause?

1. <u>**What's Wrong with My Hormones**</u>? Gillian Ford, PMS and Menopause Educator California, Desmond Ford Publications, 1992. Order from Bajamar Pharmacy, St. Louis, MO.

2. <u>**The Silent Passage: Menopause.**</u> Gail Sheehy, Random House, New York, 1991. The best-selling book that brought the M word out of the closet and into mainstream. Still a good one to provide an overview of what to expect and to read other women's experiences.

3. <u>**PMS: A Positive Program To Gain Control.**</u> Stephanie DeGraff Bender, M.A., and Kathleen Kelleher, The Body Press Div. of HP Books, Inc., Tucson, AZ, 1986. Available from Women's Health America, Madison, WI, and from The Stephanie Bender Clinic, Boulder, Colorado.

4. <u>**Depression: The Mood Disease.**</u> Francis M. Mondimore, M.D. Johns Hopkins University Press, Baltimore and London, 1990. An excellent book on the biological aspects of affective illness, although it does not address the role of female hormones.

Chapter 8: Is It Chronic Fatigue, "Yeast," or Perimenopause?

1. <u>**Chronic Fatigue and Tiredness: A Self-Help Program.**</u> Susan M. Lark, M.D., Westchester Publishing Co., Los Altos, CA., 1993. A more in-depth exploration of the role of nutrition, vitamins, minerals, and herbs in the treatment of chronic fatigue. This book has many helpful and practical suggestions for enhancing energy levels and well-being.

2. <u>**Doctor, Why Am I So Tired**</u>? Richard N. Podell, M.D., FACP, Pharos Books, New York, 1987. Although published in 1987, this book addresses unrecognized medical causes of fatigue as well as suggestions for nutritional and other mind-body approaches to reduce fatigue. Helpful approaches to discuss symptoms with physicians.

3. <u>**The Yeast Connection.**</u> W. Crook, M.D. Professional Books, Jackson, TN, 1985. Written by a leading proponent of the Candida theory, this book gives an overview of the ideas developed by Orian Truss and W. Crook. It has not been well accepted by most allergists because of the lack of adequate studies to verify the "yeast connection."

4. **"Position Paper on the Candida Yeast Theory."** American Academy of Allergy and Immunology, 611 E. Wells St., Milwaukee, WI 53202. Provides an evaluation (from a skeptical point of view) on the scientific evidence pertaining to the yeast theory.

5. **National CEBV Syndrome Association**, PO Box 230108, Portland, OR 97223. Support group organization for people diagnosed with Epstein-Barr syndrome. Write to them for information and suggested reading list.

Chapter 9: It Went Right out of My Head

I have not seen books for a non-medical audience which focus on the hormonal connections in memory function. Two prominent researchers studying estrogen effects on the brain's memory centers are Dr. Barbara Sherwin in Toronto, Canada, and Dr. Bruce McEwen at Rockefeller University in New York City. You may locate their professional publications by checking with your local reference librarian. There are a number of books which address physical, stress/psychological, lifestyle, and other factors influencing memory.

Chapter 10: Migraines in Women

1. **Help for Headaches**. Joel Saper, M.D., Warner Books, NY, 1987.
2. **Headache Relief**. Alan Rapoport, M.D., and Fred Sheftell, M.D., Simon and Schuster, New York, 1990.
3. **The Headache Book**. Seymour Solomon, M.D., and Steven Fraccaro, Consumers Union, Mount Vernon, NY, 1991.
4. **National Headache Foundation 800-843-2256**
5. **American Council for Headache Education 800-255-ACHE**
6. **Headache Centers**. I have listed the following programs because the physician directors have more experience in addressing the hormonal issues many programs overlook. There are also many medical centers with pain clinics that treat headache problems, as well as pain programs affiliated with university medical centers that have headache specialists. Either of the national organizations above can provide additional referral resources in your area.

Elizabeth Lee Vliet, M.D.
1. **HER Place: Health, Enhancement and Renewal for Women at All Saints Hospital**
   1400 Eighth Avenue, Ft. Worth, Texas 76104 Phone: 817-922-7470 FAX: 817-922-2535

2. **HER Place: Women's Center for Health, Enhancement and Renewal, Inc. (Arizona)** #64507 Desert Foothills Station, Tucson, AZ. 85728, Phone: 520-577-7709

Stephen D. Silberstein, M.D., Chief of Neurology and Co-Director, **The Comprehensive Headache Center at The Germantown Hospital Medical Center**, Philadelphia, PA

Joel Saper, M.D., Medical Director
The Michigan Neurological Institute, Ann Arbor, Michigan

Lee Kudrow, M.D., Director
California Medical Clinic for Headache, Encino, CA

Chapter 11: Fibromyalgia, Aches, and Pain

1. **American Academy of Pain Management** 209-545-0754
3600 Sisk Road Suite 2-D, Modesto, CA 95356. This organization
reviews credentials of specialists in pain management from many different professional backgounds, provides a referral resource to help
identify pain programs and specialists around the country, and will
also provide information on upcoming conferences, books, and other
resources.

2. **Fibromyalgia Network**   805-631-1950
5700 Stockdale Highway, Suite 100, Bakersfield, CA 93309

3. **Elizabeth Lee Vliet, M.D.**
    **HER Place: Health, Enhancement and Renewal for Women at All
    Saints Hospital**
    1400 Eighth Avenue, Ft. Worth, Texas 76104 Phone: 817-922-7470
    FAX: 817-922-2535

    **HER Place: Women's Center for Health, Enhancement and Renewal,
    Inc. (Arizona)**
    #64507 Desert Foothills Station, Tucson, AZ. 85728,
    Phone: 520-577-7709

These two programs are tailored to women, and include complete hormonal measurement to check this overlooked cause of fibromyalgia.
Both are outpatient programs, which provide comprehensive medical
evaluation, followed by multidisciplinary therapy approaches including
alternative therapies (such as acupuncture, myofascial release, neuromuscular therapy, massage therapy, dietary changes, biofeedback, hypnotherapy, water therapies, chiropractic, osteopathic manipulation, and
others) along with traditional medical options. Women's previous medical test results are reviewed to be certain that disorders more common
in women have not been overlooked.

Chapter 12: Interstitial Cystitis and Other Bladder Problems

1. **Alliance for Aging Research,** 2021 K Street, N.W., Suite 305, Washington, D.C. 20006, Telephone: 202-293-2856
2. **Interstitial Cystitis Association** (Vicki Ratner, M.D. , Founder) P.O. Box 1553, Madison Square Station, New York, New York 10159 Telephone: 212-725-5175
3. **The Bladder Health Council, American Foundation for Urologic Disease,** 1120 N. Charles Street, Baltimore, MD 21201, Telephone: 800-242-2383
4. **HIP, Help for Incontinent People,** P.O. Box 544, Union, SC 29379 Telephone: 800-BLADDER
5. **The Simon Foundation for Continence,** P.O. Box 835, Wilmette, IL 60091 Telephones: 800-23-SIMON (patients) 708-864-3913 (health professionals)
6. **Women Leaders in Urology:**

> Tamara G. Bavendam, M.D., Director of Female Urology
> Department of Urology, University of Washington School of
> Medicine, Seattle, WA

> Kristene E. Whitmore, M.D.
> Director, The Incontinence Center Telephone: 215-893-2643
> Chair, Department of Urology, Graduate Hospital
> Clinical Associate Professor of Urology, University of
> Pennsylvania, Philadelphia, PA

Chapter 13: Estrogen and Your Heart

1. **The Female Heart: The Truth About Women and Coronary Artery Disease**. Marianne Legato, M.D., and Carol Colman, Simon and Schuster, 1991.
2. **Nutrition, Hypertension & Cardiovascular Disease**. Ronald S. Smith, Beavertown, Oregon: Lyncean Press, 1984. Although this was published in 1984, it is clearly written, understandable explanations of hypertension and cardiovascular disease; it emphasizes risk factors and prevention.
3. **No Ifs, Ands or Butts: A Smoker's Guide to Kicking the Habit**. Julie Waltz, Northwest Learning Associates, Tucson, AZ, 1989. Available by calling: 520-299-8435. Quite simply, one of the best and most practical guides for helping "kick the tobacco habit." Full of helpful tips and very human stories of dealing with change at all levels.

4. **American Medical Women's Association (AMWA).** Continuing Education Workshop: **Coronary Heart Disease in Women** (CME credit for physicians). Contact AMWA at 703- 838-0500

Chapter 14: Breast Cancer

1. <u>**Breast Cancer: If It Runs In Your Family, How to Reduce Your Risk.**</u> Mary Dan Eades, M.D., Bantam Books, 1991. An excellent review of the known risk factors for breast cancer (even if it doesn't run in your family), and more in-depth discussions than I had space for in my book. It is thorough, very readable, and gives sound practical approaches for changes in your lifestyle. I highly recommend it for all women!

2. <u>**Dr. Susan Love's Breast Book.**</u> Susan Love, M.D., with Karen Lindsey, Addison Wesley Publishing Co., Inc., 1990, 1991. One of the most comprehensive, up-to-date books available on total breast health for women of all ages. Very detailed and well researched, I highly recommend it.

3. American Medical Women's Association (AMWA) **Breast and Cervical Cancer Education Project**, a continuing education workshop for physicians and other health professionals. For information about obtaining a speaker, contact AMWA at 703-838-0500

Chapter 15: Hormone Replacement Therapy

1. <u>**Menopause**</u>. Miriam Stoppard, M.D., Dorling Kindersley Publishing, London and New York, 1994. A beautifully illustrated book that addresses the total woman during this important transition and the years beyond. Color charts and graphs make it easier to understand difficult medical concepts and help women manage their menopause in optimal ways.

2. <u>**Menopause and Midlife Health**</u>. Morris Notelovitz, M.D., and Diana Tonnessen, St. Martin's Press, New York, 1993. Written by a pioneer in osteoporosis and menopause, this book presents accurate and up-to-date information about managing your health, including the role of healthy lifestyle habits. Discusses hormone therapies, pros and cons of gynecological procedures, issues about breast cancer and other concerns of importance to women.

3. <u>**Menopause: A Guide for Women and Men Who Love Them**</u>. Winfred B. Cuttler, Ph.D., and Celso-Ramon Garcia, M.D.,W.W. Norton and Co., 1992. Much more technical than most books on menopause, but this one is well-researched and provides a wealth of information for women who want greater depth on the physiology and medical aspects.

4. <u>Ovarian and Uterine Cancer: If It Runs In Your Family, Reducing Your Risk</u>. Sherilynn J. Hummel, M.D., and Marie Lindquist, Bantam Books, 1992.

Chapter 16: Still "Killing Us Softly" 1995 Update: Advertising's Impact on Women

1. **Cambridge Documentary Films, Inc. 617-354-3677.** Resource for rental or purchase of Dr. Jean Kilbourne's films "Killing Us Softly" and "STILL Killing Us Softly" as well as other important documentary films on significant topics of interest to women and their families. I highly recommend this film, and encourage readers to rent it for showing/discussion to community and school groups.

Chapter 17: Patient and Physician

1. <u>**The Complete Guide To Women's Health: 2nd Revised Edition.**</u> Bruce D. Shephard, M.D., F.A.C.O.G. and Carroll A. Shephard, R.N., Ph.D., New York, Penguin Group/Mariner Publishing Co., Inc., 1982, 1990.

2. <u>**Understanding Menopause.**</u> Janine O'Leary Cobb, Key Porter Books, Toronto, Ontario, 1989. Good overview of the menopause transition written by a layperson who takes a broad view of women's needs. This book has been out for several years, and the hormone information is understandably out of date, but other aspects are helpful.

Chapter 19: Fat to Fit

1. <u>**Winning the Weight and Wellness Game**</u>. Julie Waltz Kembel, Northwest Learning Associates, Inc., 5728 N. Via Umbrosa Tucson, AZ 85715, 1993, Telephone: 520-299-8435. Simply one of the best books on the subject of healthy approaches to successful weight management and changing unwanted habits. Lots of practical tips and helpful charts.

2. <u>**The Callaway Diet: Successful Permanent Weight Control For Starvers, Stuffers, and Skippers.**</u> Wayne Callaway, M.D., Bantum Books, New York, 1990. Excellent resource to explain the effects on the body from chronic diets, how to break out of the trap of "skipping and stuffing," and how to diminish problems from insulin resistance. Dr. Callaway has extensive experience in obesity treatment and provides medically sound, up-to-date information.

3. <u>The Dean Ornish Program for Reversing Heart Disease</u>. Dean Ornish, M.D., Ballantine Books, New York, 1990. This is one book that should never go out of date, since the recommendations for healthy eating, exercise, and stress management apply to all of us throughout our lives. Definitely not just for people with heart disease, I highly recommend it to women who want to maximize their health at all stages of life.

4. <u>The Bodywise Woman: Reliable Information About Physical Activity and Health.</u> The Staff and Researchers of the Melpomene Institute for Women's Health Research, Prentice Hall Press, New York, 1990.

5. <u>Outsmarting The Female Fat Cell.</u> Debra Waterhouse, M.P.H., R.D., Hyperion, 1993. Helpful insights about male-female differences in weight loss, hormonal influences, and constructive ways of eating healthy and managing weight.

Chapter 20: Take Charge!

1. <u>Imagery in Healing</u>. Jeanne Achterberg, Ph.D., New Science Library, Shambhala, Boston and London, 1985. This is a classic, well-researched book that combines the practices of traditional healers with the scientific understandings of modern medicine to show how the techniques of mental imagery can be used in serious illness as well as for enhancing wellness.

The following books are ones I have used often in my women's growth groups and seminars because I feel they offer a great deal of clarity about our lives as women, how we have reached the place we are now and the opportunities to discover the fullest dimensions of ourselves as women for the times ahead.

2. <u>Women Who Run With the Wolves</u>. Clarissa Pinkola Estes, Ph.D., Ballantine Books Div. of Random House, Inc., 1992. A powerful and moving book about women recovering the creative, spontaneous, passionate soul force within each individual woman which is too often masked by societal roles and expectations. "Full of wonderful, passionate, poetic, and psychologically potent words and images that will inspire, instruct and empower women to be true to their own nature and thus in touch with sources of creativity, humor and strength." —Jean Shinoda Bolen, M.D.

3. <u>The Crone: Woman of Age, Wisdom and Power</u>. Barbara G. Walker, Harper, San Francisco, 1985. Many women have a negative image of a "Crone." Barbara Walker's book clarifies the derivation of "crone" as being from "crown," representing "wise woman" after meno-

pause; shows the historical roots of devaluation, repression, and denial of the wisdom of older women, and offers a wealth of insights into ways women may develop the kind of constructive healing power which will benefit themselves as well as present and future generations.

4. **The Heroine's Journey: Woman's Quest For Wholeness**. Maureen Murdoch, Shambhala Publications, Inc., Boston and London, 1990. A meaningful exploration of feminine psyche and female psychological development, and a guide to help women find the spiritually alive feminine self who will be actively engaged in personal and cultural empowerment.

5. **The Road Less Traveled**. M. Scott Peck, M.D., Simon and Schuster, New York, 1978. Over ten years on the N.Y. *Times* bestseller list indicates the power of this book. It is one of the most meaningful books I have read; I continue to find new levels of thought-provoking ideas each time I read it. A classic, and highly recommended.

III. NEWSLETTERS

Women's health is now such a marketable topic that many newsletters, of varying quality, have sprung up in just the last few years. I have reviewed many of the ones available, and have been concerned about lack of depth in the articles and/or obvious bias in the information. I think the three below provide the most responsible reporting, timely topics, careful background research for the articles, and a variety of options and approaches. These are ones I subscribe to for our center library.

I have included several newsletters on other topics which may be of interest to women although they are not devoted solely to women's health.

Women's Health Access. Published bimonthly by Women's Health America (Marla Ahlgrimm, R.Ph., Founder), this cutting edge newsletter offers the latest developments concerning prevention, diagnosis, treatment, and self-help tips on a wide range of women's health topics, including menopause, osteoporosis, infertility, PMS, endometriosis, cancer, headaches, heart disease, and many others. Subscription rates $18.00/year or $30.00 for two years. **A portion of WHA profits go to support women's health research and education.** For a complimentary newsletter, call 608-833-9102, or write WHA, P.O. Box 9690, Madison, WI 53715

Harvard Women's Health Watch. The Editorial Advisory Board is composed of women physicians on the Harvard Medical School Faculty. I think the information is sound, current, very readable, and a valuable guide to modern medical approaches for women. Covers a wide variety of topics, both medical and psychological, to address the questions for women of all ages. Subscription $24.00 per year. Write Harvard Women's Health Watch, P.O. Box 420234, Palm Coast, FL 32142-0234

A Friend Indeed. Janine O'Leary Cobb, Founder and Editor. 514-843-5730. Ten issues a year of helpful discussion on a variety of menopause issues; the readers dialog and questions sections have been well-received. Write to Box 515, Place du Parc Station, Montreal, Canada H2W 2P1.

Herbal Gram, American Botanical Council, Austin, TX (512-331-8868) and the Herbal Research Group, Littleton, CO. 800-248-8552. Published four times a year. Reliable resource for information on risks and benefits of various herbs. Members of Herbal Research Group may request information searches on various herbs and topics.

Nutrition Action published by the Center for Science in the Public Interest, Washington, D.C. An excellent, progressive newletter which is NOT supported by advertising. It is hard-hitting and unbiased by commercial influences. Contains practical advice on reading food labels, selecting healthy options, and avoiding hidden sources of fat, salt, and sugar. Write to CSPI, 1875 Connecticut Ave., Suite 300, Washington, D.C. 20009.

Tuft's University Diet and Nutrition Letter. I have subscribed to this for many years and have consistently found it to provide a wealth of sound information on healthy eating, evaluating nutritional claims, types of diets, supplements, and a host of other helpful tips. Published monthly by the Tufts University School of Nutrition. For subscriptions, write to Box 57857, Boulder, CO 80322. Other correspondence should be directed to the Editor c/o 53 Park Place, New York, NY 10007.

498 / SCREAMING TO BE HEARD

IV. MENOPAUSE and Mid-Life CENTERS

All Saints Health System
HER Place: Health Enhancement and Renewal for Women
Elizabeth Lee Vliet, M.D., Founder and Medical Director
1400 Eighth Avenue, Ft. Worth, TX 76104 Phone: 817-922-7470
FAX: 817-922-2535

An integrated, wellness/preventive-medicine-oriented program for mid-life women as well as women of other ages experiencing hormonally-aggravated health concerns: PMS, menstrual migraines, fibromyalgia, pelvic pain, chronic fatigue, bladder disorders, menopause, osteoporosis, depression/anxiety syndromes, post-partum depression. Comprehensive evaluation and individualized "health plan" includes blood chemistries with hormone profiles, bone density testing, resting metabolic assessments, cardiac stress test, exercise and nutrition evaluations, physical exams, mammography, ultrasonography, psychological profile, and specialized gynecology consultations/procedures when needed.

On-site seminars, workshops, and discussion groups on a variety of women's health topics are offered, along with continuing education courses for health professionals.

This consultation program emphasizes early identification of health risks, the woman as the leader of her health team, and a written take-home health plan to use in working with her own physician and other health practitioners. When hormone therapy is appropriate, the recommendations are highly individualized to the needs of each woman using natural human hormone preparations. Alternative medicine therapies are encouraged where appropriate for the individual. For out-of town women, moderately priced hotels are nearby and there is a lower-cost, on-site option in the "Bed-and Breakfast" wing of the hospital.

Cleveland Menopause Clinic 216-442-4747
Wulf Utian, M.D., Medical Director.

Dr. Utian is well known as the founder of the North American Menopause Society and the world's first menopause clinic in South Africa. He has been a leader in this country in bringing attention to the multiple health concerns of the mid-life and menopausal woman. This program offers comprehensive gynecology and menopause services: physical examination, bone density testing, mammography, ultrasonography, and a multi-disciplinary team to provide a variety of therapies, including HRT. Specialized gynecological procedures are available when needed.

Menopause Institute of Northern California
Treatment of Male and Female Sex Hormone Disorders
Phillip Warner, M.D., Founder and Medical Director
700 W. Parr Avenue, Suite D
Los Gatos, CA 95030
Phone: 408-370-1833 FAX: 408-378-8978

Dr. Warner has extensive experience with the estradiol and testosterone implants, as well as other options to provide natural hormone therapy for men and women. He is a gynecologist with 30 years of clinical practice and a particular interest in providing quality care to menopausal women.

Women's Medical and Diagnostic Center and Climacteric Clinic
Morris Notelovitz, M.D., Ph.D., Founder and Medical Director
1-904-372-5600
Gainesville, Florida

Dr. Notelovitz is also one of the leading authorities on menopause. He founded this center in 1986 and it remains one of the few in the country where an integrated approach is offered to the evaluation and therapeutic options for mid-life women.

INDEX